Clinics in Developmental Medicine No. 152
CRYING AS A SIGN, A SYMPTOM, AND A SIGNAL

© 2000 Mac Keith Press
High Holborn House, 52–54 High Holborn, London WC1V 6RL

Senior Editor: Martin C.O. Bax
Editor: Hilary M. Hart
Managing Editor: Michael Pountney
Sub Editor: Pat Chappelle

Set in Times and Avant Garde on QuarkXPress

First published in this edition 2000

British Library Cataloguing-in-Publication data:
A catalogue record for this book is available from the British Library

ISSN: 0069 4835
ISBN: 1 898683 21 2

Printed by The Lavenham Press Ltd, Water Street, Lavenham, Suffolk
Mac Keith Press is supported by Scope (formerly The Spastics Society)

Clinics in Developmental Medicine No. 152

Crying as a Sign, a Symptom, & a Signal

Clinical, emotional and developmental aspects of infant and toddler crying

Edited by

RONALD G. BARR
Dept of Pediatrics and Psychiatry
McGill University
Montreal, Canada

BRIAN HOPKINS
Dept of Psychology
Lancaster University
Lancaster, England

JAMES A. GREEN
Dept of Psychology
University of Connecticut
Storrs, CT, USA

2000
Mac Keith Press

Distributed by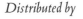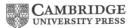

CONTENTS

AUTHORS' APPOINTMENTS   *page vii*

1. CRYING AS A SIGN, A SYMPTOM AND A SIGNAL: EVOLVING   1
   CONCEPTS OF CRYING BEHAVIOR
   Ronald G. Barr, Brian Hopkins and James A. Green

2. CAN WE HEAR THE CAUSES OF INFANTS' CRYING?   8
   Gwen E. Gustafson, Rebecca M. Wood and James A. Green

3. CRYING AS AN INDICATOR OF PAIN IN INFANTS   23
   Kenneth D. Craig, Cheryl A. Gilbert-MacLeod and
   Christine M. Lilley

4. COLIC: THE 'TRANSIENT RESPONSIVITY' HYPOTHESIS   41
   Ronald G. Barr and Megan Gunnar

5. 'CLINICAL PIES' FOR ETIOLOGY AND OUTCOME IN INFANTS   67
   PRESENTING WITH EARLY INCREASED CRYING
   Liisa Lehtonen, Siobhan Gormally and Ronald G. Barr

6. CRYING COMPLAINTS IN THE EMERGENCY DEPARTMENT   96
   Steven Poole and David Magilner

7. CRYING IN THE CHILD WITH A DISABILITY: THE SPECIAL   106
   CHALLENGE OF CRYING AS A SIGNAL
   James A. Blackman

8. TODDLER TANTRUMS: FLUSHING AND OTHER VISIBLE   121
   AUTONOMIC ACTIVITY IN AN ANGER–CRYING COMPLEX
   Michael Potegal

9. ACOUSTIC CRY ANALYSIS, NEONATAL STATUS AND LONG-TERM   137
   DEVELOPMENTAL OUTCOMES
   James A. Green, Julia R. Irwin and Gwen E. Gustafson

10. CRYING IN INFANT PRIMATES: INSIGHTS INTO THE   157
    DEVELOPMENT OF CRYING IN CHIMPANZEES
    Kim A. Bard

11. DEVELOPMENT OF CRYING IN NORMAL INFANTS: METHOD,   176
    THEORY AND SOME SPECULATIONS
    Brian Hopkins

12. THE CRYING INFANT AND TODDLER: CHALLENGES, EMERGENT   210
    THEMES AND PROMISSORY NOTES
    Ronald G. Barr, Brian Hopkins and James A. Green

INDEX   219

AUTHORS' APPOINTMENTS

Kim A. Bard

Senior Lecturer, Department of Psychology, University of Portsmouth, England

Ronald G. Barr

Professor of Pediatrics and Psychiatry, McGill University and Montreal Children's Hospital, Montreal, QC, Canada

James A. Blackman

Professor of Pediatrics, University of Virginia; and Director of Research, Kluge Children's Rehabilitation Center, Charlottesville, VA, USA

Kenneth D. Craig

Professor of Psychology, University of British Columbia, Vancouver, BC, Canada

Cheryl A. Gilbert-MacLeod

Doctoral Student, Department of Psychology, University of British Columbia, Vancouver, BC, Canada

Siobhan Gormally

Consultant Pediatrician and Neonatologist, Our Lady of Lourdes Hospital, Drogheda, Co. Louth, Ireland

James A. Green

Associate Professor of Psychology, University of Connecticut, Storrs, CT, USA

Megan Gunnar

McKnight Professor of Child Development, Institute of Child Development, Minneapolis, MN, USA

Gwen E. Gustafson

Associate Professor of Psychology, University of Connecticut, Storrs, CT, USA

Brian Hopkins

Professor of Psychology, Lancaster University, Lancaster, England

Julia R. Irwin

Postdoctoral Fellow, Yale Child Study Center, Yale University, New Haven, CT, USA

Liisa Lehtonen

Research Fellow in Developmental Pediatrics, McGill University–Montreal Children's Hospital Research Institute, Montreal, QC, Canada

Christine M. Lilley

Doctoral Student, Department of Psychology, University of British Columbia, Vancouver, BC, Canada

David Magilner

Attending Physician, Mary Bridge Children's Hospital and Health Center, University of Washington, Tacoma, WA, USA

Steven Poole

Professor and Vice-Chair of Pediatrics, University of Colorado School of Medicine, Denver, CO, USA

Michael Potegal

Postdoctoral Fellow, Pediatric Neuropsychology Clinic, Department of Pediatrics, Fairview–University Medical Center, Minneapolis, MN, USA

Rebecca M. Wood

Lecturer in Psychology, University of Connecticut, Storrs, CT, USA

1

CRYING AS A SIGN, A SYMPTOM AND A SIGNAL: EVOLVING CONCEPTS OF CRYING BEHAVIOR

Ronald G. Barr, Brian Hopkins and James A. Green

If a newborn baby undergoing a circumcision is crying forcefully, is this crying a sign of pain, or not? "Or not?"!—for the infant's parents, that option would not even be reasonable. In fact, until about 15 years ago, one of the more dramatic divergences of opinion between parents and clinicians was that the answer would have been an unequivocal "yes" for parents but a "no" for most clinicians. (One wonders how convinced the clinicians were about their "no"; but at least that is what the textbooks said, what the studies of physician attitudes and practices confirmed, and what the typical clinical practice of not providing readily available analgesia not so subtly implied.) Interestingly, the reason for this difference of opinion was not because of what the parents or clinicians heard, saw or measured, but rather because they brought different starting assumptions to bear on their interpretation of the behavior. Parents assumed that infants could experience pain, and that the crying was a sign of that pain. Clinicians, based on what was known and believed about the development and functioning of the nervous system, assumed that infants could not experience pain. The crying may have reflected distress (or even being held down), but not specifically pain.

Not so many years later, parents and clinicians share more similar starting assumptions. Now, thanks to landmark studies by Anand and his colleagues (Anand and Hickey 1987; Anand et al. 1987a,b) as well by Fitzgerald and many others (for reviews, see Chapter 3; and Fitzgerald 1991a; Barr 1992, 1994; Anand 1993; Fitzgerald and Anand 1993), clinicians are more likely to believe that infants do experience pain similar to that experienced by adults and that, if anything, more immature preterm infants experience even more pain, rather than less (Fitzgerald et al. 1988a, 1988b; Fitzgerald 1991b; Fitzgerald and Andrews 1998). Despite this change in starting assumptions, however, the question of whether crying can be interpreted as a sign of pain, and if so, what exactly it tells us about the pain or the state of the infant, will not go away. For example, reasonable arguments can be made that the crying in response to a pain stimulus can be (a) a specific sign that the infant is experiencing pain, (b) a nonspecific sign of stress (or distress) but not pain, or (c) a signal of robustness and strength (Barr 1998).

This sort of controversy provided the motivation for assembling this volume. It was apparent at the outset that definite answers would not be forthcoming, and that a single overarching theoretical synthesis was not achievable (see Chapters 9, 11). But it was also apparent that the relatively recent and impressive increases in clinical and research interest in crying behavior, aided by the variety of approaches that were being brought to bear on the phenomenon (or phenomena), were beginning to yield some interesting and challenging new ways of thinking about crying. How we think about crying, what it is, and what it might mean has evolved significantly. We wanted this volume to provide at least a venue in which these problems could be raised, articulated, and presented in ways that would be helpful for thoughtful clinicians and researchers.

To set the tone for the book, we adopted the title of *Crying as a Sign, a Symptom and a Signal*. Besides its alliterative allure (and the convenient shorthand it offered as the 'S3' volume), we hoped this might provide an heuristic organization for presenting an introduction to this disparate literature, especially since we wanted to bring findings from clinical and nonclinical fields together. We intend that these terms not be taken in a highly technical sense. The first two (crying as a 'sign' and as a 'symptom') are taken in their usual *clinical* meanings. By 'signs', clinicians are usually referring to some physical findings or biological measures that can be taken as objective evidence for a disease, typically ascertained on physical examination or testing. Signs tell us something about the patient, but they are not there for the purpose of communicating anything to anyone else. They are properties of the patient or the organism, like height and weight. Thinking of crying as a sign is thinking of crying as an objective indicator of the condition or state of the organism (like being hungry, fatigued, in pain or having central nervous system damage—see Chapters 2, 3, 9) independent of whether the infant ever 'intended' to communicate these conditions by crying. By 'symptoms', clinicians are usually referring to complaints, concerns or reports by patients that provide functional evidence for a disease, typically ascertained during history taking. In most clinical contexts, caregivers complain about crying (too much or too little, or it sounds like the infant is in pain). Crying as a symptom refers to crying as a clinical concern (as in crying complaints and colic—Chapters 4, 5; as a presenting complaint in the emergency room—Chapter 6; in the disabled child—Chapter 7; or in temper tantrums—Chapter 8). Symptoms are more subjective, and considerably more subject to varying interpretations and biases.

We use 'signals' to imply the way crying functions 'in context' but without any reference to its possible clinical significance. Considering crying as a signal implies minimally that crying has a function (or many functions), and that its function(s) can be understood only in a context that includes reception and interpretation of the signal. It need not (and for our purposes does not) entail that the signal (say, crying) is 'intentional'. Crying may function to communicate pain in an infant to her/his caregiver whether or not the infant is actually in pain and whether or not s/he intended (consciously or unconsciously) to do so. The question of what crying communicates runs throughout these chapters in both clinical and nonclinical settings, but is of particular salience when crying is considered as a developmental phenomenon and as an expression of emotion outside the clinical setting (discussed in Chapters 2, 8, 10, 11; see also Chapters 3, 7).

Of course, it is not that crying is a sign *or* a symptom *or* a signal; clearly, it can function as all three. However, different starting assumptions are brought to bear and different questions are generated depending on which it is considered as being. Indeed, much of the literature has been organized around these three perspectives on crying behavior. We wanted to bring these three perspectives together in one place, and the 'triple S' title was a convenient device for doing so.

As it turns out, these three perspectives capture the three primary themes in what might be called the 'modern era' of cry research. Furthermore, there are a number of publications that might be considered 'seminal' that were published within a few years of each other, and which provided a significant impetus to the growth of interest in crying behavior. As is often the case in science, interest in crying as a sign was stimulated by the application of a new technology to cry sounds. What has been referred to as 'the Scandinavian group' applied the technology of sound spectrograms to infant cries that, among other things, provided remarkable 'pictures' of sounds (see Chapter 9). At least part of the aim was to define cry 'types', and to determine whether cries could be used as signs in the diagnosis of a number of neonatal disorders. This work generated the first of what came to be known as International Cry Research Workshops, and a seminal volume on crying (*The Infant Cry: a Spectrographic and Auditory Analysis*, Wasz-Höckert *et al.* 1968). Indeed, this was the first volume on crying in the *Clinics in Developmental Medicine* series of which the current volume is the second (over 30 years later). Although the claim that there are meaningful cry types is not so well supported now as it seemed to be at that time (see Chapters 2, 9), the question as to whether crying can be used as a sign of clinical status continues to be an active area of investigation, both in regard to pain (see Chapter 3) and central nervous system function, and as a screen for sudden infant death syndrome (see Chapter 9).

Interest in crying as a symptom was stimulated by two articles both related to the clinical problem of early 'excessive' or 'paroxysmal' crying. In 1954, Wessel and his colleagues reported on a series of 98 infants from the Yale Rooming-In Project that offered a unique opportunity to follow infants and their families closely in the first weeks of life. From this paper was derived what has become the most widely used definition of clinically significant early crying (or as the authors said, "sometimes called 'colic'"), now usually referred to as Wessel's 'rule of threes' (Wessel *et al.* 1954). Despite a number of limitations in this definition (see Chapter 5), it has become a remarkably useful benchmark for studies on clinically significant crying. This paper was followed by another classic in 1962 from the office practice of T. Berry Brazelton in which he reported on the amounts and patterns of crying and fussing that occurred in normally developing infants as recorded by parents in daily diaries (Brazelton 1962). This was the first systematic description of the so-called 'peak pattern' of early crying, and demonstrated (among other things) that the pattern was not specific to a distinct clinical syndrome, but was characteristic of nonclinical crying as well (see Chapters 4, 5, 11).

Probably the most important early paper on crying as a signal was Wolff's study on the natural history of crying and other vocalizations in early infancy (Wolff 1969). This study was unique for a number of reasons. Not least of these were the 'naturalistic' observations of infants for hours at a time in their own homes combined with experimental manipulations to determine the necessary and sufficient conditions for terminating crying. Wolff anticipated later "multimethod, multimodal" approaches to understanding crying (and other infant behavioral states) including the use of sound spectrography. He considered crying not only as a vocalization, but also as an expression of emotion and as a behavioral

3

state of the infant, and all of this in the context of a dynamic, developing system [see especially his later book (Wolff 1987) in which the earlier studies were revisited and reinterpreted in light of subsequent research]. Indeed, there is hardly a question addressed in the current volume that was not raised, or in some cases defined, by Wolff's earlier work.

Of course, highlighting the work of any one or a few investigators runs the risks of inappropriate or biased attributions of significance and of overlooking many other significant contributions. However, our point here is not to render an objective historical judgment on the relative merits of various contributors to recent understanding of infant crying behavior. Interest in infant crying did not start with these investigators. Nor does their work encompass all of the contributions that came before (see, for example, Darwin 1872) or anticipate all of the contributions that have been made since. Rather, our point is to locate some of the recent historical antecedents that have contributed to defining the clinical and developmental themes that the reader will find reflected in different ways and from different points of view in this volume. It is probably fair to say that there has been a rapid and generative proliferation of interest and investigative work concerning infant crying since these papers were published. Furthermore, the kind of multimethod, multimodal approaches and descriptions that characterized Wolff's eloquent work are now much more common whether crying is being considered as a sign, a symptom or a signal.

These three perspectives on crying continue to be fertile and active foci of investigation and interest. However, the proliferation of studies has occurred both 'within' and 'across' these perspectives, and this intermingling has contributed to new insights into the nature of crying behavior. It seemed timely to reconsider where this work has taken us since these (and other) authors provoked and stimulated the field. As the reader will see, much has been learned, but there is still a considerable way to go.

After more than 30 years of active research on crying, there remain a number of important questions to be solved. This fact may at first seem surprising. Crying is, after all, something we have all experienced and that we all think we 'know'. It is a phenomenon of everyday life, especially with infants and toddlers. But crying presents a problem not just because of discrepant interpretations between parents and unfeeling clinicians. Even in everyday life, crying raises questions of interpretation. In the midst of the pain and effort of childbirth, that first 'birth cry' is universally welcomed by mothers the world over as a sign that their baby is alive and healthy. However, if that same infant cries interminably at 6 weeks of age because of 'colic', the crying can raise questions about whether the infant is sick or dying, can induce anxiety, guilt, or lack of confidence in caregiving skills in the mother, and even, in the extreme, result in abuse or death of the infant (see Chapter 5). Even in normal infants in everyday life, interpretation is difficult. Indeed, as the star of the television series *Murphy Brown* declared while trying to decide if her infant's crying represented hunger, fatigue or a wet diaper, it is pretty much like talking to a porpoise (see Chapter 2). If an infant is compromised by asphyxia at birth, the difficulty of trying to understand whether that infant's crying represents pain, hunger or some other need is complicated even further for already stressed parents (see Chapter 7). When a toddler has a temper tantrum, does the crying that accompanies the kicking and hitting have the same meaning as the crying that accompanies a fall and a grazed knee (see Chapters 6, 8)? Finally, does crying in humans have the same meaning as crying in other animals, especially in biologically closely related chimpanzees (see Chapter 10)? So, even though we feel we 'know' crying as an everyday experience, it turns out that knowing what it 'means' is more difficult than we might have imagined.

Understanding what crying means is one concern, but understanding, perhaps even more basically, what it 'is' is also a surprisingly difficult problem (see Chapters 4, 9, 10, 11). When we use the word 'crying', do we also intend to include 'fussing' and 'screaming', or are they something different? Similarly, when we use the word 'crying', are we referring to a single expiration that sounds 'negative', a series of connected expiratory negative vocalizations, or a 20-minute bout of crying and fussing with intermittent pauses (Barr 1990)? Indeed, are we referring to vocalizations alone, or to a complex set of behaviors that includes a typical facial expression, motor activity and flushing, and of which vocalizations are but one component? Is crying a communicative signal at all, or is it a behavioral state of the infant, like wakefulness and sleeping?

Of course, scientists and investigators whose job it is (*inter alia*) to measure this complex behavior are faced with further challenges. As will become apparent (see Chapters 9, 11), crying can be measured at microlevels of thousandths of a second in digital acoustic analyses, in 10-second bins during direct observations, with analogue rating scales by parents as to how it sounds, and by questionnaires or by diaries over hours, days or weeks. These methods each generate a plethora of measures (one system for digital analysis of cry sounds produces 88 measures for a single cry sound—see Chapter 9). As one might guess, crying 'frequency' at one level of description (*e.g.* direct observation) is not likely to be in any way equivalent to crying 'frequency' at another (*e.g.* diary description). It is a considerable challenge to decide which of these measures are important and why. In addition, trying to understand whether there are appropriate 'translation rules' between one level of description and another has hardly been addressed at all.

Finally, all these approaches and measures are scattered through a variety of literatures that include (but are not limited to) pediatrics, nursing, developmental psychology, communication sciences, speech and language and acoustic engineering. By and large, the work is disciplinary rather than interdisciplinary, complicating chances of an intergrated synthesis even further. Murphy Brown (the lead character in the series of the same name) or anyone else who wanted to 'go to the literature' could be forgiven if she remained confused and gave up in disgust at how unhelpful this all was. Although crying is an everyday life experience, what it is and what it means present a number of problems for parents, for clinicians and for researchers that are still far from solved.

When we recruited authors for this volume, we provided some broad guidelines about what we hoped they would address. On the one hand, we wanted them to address the topic of their chapter, but we did not want it to be 'simply' a review. On the other hand, all of these authors had made contributions of their own to their topic area, but we did not want them simply to report their work again here. So, our charge to them was to write an essay, as it were, that put their topic—or more accurately, their problem area—'in context', drawing where possible on the recent history of that area, defining the problems in ways that would be informative to a reflective reader, and using their own work and that of others to support current conceptualizations of the nature and meaning of crying, and to go beyond current findings by offering informed speculations about where the questions they were addressing were headed and what more needed to be known. Of course, this was not equally easy to accomplish for all topics. There are some areas (for example, the significance of crying in physically challenged infants and children—Chapter 7) about which there has been almost no systematic investigation to date. Nevertheless, whatever the 'state of the art' for any particular topic, all of the topics included were considered to present current and important challenges to our understanding of crying.

In any volume of this type, there are inevitably topics, investigators, approaches and methods that are not included or are insufficiently represented. Indeed, there are now many investigators who contribute regularly to the literature on crying behavior who could have made significant contributions to this volume. Despite these inevitable limitations, we were impressed when the contributions arrived that most of the key concepts and controversies concerning crying behavior were very well articulated and represented. Many of the chapters make it remarkably clear about where progress and evolution in our understanding have occurred. They also make it clear where critical studies are missing, where substantive problems persist, and what needs to be done to understand better the roles of crying as a sign, a symptom and a signal.

Indeed, to our delight, the chapters collectively seemed to send three additional messages. First, they compellingly illustrate the remarkable *complexity* inherent in a behavior so apparently simple as crying behavior. Second, they remind us, at one and the same time, how inherently fascinating and frustrating this very basic behavior can be. Finally, they may even evoke a little sympathy for the investigators who are trying to 'unpack' the phenomenon in the service of understanding it better. Most certainly, this volume should generate considerable sympathy for parents and caregivers everywhere who are trying to understand crying as an everyday life phenomenon that is both motivating and distressing, but is a challenge to respond to appropriately and to comprehend.

REFERENCES

Anand, K.J.S. (1993) 'The applied physiology of pain.' *In:* Anand, K.J.S., McGrath, P.J. (Eds.) *Pain in Neonates.* Amsterdam: Elsevier, pp. 39–66.
—— Hickey, P.R. (1987) 'Pain and its effects in the human neonate and fetus.' *New England Journal of Medicine,* **317,** 1321–1347.
—— Carr, D.B., Hickey, P.R. (1987a) 'Randomized trial of high-dose anesthesia in neonates undergoing cardiac surgery: Hormonal and hemodynamic stress responses.' *Anesthesiology,* **67,** A501.
—— Sippell, W.G., Aynsley-Green, A. (1987b) 'A randomized trial of fentanyl anesthesia undergoing surgery: effect on the stress response.' *Lancet,* **1,** 243–248.
Barr, R.G. (1990) 'The early crying paradox: a modest proposal.' *Human Nature,* **1,** 355–389.
—— (1992) 'Les nourissons ressentent-ils la douleur? Trois réponses possibles.' *Psychiatrie, Recherche et Intervention en Santé Mentale de l'Enfant,* **2,** 484–495.
—— (1994) 'Pain experience in children: developmental and clinical characteristics.' *In:* Wall, P.D., Melzack, R. (Eds.) *Textbook of Pain, 3rd Edn.* London: Churchill Livingstone, pp. 739–764.
—— (1998) 'Reflections on measuring pain in infants: dissociation in responsive systems and "honest signalling".' *Archives of Disease in Childhood,* **79,** F152–F156.
Brazelton, T.B. (1962) 'Crying in infancy.' *Pediatrics,* **29,** 579–588.

Darwin, C. (1872) *The Expression of the Emotions in Man and Animals*. (*Republished* 1979 by Julian Friedmann, London.)

Fitzgerald, M. (1991a) 'Development of pain mechanisms.' *British Medical Bulletin*, **47**, 667–675.

—— (1991b) 'The developmental neurobiology of pain.' *In:* Bond, M.R., Charlton, J.E., Woolf, C.J. (Eds.) *Proceedings of the VIth World Congress on Pain.* Amsterdam: Elsevier, pp. 253–261.

—— Anand, K.J.S. (1993) 'Developmental neuroanatomy and neurophysiology of pain.' *In:* Schechter, N.L., Berde, C.B., Yaster, M. (Eds.) Pain in Infants, Children, and Adolescents. Baltimore: Williams & Wilkins, pp. 11–31.

—— Andrews, K. (1998) 'Flexion reflex properties in the human infant: A measure of spinal sensory processing in the newborn.' *In:* Finley, G.A., McGrath, P.J. (Eds.) *Measurement of Pain in Infants and Children.* Seattle: IASP Press, pp. 47–57.

—— Millard, C., MacIntosh, N. (1988a) 'Hyperalgesia in premature infants.' *Lancet*, **1**, 292.

—— Shaw, A., MacIntosh, N. (1988b) 'Postnatal development of the cutaneous flexor reflex: comparative study of preterm infants and newborn rat pups.' *Developmental Medicine and Child Neurology*, **30**, 520–526.

Wasz-Höckert, O., Lind, J., Vuorenkoski, V., Partanen, T., Valanne, E. (1968) *The Infant Cry: a Spectrographic and Auditory Analysis. Clinics in Developmental Medicine No. 29.* London: Spastics International Medical Publications.

Wessel, M.A., Cobb, J.C., Jackson, E.B., Harris, G.S., Detwiler, A.C. (1954) 'Paroxysmal fussing in infancy, sometimes called "colic".' *Pediatrics*, **14**, 421–434.

Wolff, P.H. (1969) 'The natural history of crying and other vocalizations in early infancy.' *In:* Foss, B.M. (Ed.) *Determinants of Infant Behavior.* London: Methuen, pp. 81–108.

—— (1987) *The Development of Behavioral States and the Expression of Emotions in Early Infancy: New Proposals for Investigation.* Chicago: University of Chicago Press.

2
CAN WE HEAR THE CAUSES OF INFANTS' CRYING?

Gwen E. Gustafson, Rebecca M. Wood and James A. Green

In the American television series of the same name, Murphy Brown is a driven, professional news reporter who, at the age of forty-something, finds herself the mother of a newborn son. During one particularly frantic episode, she mutters that, whatever the baby books say, she herself cannot distinguish one of her son's cries from another. His 'hungry' cry sounds like his 'tired' cry, and his 'wet' cry is pretty much the same. The situation, she complains, is like trying to have a conversation with a porpoise! A vice-president of the USA once claimed in a speech that Murphy Brown typifies the shortcomings of today's mothers. Her failure to decode cries may be evidence for his contention. On the other hand, those baby books of Murphy's could be wrong.

In this chapter we entertain whether it is possible to tell, from the sound alone, the specific cause of a young infant's cry. *Are the cry sounds of human infants unique to the eliciting condition—for example, hunger, pain, startle or fatigue—and are they perceived uniformly and accurately as such by their caregivers?* Common wisdom, popular advice and pediatric lore all seem to nod in the affirmative. So too do introductory textbooks in child development and developmental psychology. The research literature, on the other hand, offers equivocal support at best. We review some key papers in this debate and speculate on why, after more than seven decades of research, the issue will not rest. Finally, we will outline an alternative position that we believe both fits the data better and gives common wisdom its due.

The 'cry types' hypothesis

The idea that cries are categorical patterns of sound, unique to eliciting conditions and specifically meaningful to caregivers, can be called the 'cry types' hypothesis. According to Murray (1979), this idea drew from, and has much in common with, the proposal that some nonhuman species communicate using discrete signals (Wilson 1975). Such signals are purported to act in an 'on' or 'off' manner, transmitting dichotomous messages such as 'yes' or 'no', and 'here' or 'there'. Discrete signals are thought to characterize the process by which animals recognize fellow members of their species, especially during courtship. For example, male fireflies of various species flash distinct patterns of light during their courtship rituals; females of each species identify conspecific males by recognizing these distinctive patterns. Another feature of discrete signals is their consistency from occasion to occasion, regardless of the potency of the eliciting stimulus. Thus, the meaning of the signal remains consistent across situations, much like a particular cry type was purported to sound the same to caregivers from one occurrence to the next (for review, see Murray 1979).

The primary research in support of cry types has come from a pioneering group of researchers in Finland and Sweden, sometimes known collectively as 'the Scandinavian cry group'. These researchers have been interested in a wide variety of questions concerning infants' cries, including sound spectrographic measures of cry characteristics and their usefulness in clinical diagnosis (for review, see Wasz-Höckert *et al.* 1985). The question of cry types occupied a series of papers in the 1960s.

A preliminary study was reported by Wasz-Höckert *et al.* (1963). One general goal was to validate the claim of nurses and pediatricians that young infants emit cries specific to eliciting conditions. A second aim was to determine whether mothers have "an instinctive ability to recognize and respond to the babies [sic] needs communicated through vocalization" (p. 9). This theoretical perspective reflected the ethological work of the era on animal communication (see Tinbergen 1951), in that the cries of human infants were hypothesized to be situationally discrete, perceptually categorical signs that triggered "innate release mechanisms" for caregivers' behavior (Valanne *et al.* 1967). The implication was that the purported cry types switched on specific and appropriate caregiving responses even in adults naïve to the care of infants (see Gustafson and Harris 1990). This initial report (1963) introduced sound spectrograms of cries deemed by the researchers themselves to be typical of cries originating from hunger, pain, birth or pleasure[1]. Indeed, there did appear to be differences among these carefully selected exemplars. However, the proportions of cries from each situation that matched these prototypes were not reported.

As a test of adults' ability to identify the cry types, Wasz-Höckert *et al.* (1964a) again used cries that "seemed typical" of four different situations. There were six 'birth' cries (recorded within the first five minutes after birth), six 'hunger' cries (recorded about four hours after feeding from infants 1 week to 8 months old), six 'pain' cries (recorded when vaccinations were administered to infants 2 weeks to 8 months of age) and six 'pleasure' cries (obtained after a meal from 4- to 8-month-olds). Rather than leave the range of possible responses to the listeners' discretion, the researchers informed their listeners (80 pediatric nurses) of the four possibilities *a priori* (*i.e.* the test was multiple choice). Overall, the listeners correctly identified an average of about 16 of the 24 cries. This result was highly significant by the binomial test, which merely compares the probability of the obtained score with the probability of chance performance (*i.e.* 6/24 correct). The correct identifications were not broken down by situation, however, so we cannot assess the likely possibility that one or two of the categories were particularly distinct (*e.g.* the birth cry of the newborn, whose respiratory tract still contains a great deal of fluid, or the contented coos and babbles that constitute the 'pleasure cries' of the older infant). The mixing of ages within and between situations further complicates interpretation of the results. Finally, we do not know the proportion of total crying in each of the situations that was consistent with the prototypes chosen for study.

---

[1]From the perspective of human behavior, pleasure cries might not seem to be cries at all. Wasz-Höckert *et al.* used the term 'cries' as it might be used in the comparative literature on communication, to refer to the calls or cries of a variety of species in a variety of situations.

A companion study (Wasz-Höckert *et al.* 1964b) examined the effects of experience with infants on adults' ability to identify these preverbal vocalizations. The participants in this second study were men and women, some experienced and some inexperienced in the care of infants. The cries were the same as in the companion study outlined above, and the previous discrimination results were essentially replicated. In addition, a modest effect of experience was reported: 1.1 more cries (out of 24) were identified by experienced *vs* inexperienced women, and 0.7 more cries were identified by experienced *vs* inexperienced men. Much greater differences apparently occurred between women and men, but these were neither tested nor interpreted.

Finally, a monograph by Wasz-Höckert *et al.* (1968) presented some analyses of the best and worst recognized exemplars of the purported cry types from the studies above. The work is important historically because it played a major role in moving the study of infant cries to the newly developed technology of sound spectography. As in the previous studies, however, the exemplars to be discriminated had been preselected by the researchers as sounding representative of the four eliciting conditions, and there were no statistical analyses of the extent to which cries emitted under any of the conditions actually adhered to the prototypes. Furthermore, even under such favorable circumstances, some of the exemplars were very poorly discriminated by the listeners.

In conclusion, these studies from the Scandinavian group offer the strongest and most frequently cited support for the idea of cry types. These reports, however, make very clear that the preselection of the exemplars as typical of their category, and the use of multiple choice rather than open-ended answer format, were steps deliberately taken to enhance the likelihood that adults would be able to discriminate the cry types. Consider the following comments from the introduction to the first (1964a) paper regarding the negative results of another researcher:

> "Sherman collected some empirical data that led . . . to the conclusion that the situational content of preverbal infant vocalizations cannot be recognized by graduate students in psychology, medical students and nurses. The cries used by Sherman were actual vocalizations obtained in the course of the experiment, in situations of hunger, dropping the infant towards the table, restraint of the face of the infant towards the table, and sticking with a needle. . . By our preliminary studies, we found some evidence that the negative results of Sherman – extensively referred to in various textbooks – could possibly be disconfirmed by using recorded vocalizations typical to the situations of birth, pain, hunger, and pleasure, and by giving these response categories in advance to the subjects (multiple choice technique)." (p. 154)

Along these same lines, the reader is cautioned in the discussion section of the second report (1964b) that one should not carry out a cry discrimination study "simply by recording a few cries and using these as items"; instead, one should control "for the representativeness of the signal proper" (p. 395). Thus, at best, these studies allow the conclusion that adults may sometimes be able to hear the causes of crying *if* the range of eliciting conditions is sufficiently limited, *if* the cry exemplars are carefully preselected, and *if* the range of possible interpretations is narrowly constrained. We submit that the results are perhaps better interpreted as indicative of what people (both the researchers and the listeners) thought sounded most and least like a hunger cry, a birth cry, and so on. A crucial question in the debate over cry types remains unanswered: namely; does all, or even most, of the crying emitted by the infants in the various eliciting conditions actually conform to these ideals?

Crying as undifferentiated noise

In direct opposition to the cry types hypothesis stands the possibility that early cries are nothing more than random noisemaking, uninformative with respect to specific motivating condition or caregiving need (for review, see Wasz-Höckert *et al.* 1968). Two reports by Sherman (1927a,b), both concerned with the differentiation of emotional responses in human neonates, have long been cited as the primary support for this position. Sherman's studies were remarkably thorough, although they necessarily suffered some limitations of the era: motion pictures were still silent, the computer and the sound spectrograph had yet to come into use, and statistical techniques were relatively primitive. The results were not at all favorable to the notion of categorical cry types.

The first paper (Sherman 1927a) addressed adults' ability to name and differentiate the reactions of neonates (less than 8 days of age) "to stimuli which presumably elicit distinctive emotional responses" (p. 265). Four types of stimuli were employed: hunger (a 15 minute delay in a scheduled feeding); dropping suddenly from a height of 2–3 ft (60–95 cm); restraint of head and face; and a series of four pricks on the face with a needle. Adults were asked to watch infants' responses (sometimes live and sometimes on film) to the various stimuli and to name the emotion that each infant was experiencing, as well as the probable eliciting stimulus. Their responses were not constrained (that is, they were not multiple choice)[1]. The various studies permuted listener experience and knowledge of the eliciting stimuli. In some of the conditions, the participants viewed the silent film not only of the emotional responses, but also of the (actual or alleged) eliciting stimulus. In other conditions, they were allowed to see the crying infant just after the stimulus had been applied. The participants included graduate students in psychology, medical students, neonatal nurses and normal school pupils. The primary questions concerned how well the observers agreed, and on what basis—differences in infant responses (on film), or knowledge of the stimuli themselves? Additional questions concerned the effects of experience and training related to infants.

In general, when the eliciting stimuli were not shown, the respondents' answers were nonsystematic with respect to actual cause. The results became far more systematic when the eliciting stimuli were shown, but still there was a great deal of attribution. To needle pricks, for example, some said pain, but others said anger or fear. To hunger, many said anger. The results became systematically erroneous when stimuli and reactions were mismatched experimentally. Sherman concluded that there was a considerable lack of

---

[1]Sherman's concern about selection bias led him to allow participants to hear whatever crying ensued in the cry-eliciting contexts rather than just preselected samples (see Sherman 1928). They were given an open-ended rather than a multiple-choice response task because of his concern that specifying and limiting the range of possibilities might spuriously enhance accuracy. Recall that the 'cry types' papers from the Scandinavian group employed carefully selected prototypes and a multiple-choice response task.

agreement when respondents were not privy to the eliciting stimulus, and that the stimulus that seemed immediately to precede the responses (whether truly the initiating stimulus or not) was the best predictor of the adults' judgments.

This first series of studies was concerned with global emotional reactions, not purely with the information value of cry sounds. When observing infants live, the adults had access not only to the cry itself but also to other cues (*e.g.* body movements and changes in facial coloration); furthermore, it is not clear that crying was always part of the emotional response. Participants in the motion picture condition complained that they might have done better at judging infants' emotions if they had been able to hear the cry; on the other hand, those allowed to see the infants themselves said that they had been observing the infants rather than listening to the cries.

A different procedure was employed in the second series of studies, in order to examine the effects of cries *per se* (Sherman 1927b). The listeners (graduate students in psychology, medical students and student nurses) sat in small groups in front of a screen, behind which infants were placed one at a time on a table and subjected to one of the four stimuli described above. Again, the range of possible stimuli was not provided to the listeners. All in all, the listeners were remarkably unsuccessful at naming either the eliciting stimuli or the underlying emotions for the cries.

In summary, Sherman's results were indeed unfavorable to the notion of cry types. Unfortunately, he was misinterpreted early on as favoring the notion that cries show no systematic variations, an error that continues to be perpetuated even today. We shall return in the next section to Sherman's remarkably modern position on the existence and causes of variations in cry sounds.

That crying might be undifferentiated noise was the conclusion of another careful empirical report that appeared just a few years after the Scandinavian studies. Müller *et al.* (1974) were concerned that the question of cry types come under tighter experimental control. They examined adults' discrimination of cries elicited from 3- to 5-month-old infants under three different conditions: 'pain' (rubber band snap), 'hunger' (removal of the nipple early in a feeding), and 'startle' (a clap of wooden blocks close to the ears). All of the participants were mothers[1]; some rated the cries of their own infants as well as those of other infants. The participants could not differentiate the crying, regardless of whether the infants were their own, and regardless of whether the crying had just begun (1–15 seconds of crying) or had been going on for a little while (31–45 seconds of crying). In fact, they tended to attribute all the cries to hunger. Müller et al. (1974) concluded:

> "These results support the contention that the acoustic characteristics of the cries of the normal infant appear to carry little perceptual information to the mother with respect to the cry-evoking situation. It might be hypothesized, therefore, that within the normal home situation the cry generally acts simply to alert the mother, and that any of her suppositions concerning the situation that evoked the crying behaviour must be based upon additional environmental cues." (p. 95)

---

[1]Apparently, neither Wasz-Höckert *et al.* nor Sherman included infants' own mothers as participants in their studies of possible differentiation of cry sounds by cry cause.

These results are, however, subject to at least two considerations. First, the eliciting conditions for the stimuli were different from those employed in the studies either of Wasz-Höckert *et al.* or of Sherman. For example, Müller *et al.* elicited 'hunger' cries by pulling the nipple from the mouths of nursing babies, whereas the other researchers used 'hunger' cries emitted spontaneously from infants whose feeding time was near (Wasz-Höckert *et al.*) or delayed (Sherman). Whether all of these should be considered hunger cries is debatable. Second, all three of the conditions of Müller *et al.* are in a sense similar, and thus the cries themselves might have been similar. When one pulls the nipple from the mouth during a feeding, snaps the infant's foot with a rubberband, or claps wooden blocks loudly near the infant's head, one causes a sudden interruption of the infant's current state and ongoing behaviors. Whether the resulting crying can be assumed to be due to 'pure' and independent causes of, respectively, hunger, pain and startle is debatable.

The case of crying is no exception to the adage that the null hypothesis (demonstrating that there is no difference) is difficult to confirm. Empirical support for the notion of cry types was unconvincing, but so too, is evidence for the argument that there is *no* information in the sound. We propose that controversy endures precisely *because* the question of context-related differentiations in cries has traditionally been posed as a dichotomy of extremes, neither of which is wholly accurate or wholly inaccurate. It will always be possible to design highly constrained situations in which adults can discriminate reliably on the basis of sound alone, and it will always be possible to cast legitimate doubt on whether they can do so in the real world. It will always be possible to argue whether statistical techniques were appropriate. After more than seven decades of controversy, the one thing that is clear is that neither of these extremes is likely to prevail on the basis of data. We now turn, therefore, to a different paradigm entirely.

Toward a resolution: crying as a graded signal

An alternative both to the 'cry types' view and to the view that the cry is undifferentiated noise is the emerging view that crying is a graded signal (*e.g.* Murray 1979, Zeskind *et al.* 1985, Porter *et al.* 1986, Gustafson and Harris 1990). In the comparative literature on communication, graded signals have been described as variable in duration, intensity and meaning across contexts (Wilson 1975, Masataka and Symmes 1986, Newman and Goedeking 1992). In contrast with *discrete* signals, which show little variation in duration or intensity, graded signals are proposed to change according to the motivational state of the animal (Green 1975) or to the difficulty of the task it is performing. In general, the more motivated the animal or the greater the task demand, the more intense and prolonged the message (Wilson 1975). A considerable shift in the intensity of a graded signal can change its qualitative meaning (*e.g.* Green 1975), but a graded signal does not carry a unique, symbolic meaning for receivers (Brown 1975).

Although the issue of discrete *vs* graded signaling remains a point of some debate in the comparative literature, there have been several demonstrations suggestive of communication via graded signals among nonhuman primates. For example, Green (1975) identified 10 different call types used by Japanese macaques on the basis of acoustic parameters such as minimum, maximum and dominant frequency, and total duration of the vocalizations.

The monkeys were shown to prefer using certain vocalizations in contexts that could be categorized in terms of the "demeanor, arousal, social spacing, and orientation of the animal" (p. 72). Such contexts included subordination, threat, and flight from an attacker. More difficult was the assignment of call preferences to functional contexts such as asocial (*i.e.* no contact with other monkeys), mating, and agonistic (both defensive and aggressive) contexts. Furthermore, monkeys' prolonged vocalizations seemed to change as a function of their internal states, becoming noisier with increased agitation.

In a study of Barbary macaque calls, Hammerschmidt and Fischer (1998) used discriminant function analysis to identify seven graded configurations of acoustic values (these values included peak frequency and call duration). Several of the configurations occurred in more than one type of situation (*e.g.* agonistic, foraging, play), indicating that they could not be considered 'discrete'. Masataka and Symmes (1986) showed that the 'isolation calls' of infant squirrel monkeys grew systematically longer with increases in distance from the natal group. In turn, natal group members lengthened their response calls as a function of distance from the infant. Finally, Jürgens (1979) used the self-cerebral-stimulation rates of squirrel monkeys to identify brain areas associated with various degrees of 'aversive' and 'pleasurable' sensations, and to describe the corresponding vocalizations. The type and number of vocalizations produced by the monkeys depended on which brain structure was stimulated, as well as on the length, pulse frequency and intensity of the stimulation. In general, the acoustic frequency ranges of the vocalizations became higher as the aversiveness of the sensations increased.

There are theoretical reasons to propose that human infants might also use graded signals. Lieberman (1973) has noted that the human infant's vocal tract is similar to the tracts of nonhuman primates that communicate using graded signals. Furthermore, according to Bastian (1965), most variations that occur within an infant's cry are due to changes in the lower, rather than the upper, vocal tract. This lower portion controls the pitch, timing and intensity of vocalizations, and is heavily influenced by the autonomic nervous system. Several models of cry production also discuss the influence of the autonomic nervous system on the acoustic quality of the cry (Lester and Zeskind 1982, Porges 1983, Lester *et al.* 1988, Porges *et al.* 1994). According to Porges *et al.*, the primary mechanism for this influence is the vagus (cranial nerve X). The vagus has a right and left branch, each of which has fibers that stem from either the dorsal motor nucleus or the nucleus ambiguus. The portion of the right vagus that originates from the nucleus ambiguus affects heart rate by way of the sino-atrial (S-A) node, and vocal intonation via the larynx. When an emotional response is triggered, whether by an outside event or by internal discomfort, the amygdala stimulates the nucleus ambiguus. The nucleus ambiguus, in turn, affects the S-A node of the heart and the right side of the larynx via the vagus. The vagus, therefore, is responsible for changes in heart rate and vocal intonations that are associated with variations (gradations) of emotion states.

This model (Porges *et al.* 1994) predicts that vagal tone should decrease under stressful conditions, and that this decrease should affect the cry. In a relevant experiment, Porter *et al.* (1986) collected cries elicited by unanesthetized circumcision, a series of steps that become progressively more intrusive and presumably painful for the infant. Cries elicited by the most intrusive surgical procedures had higher maximum fundamental frequencies, shorter and more frequent wails within each bout, and shorter intervals between bouts than cries recorded during less intrusive procedures. A later study showed that a measure of vagal control of the heart's S-A node (vagal tone) decreased during circumcision surgery, suggesting lower inhibition by the vagus on contraction of the laryngeal muscles (Porter *et al.* 1988). In other words, gradations in infant distress seemed to manifest in gradations of cry acoustics.

Sherman's comments on crying (*e.g.* Sherman 1928) did not refer specifically to the notion of graded signals, but the similarities are quite remarkable. Having concluded that the emotional displays, including the cries, of neonates were not categorically differentiated by specific cause, Sherman went on to note:

> "The character of the cry . . . depended directly upon the manner with which the stimulus was applied. When a stimulus such as restraint or pain was applied with little intensity and gradually, the ensuing cry was low pitched and of short duration. On the other hand, when the stimulus was applied suddenly and with great intensity the ensuing cry began suddenly, was of longer duration, and was high pitched. This indicates that the character of the cry during an emotional reaction is dependent not upon the "type" of the emotional response elicited but upon the character of the stimulus eliciting the reaction." (p. 388)

> The spasmodic breathing and the holding of the breath, so often described as a characteristic only of certain emotions, were also found to be factors of the intensity of the stimulus. This was illustrated in the reaction to sticking with a needle. When this stimulus was applied lightly and repeated but once or twice the infant often puckered its lips and cried but a few seconds. However, when this stimulus was applied with some intensity and repeated quickly several times the infant cried spasmodically, and held its breath between the "spells" of crying. These characteristics, that is, the spasmodic breathing and the holding of the breath, are therefore related to the intensity of the crying which is in turn directly influenced by the intensity of the stimulating condition." (p. 390)

Self-report measures indicate that adults can hear gradations in infants' crying. Participants in the Porter *et al.* (1986) study rated cries emitted during the most intrusive parts of the circumcision procedure as sounding more urgent than cries recorded either before or after the surgery. Indeed, the infants' vagal tone decreased during these cries (presumably indicating greater distress), fundamental frequency increased, and cry duration decreased. Other studies have related cry ratings (*e.g.* of urgency, of arousing quality) to variations in acoustic measures of the sounds, such as: (1) the length of pauses between cries (Zeskind *et al.* 1992); (2) dysphonation or arrhythmic vibration of the vocal folds (Gustafson and Green 1989); (3) the number and duration of wails within a bout (Zeskind *et al.* 1985); and (4) fundamental frequency (Porter *et al.* 1986).

Might gradations in cry acoustics be somehow informative with respect to the specific cause of crying? Sherman (1928) seemed to be entertaining this possibility when he noted that some listeners thought that they could sometimes differentiate specific responses on the basis of their intensities. Data from our own laboratory (Gustafson and Harris 1990) suggest that gradations may help a listener to whittle down the range of possible causes. Mothers of infants and young women who were not mothers listened to segments of cry

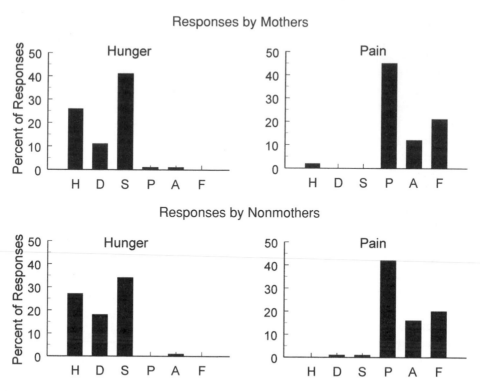

Fig. 2.1. Percentage distributions of answers from mothers (N = 20) and nonmothers (N = 20) to the question "Why is this baby crying?" H = hungry; D = in need of a diaper change; S = sleepy; P = in pain; A = angry; F = frightened or startled. The heading at the top of each graph indicates the actual context in which the crying occurred.

bouts elicited in two different situations. In one situation, 1-month-old infants were waiting to be fed, and in the other, newborn (male) infants were being circumcised. From audiotape recordings of two infants in each eliciting condition, two 15-second segments from early (minute 1) in the episode were randomly selected along with two 15-second segments from later (minute 3) in the episode. Thus, there were 16 different segments, four early and four late from each infant, from both the pain and hunger conditions. For each segment, participants answered the question "Why is this baby crying?" by choosing one of the following explanations: the baby is hungry, the baby is sleepy, the baby needs a diaper change, the baby is in pain, the baby is angry, or the baby is frightened or startled. The results showed that responses to early cries were correct more often than responses to late cries, and that mothers were somewhat more accurate than nonmothers (Fig. 2.1). Even the mothers, however, were far from accurate in absolute terms.

The distributions of these responses are particularly interesting. For both mothers and nonmothers, when an early segment of crying was heard from infants actually in pain, almost all of the answers were for pain, anger or fright; these are causes that would be associated with sudden onset of crying and with crying at high intensity. We surmise, therefore, that the main message here is not pain specifically, but rather, sudden and intense distress. On the other hand, hunger cries from early in the episode were attributed almost always to causes that begin at low intensity and grow—hungry, in need of a diaper change, or sleepy[1]. Thus, the early cries from the two kinds of eliciting conditions (pain and hunger) appeared to be readily discriminated along one global dimension of distress. To the extent that the listeners associated different discrete causes with different points along this dimension, they heard something relevant to the likely causes of crying.

As the bouts of crying continued, however, the distributions of interpretations became unsystematic. In another study (Green *et al.* 1998), we presented results consistent with the proposal that a bout of crying from hunger may settle into a 'basic' or regular cry over time (see also Wolff 1969). If the same is true of crying initiated by transient pain, then the two cries may have become indistinguishable as time went on. The more general point is that cry bouts appear to change in acoustic organization as they continue (see also Thodén and Koivisto 1980, Porter *et al.* 1986), and the level of perceived distress should change accordingly (Green *et al.* 1998). Wiedenmann and Todt (1990) have shown that adults rate some points in a prolonged cry bout more than others as especially intense and motivating to a caregiver. In other words, crying is a dynamic event, both in production and in reception. A bout of crying is much richer and more variable than the isolated snippets of sound used in typical cry studies.

If graded signals do not convey specific messages, how do they affect the interpretations and behaviors of caregivers? The cry types position, it will be recalled, borrowed ideas from early ethology and thus presupposed a direct link between a categorical stimulus and specific caregiving behaviors. The 'hunger cry', for example, 'released' feeding behavior. The graded signal view is far less specific in its predictions. It simply proposes that a listener's motivation to respond to the signal (in this case, crying) will vary as a function of (a) the amount of emotion (in this case, distress) reflected in the sound itself (Bastian 1965), and (b) the context in which the sound occurs (Wilson 1975). Thus, the graded signal view predicts variations in latency and probability of caregivers' responses to crying. Implications for specific caregiving behaviors are less clear.

The predictions that caregivers would show higher response probabilities and shorter response latencies to cries that reflect high levels of infant distress were addressed in a study by R.M. Wood (unpublished master's thesis 1997). Participants heard nine cries from a 1-month-old infant, three of which had been judged by experienced caregivers to reflect low distress, three moderate distress, and three high distress. The participants were asked to identify, by raising a hand, the point in each cry when they thought they would initiate caregiving. A loglinear analysis showed that they were more likely to respond to cries of medium and high distress than to show any other response pattern. The possible response patterns, and their observed frequencies, were: responses to medium and high only (n = 23); responses to medium only (n = 0); responses to high only (n = 5); responses to low, medium and high (n = 5); responses to low only, low and medium only, low and high only

---

[1] These are, coincidentally, the same three 'types' of cries that Murphy Brown (see p. 8) thought sounded alike.

(n = 0); and no response (n = 1). The results also showed that the participants responded most quickly to cries of high distress and waited longest to respond to low distress cries.

Another study from our laboratory (see first experiment in Gustafson and Harris 1990) also demonstrated an effect on latency to respond. In a simulated babysitting situation, women were asked to care for an infant mannequin that began to cry. Clearly, the women did not know why our mannequin was crying. Regardless of whether they were hearing cries from a hungry baby or a baby being circumcised, they first sampled from the same set of soothing behaviors (pick up, hold to the shoulder, talk, and provide tactile and vestibular stimulation) before they tried specific caregiving ministrations such as feeding, diapering, or checking for the source of pain. Those hearing the baby in pain fed the mannequin sooner than did those hearing the baby who was actually hungry! They were not responding to 'cry types'; instead, they seemed to be responding to the distress level reflected in the crying from the two situations (see also Gustafson *et al.* 1987). It is interesting to note that the women also offered a pacifier sooner when they heard cries of the hungry infants than when they heard cries from the infants in pain. Perhaps this attempt to soothe (offering a pacifier rather than feeding) would be sufficient to calm a baby who emitted these lower intensity cries.

According to the graded signal view, the context in which the signal is emitted can change its meaning (*e.g.* Wilson 1975, Murray 1979). Thus, a conspecific's response to a graded signal will depend in part upon the context in which the signal occurs. One kind of context is the signaler's own behavior. For example, an aggressive display by a rhesus macaque (that becomes increasingly threatening over time) can be menacing or not, depending upon whether it is coupled with playful behavior (Wilson 1975). In an experimental study of adults' interpretations of human infants' vocalizations, J.R. Irwin (unpublished doctoral dissertation, 1998) demonstrated that facial expressions and bodily movements affected whether the cry sound was interpreted as a cry or a noncry vocalization.

Contextual information relevant to caregiving also influences adults' responses to crying. For example, when Sherman's (1927a) participants were asked to assign an emotion to a cry without knowledge of the eliciting condition, their responses were unsystematic and incorrect. Their responses became *systematically* incorrect when they were given incorrect information about the situation that caused the crying, showing that contextual information can be a powerful determinant of cry interpretations. In a naturalistic study of caregiving behavior, Bernal (1972) found that mothers waited longer to respond to cries if their infants had just been fed. R.M. Wood (unpublished mater's thesis1997) demonstrated experimentally an effect of context on caregiving responses. In this study, adults who were told that infants needed a nap waited longer to respond to even highly distressed crying than those who had no contextual information. As predicted by the graded signal view, context appears to influence adults' interpretations of, and responses to, crying.

Conclusions
We return now to the question asked at the outset: *Are the cry sounds of human infants unique to the eliciting condition—for example, hunger, pain, startle, or fatigue—and are they perceived uniformly and accurately as such by their caregivers?* Such notions are widely shared in the clinical, research and popular literatures on infant crying, and many

parents and other caregivers believe the answers to be "Yes".[1] Nonetheless, we have found little empirical support for such notions, and a great deal of evidence against them. The fundamental problem is that the sounds themselves appear not to be unitary and isomorphic with respect to discrete causes. It follows that adults are unable to perceive them uniformly and accurately on the basis of the sound alone. Infant crying fits much better with notions of graded signals that convey degrees of distress and that reflect the intensity and duration of the eliciting stimulus.

We are not saying, however, that cry acoustics are uninformative or random noise. Crying is different from other soundmaking and thus alerts the caregiver to the infant's distress (Müller et al. 1974). It is so salient in this regard that it has been called a biological alarm and compared to a siren (Ostwald et al. 1968). Beyond alerting the caregiver, the sounds of crying convey level of distress or urgency of need. The probability and latency of a caregiver's response are thus affected. Level of distress per se appears to offer some clue as to the specific cause of crying. Coupled with contextual information[2]—the infant's facial expression and bodily movements, surrounding events and caregiving schedule—the sounds of crying may be highly informative with respect to a discrete cause. Thus, the suggestion that crying is a graded rather than a discrete signal does not obviate the possibility of accurate interpretation. Instead, it makes interpretation a complex process worthy of the remarkable perceptual and problem-solving capabilities of the human adult. Rather than respond more or less automatically to a handful of discrete causes, the caregiver integrates multiple sources of information and decides whether and how to respond. Such a communication system is very adaptable, in that it allows a wide variety of messages and a wide variety of responses.

Nonetheless, it may be that not all crying has definable causes even with the help of contextual information. Aldrich et al. (1945) tabulated the number and duration of "spells" of crying that were due to several obvious causes (e.g. hunger, soiled diapers) and to unknown causes. They concluded that "the most clear-cut result of our study of the causes of neonatal crying is the demonstration of the importance of unknown responses. In total minutes of crying this group of reasons closely approaches the amount for hunger and in the number of crying spells it exceeds it" (p. 96). Spock and Rothenberg (1985) note that almost all young infants get into "fretful periods" that cannot be precisely explained. They delineate a series of questions, essentially trial-and-error, for figuring out what to do when the cause of crying is unclear.

The graded signal view is invoked with increasing frequency to characterize infant crying. As noted earlier, this view comes from the comparative literature on communication, particularly among nonhuman primates. It has great intuitive appeal, but there are still questions of conceptual and operational definition, and there is the ongoing process of

[1]Wasz-Höckert et al. (1963) noted that they undertook their studies in part because of the claims of nurses and pediatricians regarding the existence of cry types. Sherman (1927a) noted that the neonatal nurses in his study were confident that they could hear the causes of crying, even when their judgments were erroneous.

[2]Such contextual factors have always been the basis for labeling the causes of cries, even in studies of cry types. We know of no attempts to measure discrete internal states of the infant vis-à-vis crying.

discovering which species use graded signals and how exclusively they do so. A critical review of the current status of the graded signal notion in the comparative literature, coupled with a detailed analysis of where it fits and fails to fit the cries of human infants, would a useful contribution to the literature on infant crying.

An important question in the study of cries as graded signals is how to conceptualize their effects on caregivers. One possibility is that variations in the emotional nature of graded signals may modify the motivational state of the receiver (Bastian 1965). Along these lines, Zeskind *et al.* (1985) have proposed that manifestations of physiological arousal in the infant's cry are paralleled by physiological changes in the adult, a process they call a "synchrony of arousal". Although the synchrony of arousal hypothesis has not been tested directly, there is evidence that, in some situations, adults' physiological arousal is affected by infant crying. For example, Murray (1985) reported that listeners responded to infants' cries with decreased pulse amplitude and blood volume, and accelerated pulse rate. These physiological changes (which indicate sympathetic arousal) apparently did not occur in response to equally aversive animal and mechanical sounds. Wiesenfeld *et al.* (1981) assessed parents' physiological reactions to the "pain" and "anger" cries of their own and unfamiliar infants (4–6 months of age). The pain cries were elicited by a rubber band snap to the heel, and the anger cries occurred in response to withdrawal of a sucrose-flavored pacifier, or restraint of the infant's movement. Mothers and fathers responded to their own infants' pain cries with increased skin conductance, but did not exhibit the increase upon hearing their own infants' anger cries, or the pain and anger cries of unfamiliar infants. These findings suggest that the physiological arousal of the listener can change as a function of the aversiveness of the sound (see also the review by Donovan and Leavitt 1985).

The synchrony of arousal hypothesis ties perception, motivation and caregiving decisions all into one. We submit that it might be useful, at least for now, to separate these issues in research. Perceiving the temporal patterns of sound relevant to degree of distress or urgency in the infant may be a rather direct and universal process[1]. Its basis may be patterns of sound that specify, for example, energy expenditure or force across all sorts of stimuli, from human infants to hurricanes to engines to porpoises (thank you, Murphy Brown!). Becoming motivated to respond, and deciding whether and when to respond, might involve very different processes.

Finally, there remains debate over what is in the black box (*i.e.* the infant) that connects the graded characteristics of the eliciting stimulus with gradations in the crying response. To think simply of output that mirrors input has been less attractive than to invoke internal events such as degree of arousal, amount of distress or urgency of need. Rather little is known at present about such internal events during crying. Little is known, too, about the range of stimulus parameters within which cry gradations can mirror quantitative aspects of the stimuli. Are there thresholds below which crying is not initiated, and are there levels of intensity too great to be mirrored in crying? Is there a point beyond which the infant ceases to cry and 'shuts down'? Future research might collect infant measures concurrent with crying, both across systematic variations in stimulus intensity and duration, and across contemporary

[1]Note the great similarities between the responses of mothers and those of nonmothers in Figure 2.1.

and developmental time. These concurrent measures might include facial expression, vagal tone, cortisol level, gross bodily movement, EEG and so on, for the purpose of assessing how uniformly they parallel cry acoustics. Such a data matrix would aid in the clarification of underlying processes. Furthermore, developmental changes in this matrix are to be expected, and they might have tremendous importance for our understanding of what is communicated by crying.

ACKNOWLEDGEMENTS

Most of our research cited in this chapter was supported by Grant #HD22871 from the US Public Health Service/National Institutes of Health. We thank Julia R. Irwin, Ph.D., and Ronald W. Kelly, M.D., for several helpful discussions on infant crying.

REFERENCES

Aldrich, C.A., Sung, C., Knop, C. (1945) 'The crying of newly born babies. II: The individual phase.' *Journal of Pediatrics*, **27**, 89–96.
Bastian, J.R. (1965) 'Primate signaling systems and human languages.' *In:* DeVore, I. (Ed.) Primate Behavior: Field Studies of Monkeys and Apes. New York: Holt, Rinehart & Winston, pp. 585–606.
Bernal, J. (1972) 'Crying during the first 10 days of life, and maternal responses.' *Developmental Medicine and Child Neurology*, **14**, 362–372.
Brown, J.L. (1975) *The Evolution of Behavior*. New York: W.W. Norton.
Donovan, W.L., Leavitt, L.A. (1985) 'Physiology and behavior: Parents' response to the infant cry.' *In:* Lester, B.M., Boukydis, C.F.Z. (Eds.) *Infant Crying: Theoretical and Research Perspectives*. New York: Plenum, pp. 241–261.
Green, J.A., Gustafson, G.E., McGhie, A.C. (1998) 'Changes in infants' cries as a function of time in a cry bout.' *Child Development*, **69**, 271–279.
Green, S. (1975) 'Variation of vocal pattern with social situation in the Japanese monkey (*Mucaca fuscata*): A field study.' *In:* Rosenblum, L.A. (Ed.) *Primate Behavior: Developments in Field and Laboratory Research. Vol. 4*. New York: Academic Press, pp. 1–102.
Gustafson, G.E., Green, J.A. (1989) 'On the importance of fundamental frequency and other acoustic features in cry perception and infant development.' *Child Development*, **60**, 772–780.
—— Harris, K.L. (1990) 'Women's responses to young infants' cries.' *Developmental Psychology*, **26**, 144–152.
—— Cleland, J.W., Harris, K.L. (1987) 'Infant crying and social interaction: Studies of the process.' *In:* Kirkland, J., Wasz-Höckert, O., Michelsson, K. (Eds.) *Proceedings of the 2nd International Workshop on Infant Cries, Helsinki, 1986*. Palmerston North, New Zealand: Massey University Press, pp. 31–34.
Hammerschmidt, K., Fischer, J. (1998) 'The vocal repertoire of Barbary macaques: A quantitative analysis of a graded signal system.' *Ethology*, **104**, 203–216.
Jürgens, U. (1979) 'Vocalization as an emotional indicator: A neuroethological study in the squirrel monkey.' *Behaviour*, **69**, 88–117.
Lester, B.M., Zeskind, P.S. (1982) 'A biobehavioral perspective on crying in early infancy.' *In:* Fitzgerald, H.E., Lester, B.M., Yogman, M.W. (Eds.) *Theory and Research in Behavioral Pediatrics. Vol. 1*. New York: Plenum, pp. 133–180.
—— Corwin, M., Golub, H. (1988) 'Early detection of the infant at risk through cry analysis.' *In:* Newman, J.D. (Ed.) *The Physiological Control of Mammalian Vocalization*. New York: Plenum, pp. 395–411.
Lieberman, P. (1973) 'On the evolution of language: A unified view.' *Cognition*, **2**, 59–94.
Masataka, N., Symmes, D. (1986) 'Effect of separation distance on isolation call structure in squirrel monkeys (*Saimiri sciureus*).' *American Journal of Primatology*, **10**, 271–278.
Müller, E., Hollien, H., Murry, T. (1974) 'Perceptual responses to infant crying: Identification of cry types.' *Journal of Child Language*, **1**, 89–95.
Murray, A.D. (1979) 'Infant crying as an elicitor of parental behavior: An examination of two models.' *Psychological Bulletin*, **86**, 191–215.
—— (1985) 'Aversiveness is in the mind of the beholder: Perception of infant crying by adults.' *In:* Lester,

B.M., Boukydis, C.F.Z. (Eds.) *Infant Crying: Theoretical and Research Perspectives.* New York: Plenum, pp. 217–239.

Newman, J.D., Goedeking, P. (1992) 'Noncategorical vocal communication in primates: the example of common marmoset phee calls.' *In:* Papousek, H. Jürgens, U. Papousek, M. (Eds.) *Nonverbal Vocal Communication: Comparative and Developmental Approaches.* Cambridge: Cambridge University Press, pp. 87–101.

Ostwald, P.F., Phibbs, R., Fox, S. (1968) 'Diagnostic use of infant cry.' *Biologia Neonatorum*, **13**, 68–82.

Porges, S.W. (1983) 'Heart rate patterns in neonates: A potential diagnostic window to the brain.' *In:* Field,T., Sostek, A. (Eds.) *Infants Born at Risk: Physiological, Perceptual, and Cognitive Processes.* New York: Grune & Stratton, pp. 3–22.

—— Doussard-Roosevelt, J.A., Maiti, A.K. (1994) 'Vagal tone and the physiological regulation of emotion.' *In:* Fox, N.A. *The Development of Emotion Regulation: Biological and Behavioral Considerations. Monographs of the Society for Research in Child Development, Serial No. 240, Vol. 59, Nos. 2–3.* Chicago: Chicago University Press, pp. 167–186.

Porter, F.L., Miller, R.H., Marshall, R.E. (1986) 'Neonatal pain cries: Effect of circumcision on acoustic features and perceived urgency.' *Child Development*, **57**, 790–802.

—— Porges, S.W., Marshall, R.E. (1988) 'Newborn pain cries and vagal tone: Parallel changes in response to circumcision.' *Child Development*, **59**, 495–505.

Sherman, M. (1927a) 'The differentiation of emotional responses in infants. I. Judgments of emotional responses from motion picture views and from actual observation.' *Journal of Comparative Psychology*, **7**, 265–284.

—— (1927b) 'The differentiation of emotional responses in infants. II. The ability of observers to judge the emotional characteristics of the crying of infants, and of the voice of an adult.' *Journal of Comparative Psychology*, **7**, 335–351.

—— (1928) 'The differentiation of emotional responses in infants. III. A proposed theory of the development of emotional responses in infants.' *Journal of Comparative Psychology*, **8**, 385–394.

Spock, B., Rothenberg, M.B. (1985) *Dr. Spock's Baby and Child Care.* New York: Pocket Books.

Thodén, C.J., Koivisto, M. (1980) 'Acoustic analysis of the normal pain cry.' *In:* Murry, T. Murry, J. (Eds.) *Infant Communication: Cry and Early Speech.* Houston: College Hill, pp. 124–151.

Tinbergen, N. (1951) *The Study of Instinct.* New York: Oxford University Press.

Valanne, E.H., Vuorenkoski, V., Partanen, T.J., Lind, J., Wasz-Höckert, O. (1967) 'The ability of human mothers to identify the hunger cry signals of their own new-born infants during the lying-in period.' *Experientia*, **23**, 768–769.

Wasz-Höckert, O., Valanne, E., Vuorenkoski, V., Michelsson, K., Sovijarvi, A. (1963) 'Analysis of some types of vocalization in the newborn and in early infancy.' *Annales Paediatriae Fenniae*, **9**, 1–10.

—— Partanen, T.J., Vuorenkoski, V., Michelsson, K., Valanne, E. (1964a) 'The identification of some specific meanings in infant vocalization.' *Experientia*, **20**, 154–156.

—— —— —— Valanne, E., Michelsson, K. (1964b) 'Effect of training on ability to identify preverbal vocalizations.' *Developmental Medicine and Child Neurology*, **6**, 393–396.

—— Lind, J., Vuorenkoski, V., Partanen, T., Valanne, E. (1968) *The Infant Cry: A Spectrographic and Auditory Analysis. Clinics in Developmental Medicine No. 29.* London: Spastics International Medical Publications.

—— Michelsson, K., Lind, J. (1985) 'Twenty-five years of Scandinavian cry research.' *In:* Lester, B.M., Boukydis, C.F.Z. (Eds.) *Infant Crying: Theoretical and Research Perspectives.* New York: Plenum, pp. 83–104.

Wiedenmann, G., Todt, D. (1990) 'Discrete responses of adult subjects during exposure to infant cry sequences.' *Early Child Development and Care*, **65**, 179–188.

Wiesenfeld, A.R., Malatesta, C.Z., DeLoach, L.L. (1981) 'Differential parental response to familiar and unfamiliar infant distress signals.' *Infant Behavior and Development*, **4**, 281–295.

Wilson, E.O. (1975) *Sociobiology: The New Synthesis.* Cambridge, MA: Belknap.

Wolff, P.H. (1969) 'The natural history of crying and other vocalizations in early infancy.' *In:* Foss, B.M. (Ed.) *Determinants of Infant Behaviour IV.* London: Methuen, pp. 81–115.

Zeskind, P.S., Sale, J., Maio, M.L., Huntington, L., Weiseman. J.R. (1985) 'Adult perceptions of pain and hunger cries: A synchrony of arousal.' *Child Development*, **56**, 549–554.

—— Klein, L., Marshall, T.R. (1992) Adults' perceptions of experimental modifications of durations of pauses and expiratory sounds in infant crying.' *Developmental Psychology*, **28**, 1153–1162.

3
CRYING AS AN INDICATOR OF PAIN IN INFANTS

Kenneth D. Craig, Cheryl A. Gilbert-MacLeod and Christine M. Lilley

Recognition of the serious impact of unrelieved pain in infants, and advances in knowledge concerning safe and effective means of alleviating pain in the early years of life are recent major accomplishments (Anand and McGrath 1993). Both immediate suffering and the enduring physiological damage and destructive behavioural patterns that can be the product of episodes of pain are recognized as long term consequences that can be prevented with available pharmacological and non-pharmacological interventions (Anand 1997). To benefit from these advances, clinicians, parents and other caretakers must recognize and confront the pivotal task of isolating expressions of pain from other expressions of emotional distress in individual infants. Only then can they select, deliver and evaluate appropriate interventions.

The challenge is not insurmountable. Crying, along with facial expressions, body movements and physiological activity, has been recognized as an important source of evidence concerning the subjective state of the infant. Both parents confronting the challenges of child-rearing and professionals in health care settings recognize this to be the case. To date, however, the potential remains largely untapped. Concerns remain about whether behaviour can sensitively disclose pain, and whether there are patterns of behaviour that are particular to pain. As well, relationships among various vocal and nonvocal cues as indices of pain continue to require study. This chapter examines the usefulness of cry as an index of infant pain and investigates the association between features of cry and other behaviour associated with pain.

Bioevolutionary perspectives on the functional value of cry

A capacity to communicate needs and states has substantial adaptive and survival value for infants, given their considerable vulnerability and dependence upon caretaking adults. The optimal model for effective childcare would combine a capacity for the infant to convey a high degree of specific information about personal needs with considerable empathic sensitivity and readiness to respond in caretakers. The manifest distress of infants attributable to pain, hunger, fatigue and other sources of physical discomfort, and the distress adults usually experience when encountering upset children attest to the presence and importance of inherent expressive and receptive communicative predispositions (Craig *et al.* 1996). However, the confusion often experienced by concerned adults when confronting a crying or otherwise stressed child speaks to the less than perfect nature of the infant's capacity to make her/his subjective states known and to limitations in adults' skills in divining the meaning of children's distress.

Theories of emotional expression generally postulate that the communication of affect is adaptive, because expressive individuals are more likely to survive and propagate (*e.g.* Lewis and Michalson 1983, Malatesta *et al.* 1989). Emotional displays usually provide important information about the child's state and immediate situation, serve to evoke empathic responses, and may rouse helping or other adaptive behaviour in an adult (Lewis and Michalson 1983). For example, in both humans and other species, a display of fear will alert conspecifics to possible danger. In humans, an infant's display of joy has a capacity to facilitate pair bonding. Current theories of altruism posit that the observed tendency for close relatives to assist one another during occasions of emotional distress reflects natural selection. A genotype for promoting the survival of others in need who share genetic material would have a greater probability of being represented in future generations (Cosmides and Tooby 1989, Alcock 1993). An alternative point of view is that observable distress is asocial. For example, Solter (1995) suggests a homeostatic theory of adult crying whereby tears serve to excrete stress hormones or to relieve stress hormone build-up. However, evidence dating to Darwin (1872) indicates that expressions of distress function to enlist help in altering distress circumstances (Fridlund 1994, Gross *et al.* 1994).

Crying, facial expression and other actions conveying information about subjective states are thought to have evolved through natural selection (Fridlund 1994), but they need not have served a communicative role in the first instance. For example, various facial actions may have been associated with the regulation of breathing, the protection or lubrication of the eyes, enhanced hearing, or orientation of attention (Fridlund 1994). Crying could have had its basis in the sounds associated with regulatory breathing changes. Alternatively, actions initially may serve as components of other complex chains of behaviours. For example, baring the teeth would protect the lips and gums preparatory to a biting attack. These and other movements could have been coopted by communication systems because they provided for effective transfer of information about states.

In contrast to many other species, the signalling system is particularly important for human infants because they remain vulnerable and dependent upon adult caretakers for a relatively lengthy period following birth. Older children and adults usually can act on their own behalf, but infants can do little to control or extricate themselves from problematic situations, other than to convey their distress to others. Crying represents the most conspicuous attention provoking signal available to command attention when an infant's needs are not being met (Lester 1985). Its role in signalling hunger and in eliciting maternal feeding perhaps best illustrates its communicative importance.

Like hunger, pain provides a prototypical example of the functional value of expressions of distress. Pain is a highly salient event for infants, despite their limited capacity for understanding its significance. Its association with the potentially devastating consequences of tissue damage assigns it biological priority as a sensory event that preempts attention. While painful injuries and diseases are often not life-threatening, the distinction is not available to the infant. One would expect relatively vigorous displays of distress to events deemed of lesser significance to the adult observer.

While crying is functional in many situations, it has its dangers. Barr (1999) notes that the cry of an infant might disclose her/his location to predators putting the child at risk of greater injury. As well, inconsolable crying is known to be a proximate risk factor for child abuse (Barr 1999), but these strategic risks do not repudiate the argument that communicative crying has evolved through natural selection. An adaptation need not guarantee fitness in all situations: emotional adaptations may be thought of as algorithms or decision rules that link perceptual information with the behaviour that has been most successful on average in similar situations in the past (Cosmides and Tooby 1990).

While most theories of emotional development agree on the adaptive nature of cry as a signal, they differ on an important point. Some theorists (*e.g.* Malatesta *et al.* 1989) believe that the infant's facial displays contain categorical information; that is, expressions allow observers to recognize the type of internal state experienced by the child. According to this view, cry, facial expression, body movements and other signals of emotional arousal allow infants to broadcast that they are "Hungry!" "Startled!" or "Suffering Physical Pain!" Other theorists (*e.g.* Zeskind *et al.* 1985) have proposed that infants' expressions encode only the distinction between positive and negative states, with representations of the latter encoding the degree of distress, rather than the nature of the distress. In this framework, the information contained in the infant's emotional display might be construed as "Distressed!" "Really Distressed!" or "Extremely Distressed!" This controversy has the potential to be resolved through empirical study and has stimulated considerable research on infants' behavioural expressions of affective experience (see also Chapter 2).

For the purpose of the following review, we have referred to 'the pain cry', which will be operationally defined as a cry emitted in response to a presumed painful stimulus. However, the categorical nature of cry sounds, and of infants' physiological and emotional states, is not presumed by the use of this term. Indeed, the data remain ambiguous on these points, as the following review indicates.

Description of the pain cry

Infants cry for a variety of reasons, including hunger, fatigue, anger and pain. Discrimination of these cries requires that we should be able to accurately describe their unique features. A variety of measurement strategies have been developed in the past 15 years to discover distinctive characteristics of pain cries. In general, they can be divided into two main approaches: (1) computer-based acoustic and temporal analyses focusing on characteristics such as pitch, rhythm, latency and duration; and (2) subjective analyses which utilize the human capacity to interpret the significance of the cry and to characterize it using descriptive language such as 'pleasing', 'distressing' or 'arousing'.

ACOUSTIC AND TEMPORAL ANALYSES OF PAIN CRIES

Studies of the acoustic attributes of the pain cry to date typically have examined pitch (fundamental frequency), formants, intensity, rhythm, quality, melody type, continuity, voicing, and temporal qualities including latency and duration (see also Chapters 9 and 11). These, in turn, reflect specific configurations of the larynx, the length and mass of the vocal chords, combinations of air pressure and tension of the vocal chords, and resonance in the chest, throat and cavities of the mouth. As the infant matures, articulating mechanisms comprising the lips, tongue, teeth, jaw and palate relating to voice come into play. Acoustic analyses of pain cries have described them as associated with increases in fundamental frequency and physical qualities of the tenseness of the cry, as well as altered formants (a reflection of the vocal tract shape) (Johnston and O'Shaughnessy 1988, Fuller 1991). Pain-induced cries also have a falling melody (Wasz-Höckert *et al.* 1968).

Temporal analyses, when combined with the variations in pitch and structure, have established a characteristic pattern of crying following exposure to a noxious stimulus (Johnston and Strada 1986). The first high-pitched cry cycle, or inspiration and expiration, has a rapid rise time, is extended in duration, and is followed by a period of apnea. Thereafter, the pitch becomes lower, dysphonated (*i.e.* more effort is exerted and the harmonies of the cry pattern are obscured by overloading at the larynx), and cry cycles are of shorter duration. Finally, the cry remains at a lower pitch, while becoming more rhythmic with a rising–falling pattern that is mostly phonated. This seems to be a stable pattern. Pain-induced bouts of crying tend to persist in duration in comparison to cries that reflect lower levels of arousal (Wasz-Höckert *et al.* 1968).

Latency to cry after invasive procedures and cry duration, *i.e.* total amount of time that the infant is engaged in crying behaviour, has served as a useful outcome measure for analgesia. For example, Taddio *et al.* (1994) demonstrated that a topical anaesthetic (EMLA) increased the latency between intramuscular needle injections and the first cry, and reduced overall cry duration. Similarly diminished cry duration has served as an effective index of reduced pain in newborns (*e.g.* Blass *et al.* 1991), preterm infants (Ramenghi *et al.* 1996) and older infants (*e.g.* Barr *et al.* 1995) given oral sucrose prior to painful procedures (reviewed by Abu-Saad 1997).

Acoustic features also appear to be sensitive to the severity of pain the infant is experiencing. Porter *et al.* (1986) demonstrated that with presumed increases in pain, neonatal cry cycles typically become briefer, more frequently emitted in a longer series, and higher pitched, with less distinct harmonies. For example, the more painful components of circumcision surgery were associated with cries of a higher pitch. It is these changes in pitch, temporal patterning and harmonic structures that suggest that cry reflects the degree of pain experienced by the infant.

While acoustic and temporal analyses have been productive, restricting investigations to the qualities described above leaves the possibility that other unidentified or inadequately studied features would provide more precise markers of infants' subjective states. Signal processing technologies derived from speech processing/recognition research represent alternative approaches. For example, Xie *et al.* (1996) automated infant cry analysis using a variety of mathematical and analytic strategies (*e.g.* cepstrum analysis, vector quantization and hidden Markov modeling) to characterize the time-frequency variations in normal infant cry signals. The most satisfactory cry analysis strategy used hidden Markov models. These yielded an account of 10 cry modes or 'phonemes', consistent with linguistic analysis. Both the cry modes and a composite index of distress calculated from the cry signal were validated against parent perceptions of the level of distress represented by the cries when the infants were experiencing painful needle injections and other aversive events. Cry modes characterized as "trailing, dysphonation and inhalation" were positively correlated, and "flat, falling, rising, vibration, and weak vibration" showed negative correlations with

TABLE 3.1
Spectrographic/temporal acoustic characteristics of pain cries

Study	Spectrographic/temporal characteristics
Wasz-Höckert *et al.* (1968)	Falling melody and longer duration
Johnson and Strada (1986)	Higher pitched, extended in duration, followed by a period of apnea
Porter *et al.* (1986)	Higher pitched with less distinct harmonies
Fuller (1991)	Increases in fundamental frequency
Johnston and O'Shaughnessy (1998)	Altered formants

the distress attributions, with hyperphonation showing the strongest positive correlation. The strong correlation ($r = 0.78$) between the averaged subjective observations of the parents and the computer extracted index of distress suggests a potential for developing practical applications using signal analysis techniques. While this study focuses upon levels of distress rather than the sources in specific states of pain, hunger, etc., it demonstrates the merit of studying understudied acoustic features to mark subjective states.

These descriptive studies support the utility of intensive study of the acoustic signal for describing infants' pain cries. There are consistent data from a variety of different research laboratories illustrating how a pain-induced cry 'sounds' or 'looks' on intensive analysis of the sound signal (see Table 3.1 for a summary of the findings; see also Chapter 9 for examples of sound spectrographs). As well, these methodologies offer clinicians and investigators valuable evaluative and diagnostic possibilities (Raes *et al.* 1990). However, acoustic analysis requires expensive equipment (*i.e.* sophisticated recording devices and computers) and technical expertise, making them an expensive and time consuming undertaking for the health care practitioner or caregiver, albeit worthwhile pursuing because of the numerous potential practical applications. The possibility that human listeners provide a clinically relevant and feasible means of subjectively identifying key features of the pain cry has also been pursued.

SUBJECTIVE ANALYSES OF PAIN CRIES
A number of investigators have used descriptive, subjective analyses to characterize pain cries. Brennan and Kirkland (1982) developed several semantic differential scales requiring quantitative judgments between polar opposites on qualitative dimensions, *e.g.* urgent/not urgent, soothing/arousing, aversive/nonaversive, that collectively have been successful at producing a reliable and consistent portrait of the pain cry. Mothers' ratings of infant pain cries on 50 seven-point bipolar, adjectival scales indicated that these caregivers construed the pain-induced cries as heavy, long, distressing, unsociable, violent, unpleasant, fast and strong.

Subsequent studies (Brennan and Kirkland 1983) sought to simplify the use of the numerous semantic differential scales by examining possible factor structures underlying them. This was an attempt to increase the clinical applicability of the 50 adjective scales, as few health care practitioners or caregivers would or could use them as originally designed.

TABLE 3.2
Subjective acoustic characteristics of pain cries

Study	Subjective characteristics
Brennan and Kirkland (1982)	Heavy, long, distressing, unsociable, violent, unpleasant, fast and strong
Brennan and Kirkland (1983)	Unpleasant, strong and important
Zeskind et al. (1985)	Urgent, arousing and aversive

Factor analysis revealed three different perceptual dimensions that could be used to detect and describe infant pain cries without the need of a recording apparatus, thereby increasing the clinical usefulness of the semantic differential scales. The first factor was comprised of scales that predominantly refer to affective qualities (*e.g.* pleasant, tense, agitated), the second addressed potency (*e.g.* heavy, shallow, weak, small, thin), while the third accounted for the rater's evaluation (important, unintentional, meaningful, insincere). Mothers in this sample typically characterized pain cries as unpleasant, strong and important.

Zeskind *et al.* (1985), using four different Likert scales (urgent/not urgent, aversive/not aversive, arousing/soothing and sick/healthy), found that pain cries in response to a brief, noxious stimulus were rated as urgent, arousing and aversive. However, the ratings decreased with repeated exposure, suggesting that an infant's presumed level of arousal to the pain stimulus does in fact diminish. Preliminary work on cry psychophysics, defined by Green *et al.* (1987) as the relation of the acoustic features of cry to cry perception, have suggested that subjective ratings similar to those described above are directly related to temporal and acoustic features of crying. In particular, increasing scores on the subjective dimension of overall unpleasantness or aversiveness are assigned to longer cries with more dysphonation and more energy at higher frequencies (Gustafson and Green 1989). Indeed, adults, regardless of caregiving experience, gender or ethnic background, will rate perceptually higher pitched cries as more aversive (Zeskind and Lester 1978). When judging cry similarity, adults are also sensitive to changes in peak frequency over time (*i.e.* rising *vs* falling patterns—Green *et al.* 1987).

Cumulatively, this line of research suggests that subjective analysis may provide a quick, inexpensive means of tapping into the same sound qualities indexed by cumbersome acoustic methods (see Table 3.2 for a summary of these findings). However, a decision to this effect should be made in the context of other research suggesting that clinical judgments or parental reports of excessive or problematic crying may not be isomorphic to objective characteristics of crying such as overall duration or duration of the average bout of crying (Barr *et al.* 1992). Unfortunately, accurate assessment is not always as simple as asking for parents' perceptions of crying. Cry psychometrics and issues of potential bias deserve further examination (Donovan *et al.* 1997).

Discrimination of pain from other emotion-laden cries
When an infant cries because of an invasive procedure such as a surgical incision, caregivers

and health care professionals have the added benefit of procedural information to infer that the cry most likely represents pain. However, instigating events often are not known, thereby making it difficult to discern if the infant is crying because of pain, hunger or another state. This provokes the question, does knowing what a cry 'looks' and 'sounds' like on a spectrograph or on semantic differential scales help in determining the type of cry and its associated psychological meaning? Several investigators have characterized the variation among a variety of emotion-laden vocalizations such as pain, hunger, birth and pleasure cries (*e.g.* Franco 1984, Fuller and Horii 1988, Johnston and O'Shaughnessy 1988), using the acoustic, temporal and subjective judgement methodologies described above.

ACOUSTIC/TEMPORAL CONTRASTS OF DIFFERENT CRY STATES

Franco (1984) examined phonation differences in infant cries to determine whether a relationship to communicative context exists, *i.e.* are 'noises', voice changes and phonations used in a communicative manner? She concluded that systematic analyses were warranted because "phonations constitute a means of differential characterization of vocalizations with different emotional implications and communicative functions." Armed with this perspective, the quest for discrimination between pain and other emotional cries began.

Johnston and O'Shaughnessy (1988) contrasted pain, fear and anger cries on four parameters. In pain-induced cries, the frequency of the second formant was higher, the intensity was relatively greater, the cries were longer, and there was more dysphonation or blurring of harmonics than in either fear or anger cries. Fuller and Horii (1988) ascertained three features that were the most reliable at distinguishing among children who were in pain, fussy, hungry, or engaged in cooing vocalizations, *viz.* amplitude levels of the high-frequency components, average fundamental frequency, and overall spectral power levels. In addition, they found that pain cries had significantly less difference between the amplitude of the various frequency locations and the maximal amplitude than did fussy and hungry cries. The study also demonstrated a difference in terms of tenseness, *i.e.* pain-induced cries were more tense than the other two cries, which, in turn, were more tense than cooing.

Fuller (1991) also investigated whether acoustic characteristics that separately differentiate between pain and other cries (*e.g.* formants, tenseness) could be used in a linear combination to accurately classify cry types. Findings suggested that when these characteristics are used together, one can correctly classify the majority (74 per cent) of pain-induced cries.

Although it appears that pain can be discriminated reliably from other cry types, the issue remains unresolved as to whether the differences are qualitative or quantitative in nature. It is possible that crying differences would best be understood as being on a continuum. For instance, Johnston and O'Shaughnessy (1988) proposed that pain-induced cries reflect greater levels of arousal than cries made in response to fear/startle and/or anger/frustration situations. Pain cries may be longer in duration and more dysphonated or blurred because of the greater level of associated arousal. Hence, these acoustic differences may not reflect actual qualitative differences between cry types. This is compatible with Fuller's view (1991, p. 159) which hypothesizes that "crying signals a qualitative gradient along a single continuum of infant distress–arousal rather than signaling discrete, qualitatively different internal states." Fuller based her view on the finding that the linear combination of acoustic characteristics, namely formants and tenseness, could account for only one-third of the variance between pain-induced, hungry or fussy cries, suggesting that any discrete differences may not be overly large. Gustafson and Green (1989) also propose "a single underlying dimension", and Zeskind and Lester (1978) refer to the unpleasant quality or aversiveness of the pain cries of high-risk infants.

Many of the criticisms levied at the clinical relevance of acoustic and temporal descriptions of pain cries have been directed at the inadequacies of research attempting to discriminate unique features of the pain cry. The cost/effectiveness of determining the biological state underlying an infant's communications of distress has not been demonstrated. For example, although infants with brain damage often have cries with abnormal characteristics, the relationships between cry sounds and health are often too weak to support the utility of intensive analysis of cry alone as a screening tool (for a review of this literature, see Chapter 9). Hence, health care professionals and/or caregivers rarely devote resources, nor have the inclination, to perform acoustic analyses. However, the clinical usefulness of semantic differential scales in distinguishing cry types has also been investigated.

SUBJECTIVE ANALYSES OF A VARIETY OF CRIES
Semantic differential scales identify perceptually similar cries such as the ones evident at birth or when a child is hungry or in pain. As described above, these adjectival scales produced a reliable and consistent description of the pain cry, *e.g.* heavy, long, violent, fast and strong. They are also useful for characterizing hunger cries (*e.g.* fairly weak, light, shallow, thin, small and short), birth cries (*e.g.* uneven, coarse, angular and high) and pleasure cries (*e.g.* comforting, sociable, gentle, relaxed, happy and calm). These cries also appear to have at least some distinctive qualities when examining the results of factor analyses (Brennan and Kirkland 1983). Pain-induced cries were rated as more unpleasant, strong and important than hunger cries which were described as only slightly unpleasant, weak, and neither important nor unimportant. Finally, pleasure cries are characterized as pleasant, neither strong nor weak, and neither important nor unimportant. Therefore, it appears that the semantic differential technique provides a viable means of classifying and describing perceptually similar, or dissimilar, infant cries.

As with the acoustic analyses, there is some debate about whether these subjective differences are indeed qualitative. Brennan and Kirkland's research (1982) suggests that cry may be a graded signal with a pleasure cry anchoring one end, the pain/birth cry closer to the opposite end, and the hunger cry near the center. If this were the case, then the possibility exists that health care professionals and caregivers can be trained to identify infant cry signals. The effects of training on an individual's ability to correctly identify four infant cry sounds (birth, hunger, pain and pleasure) have been studied (Gladding 1978). Training made it possible for inexperienced caregivers to recognize cry signals accurately. The discriminatory task is perhaps easier for parents and others who have ongoing contact with a specific infant and do not have to contend with the substantial individual differences in crying across infants. Experience with intraindividual variations associated with particular events would allow them to become adept at identifying varying sources of their child's distress (Murray 1979). They would also have the benefit of information that would provide context to their judgments, *e.g.* knowledge of the child's behavioral dispositions, health status or time since feeding. Wasz-Höckert *et al.* (1968) found that women with more child-rearing experience were more effective that nonmothers at identifying different types of cries. Coupling training with the experience available to most clinicians and caregivers should help to increase the precision with which care-related decisions are made.

In summary, it appears that acoustic, temporal and subjective analyses are all dependable methods for picking up variation among cries. However, their value as a means of classifying cries into discrete categories has not been wholly established. Several investigators have attempted to increase the clinical feasibility of cry analysis through technological innovations (*e.g.* Xie *et al.* 1996); however, a useful diagnostic/discriminatory tool has not yet emerged. This effort is complicated by the methodological, scientific and ethical challenge of generating provocative situations that elicit distinct emotions at similar levels of intensity. For many of the studies, it remains unclear whether the findings document differences in the type or degree of emotion experienced.

Other signals of pain in infants
Crying does not occur in isolation. Other behavioural cues of pain may be available. An important early study (Johnston and Strada 1986) documented other components of the neonate's immediate behavioural response to pain, *viz.* a drop in heart rate, followed by a period of apnea, rigidity of the torso and limbs, and a facial expression of pain. This was followed by a sharp increase in heart rate and less body rigidity. The facial expression of pain persisted. After 30 seconds, heart rate remained elevated. Body posture returned to normal, and facial expression returned to the at rest configuration. In summary, pain was communicated through cry, facial expression, body movement and physiological parameters. These modes of expression have been quantified in multidimensional pain rating systems intended for clinical use (McGrath 1996), such as the Neonatal Infant Pain Scale (NIPS—Lawrence *et al.* 1993), the Modified Behavioral Pain Scale (MBPS—Taddio *et al.* 1995b), and the Premature Infant Pain Profile (PIPP—Stevens *et al.* 1996). The selection of behaviors for inclusion in these scales should be based upon demonstrated evidence that they are sensitive and specific to infant pain to minimize false positive and false negative error rates (Abu-Saad *et al.* 1998).

FACIAL EXPRESSION OF PAIN IN INFANTS
Facial expression plays a major role in infant communication with adults (Fridlund 1994). In fact, the psychological literature on the development of emotional expression is almost entirely focused on infants' facial displays (Fogel and Reimers 1989), reflecting the maturity and functionality of the facial musculature at birth, its dynamic plasticity, and the range of displays that are meaningful to adults.

Research has consistently demonstrated the usefulness of facial expression in the study of pain during infancy (Craig 1998) and adulthood (Craig *et al.* 1992), and has identified a number of specific facial actions associated with painful distress. The Neonatal Facial Coding System (NFCS—Grunau and Craig 1987, 1990), an adaptation of components of the adult-oriented Facial Action Coding System (FACS—Ekman and Friesen 1978), scores

10 actions, with six consistently responsive to invasive procedures, *viz.* brow bulge, eye squeeze, deepened nasolabial furrow, open lips, vertical stretch mouth, and taut tongue, although there are minor variations described in different studies. The measure has reflected infant pain response in healthy and ill newborns (Stevens *et al.* 1994), preterm newborns (Craig *et al.* 1993), and older infants (Lilley *et al.* 1997) and has been examined in response to scalpel incisions (Grunau and Craig 1987), intramuscular needle injections (Grunau *et al.* 1990; Johnston *et al.* 1994), and circumcision (Taddio *et al.* 1995a). It has served as a valid outcome measure of analgesic efficacy for EMLA during circumcision (Taddio *et al.* 1997), morphine during heel lance in preterm neonates (Scott *et al.* 1999), and sucrose as a palliative for procedural pain in infants (Johnston *et al.* 1997). Facial activity also discriminated an intramuscular injection from two other noninvasive tactile events (Grunau *et al.* 1990), but studies contrasting facial activity during pain with facial activity during other aversive states have not been undertaken. In an investigation with preterm infants (Craig *et al.* 1993), facial activity was found to be more specific to the heel lance than were measures of bodily activity and physiological responses.

OTHER SIGNS OF PAIN

Body movements also provide important information. Vigorous movement of the hands, feet, arms, legs, head and torso are evident when infants' heels are lanced for blood sampling (Craig *et al.* 1993). Other bodily responses to pain include withdrawal, thrashing, jerking, wiggling, and rigidity of the limbs and torso, as well as changes in breathing patterns and state of arousal (Lawrence *et al.* 1993, Taddio *et al.* 1995a).

PHYSIOLOGICAL INDICATORS OF PAIN

A number of physiological indices have been used in the study of infant pain. Heart rate is a common measure, since it increases due to activation of the sympathetic nervous system (Craig and Grunau 1993). Cardiac vagal tone, an indication of parasympathetic action, decreases as the body devotes more resources to the stress response (Porter *et al.* 1988). Respiration rate and transcutaneous oxygen levels decrease (Craig *et al.* 1993). Oxygen saturation typically decreases in response to painful events, and intracranial pressure shows substantial fluctuation (Stevens and Johnston 1991, 1994). Variability in physiological indices may carry as much information as changes in the mean value (MacIntosh *et al.* 1993). The use of physiologic measures is somewhat problematic as these response systems are likely to reflect stress in general rather than pain (McGrath 1990, Stevens *et al.* 1994). Accordingly, physiological measures are most informative when combined with behavioural signs of distress.

Differences between cry and other modalities of emotional expression

There is no reason to expect characteristics of the emotional display to be invariant across different modes of expression. The potentially numerous sources of inference concerning subjective experiences available in crying, other vocalizations, facial activity, other nonvocal actions and physiological activity appear to share common variance, but given that they are only partially correlated they are best seen as complementary rather than as surrogates for each other. Different modalities serve different organismic needs; hence they are not redundant and the use of several modalities can add information of great interest and use to the observer, whether parent or clinician.

Sound can be conveyed with substantial fidelity over long distances (see Gustafson *et al.* 1994) and it wraps around barriers to sight. Crying may function as a distant early warning signal or "biological siren" (Zeskind and Marshall 1988) that engages the caregiver's attention and demands her/his return to the infant's side. Crying also may be most efficient at triggering the alarm of others, whether those explicitly dedicated to the child or bystanders whose concern can be provoked. Its alarming capacity appears inherent (Murray 1979, Cosmides and Tooby 1989) and difficult to inhibit. It appears to convey graded information about the degree of distress, but the signal to noise ratio for explicit information concerning the state of the child appears minimal, although, as noted above, there is some specificity in the cry pain signal. There may be adaptive features to this in that ambiguity would be alarming in its own right and would add to the sense of urgency and need to engage in visual inspection. Indeed, there may be merit to a random generator for infant crying in the absence of aversive states, thereby instigating the attention and relatively noncontingent attention and ministrations of mothers, fathers and other adults, a process that is generally agreed to be desirable and constructive. But this proposition needs to be balanced by recognition of the potentially adverse consequences of noncontingent crying. Since crying is perceived unfavourably, it has the potential to disrupt infant–caregiver relationships. In the less protected past, it also may have had the maladaptive function of alerting predators to the infant's location (Barr 1999).

Once alarmed and directly attending to a child, other sources of information can be scanned, with some pain-specific and other nonspecific indices providing supplementary meaning. These include immediate evidence of tissue damage (*e.g.* physical trauma or vital signs of physiological stress) or a source of distress (*e.g.* dangerous objects, aggressive others, predatory creatures), with these in turn evaluated in the context of the setting (*e.g.* hospital, safe comfortable home, playground) and specific knowledge of the child (age, health history, immediate antecedent events), as well as behavioural information beyond crying as to the child's physical status (Hadjistavropoulos *et al.* 1997).

Of the behavioural signs of pain and other affective and psychological states available on direct inspection of young infants, the facial display appears to provide the most distinctive information about pain (Malatesta *et al.* 1989, Grunau *et al.* 1990, Craig *et al.* 1993), although the degree of specificity has been questioned (Barr 1992). When both cry and facial expression are available via videotaped recordings of newborn's reactions, it is the facial activity that primarily determines the observer's judgment about the severity of pain the infant is experiencing (Hadjistavropoulos *et al.* 1994). This coheres with a bioevolutionary framework in that crying serves as a salient stimulus at a distance, while the information conveyed by facial and other behavioural expression would be useless unless the caregiver were in close proximity to the infant. Once present, visual inspection would provide key evidence as to whether pain were the source of expressions of discomfort and the infant's upset could be alleviated by corrective actions, such as feeding or removing a source of pain (Birns *et al.* 1966, Grossman and Lawhon 1993).

As would be expected from this complex model for processing information concerning a child's pain, the usefulness of auditory and visual information varies with the age of the child. Vocalizations of infants increasingly provide more information about eliciting conditions as they become older (Green *et al.* 1995). For example, adults used the information from visual cues, *i.e.* the face, to determine the stress level of a 3-month-old infant in the presence of conflicting information, but used cry sounds with older infants. This indicates that visual cues help disambiguate the auditory sounds of young infants, with cry sounds providing more differentiating information in older infants (Green *et al.* 1995).

Despite variations in the types of information implicit in various behaviours, the most accurate judgments of infant pain are likely to be produced by considering all available indicators of pain, including contextual information, weighted as to the degree of value implicit in each. If a sensitive and specific index of infant pain were to become available, the focus could be restricted to it. At present, the most successful caretaking strategies entail the progressive screening of increasingly specific information in the several sources available.

Developmental changes in the pain expression

Crying appears to be more developmentally specific than facial expression, bodily movement or physiological indices of pain. That is, the full-throated howl of pain is a common means of expressing discomfort in infants, but it is rarely heard among adults, probably because the cry transforms as emergence of language permits more specific expressions of distress. In contrast, the infant's pain face is similar to that of older children and adults (Grunau and Craig 1990, Craig *et al.* 1994, Lilley *et al.* 1997). The developmental changes in crying reflect both ontogenetic, neuromuscular maturation and learning, the latter accomplished through the association of cry with environmental events, internalization of display rules and the acquisition of new capacities for self-soothing, active problem-solving, and expression of distress through language. In this respect, crying and facial expressions of pain differ substantially in that the form of crying is more likely to be modified by social learning, whereas the facial display remains relatively stereotypical and is influenced more by cultural and societal norms as to when the display is appropriate. As well, neuroregulatory constraints dictate that facial displays are not as amenable as vocalizations to conscious control and conscious or unconscious display rules (Rinn 1984, Ekman 1985). Societal rules for verbal and vocal expression are generally much more explicit than standards for nonverbal behaviour. For instance, inhibition of crying becomes a focus for socialization attempts very early in life (Brooks-Gunn and Lewis 1982). Toddlers are frequently told not to cry, but less often told not to make expressive faces. Young children quickly learn the negative consequences of being labelled a crybaby, but there is no equivalent term for a child who expresses distress through facial expression.

The behavioural expression of pain shows notable continuity across the lifespan, but significant developmental changes are also evident. The preterm infant expresses pain with a high pitched cry, and a characteristic facial expression in which the eyes are squeezed tightly shut, the brows are drawn together and down, the nasolabial furrow is deepened, the mouth is open and may be stretched horizontally or vertically, and the tongue is taut and cupped (Craig *et al.* 1993, Johnston *et al.* 1993). Movements of the hands, feet, arms, legs, head and torso are also evident (Craig *et al.* 1993). A physiological stress response is apparent from changes in heart rate, respiration rate and oxygen saturation (Craig *et al.* 1993, Stevens *et al.* 1994). The term newborn displays the same constellation of behavioural signs (Grunau and Craig 1987), although there is more activity in the face and body in term infants (Craig *et al.* 1993), and certain actions appear more or less prominent at different ages (Johnston *et al.* 1993). With increasing postconceptional age, the duration of cry signals lengthens, the pitch of signals decreases (Michelsson *et al.* 1983), and cry sounds become less ambigous (Green *et al.* 1995). For example, mothers are better able to discriminate hunger and pain cry types in term than in low birthweight, preterm infants, attesting to the availability of more information in the cries of the term infant (Worchel and Allen 1997).

The essential elements of the neonate's facial display of pain are also present in older infants and toddlers (Lilley *et al.* 1997). However, as children reach the second year of life, behavioural manifestations of distress lessen in duration (Izard *et al.* 1983, Jay *et al.* 1983, Craig *et al.* 1984, Izard *et al.* 1987), and older children tend to squint their eyes instead of squeezing them shut (Izard *et al.* 1983, Izard *et al.* 1987), perhaps because visual information becomes useful in coping with pain. This is consistent with the narrowing of the eyes seen in adults. Pain responses also become more localized and goal-directed. For instance, toddlers orient towards the site of an injection and attempt to protect themselves by pulling away or guarding the site with their arms and hands (Craig *et al.* 1984). They also usually become capable of using language to protest or solicit help (Craig *et al.* 1984). As children age and become more capable of producing words, crying is replaced by pain vocalizations such as "ouch" or "owie" (Jay *et al.* 1983).

Certain patterns become evident in the developmental progression of the pain expression. Behaviour becomes less diffuse and disorganized as the child develops the capacity to self-soothe and eliminate the source of pain (Mangelsdorf *et al.* 1995). Within the first few months of life, infants' cries take on more of the features of an interactive communication system, foreshadowing the acquisition of language (Gustafson and DeConti 1990, Gustafson and Green 1991). Eventually, the role of crying diminishes as more complex verbalization emerges and expressive displays become more sensitive to environmental and contextual features, such as the presence of a parent (Gross *et al.* 1983, Gonzalez *et al.* 1987). Thus, while crying is an important indicator of pain in infants and toddlers, it must always be considered in the context of other modes of expression and the child's developmental status.

Future research
Cry is a formidable communication mechanism for infants in pain; however, several questions regarding whether distinct cry characteristics for varying negative affects exist. If they do, the question of their specific clinical utility remains unanswered. Research needs to address whether cry sounds can be specifically linked to the nature of distress in infants, or whether the more appropriate distinction is between positive and negative emotional states. However, the sole reliance on acoustic information to answer this question would seem inappropriate. Crying must always be considered in the context of other modes of expression,

including facial expression and global behavior (*e.g.* holding the sore spot, guarding). Unraveling the significance of various communication modalities is of great importance to understanding health care decision-making.

The need to determine if differences exist between negative affective states is highlighted in the following example. Infants and young children undergoing painful medical procedures are often also subjected to anxiety-provoking events. Children are removed from their parent's presence prior to surgery, and until recently, parents were rarely allowed to enter the post-anesthetic care unit following surgery. This separation in a new and scary environment is undoubtedly anxiety-provoking for infants and children, and when this is coupled with the pain of surgery, health care providers often face the formidable task of deciphering ambiguous emotional states. Arming caregivers with specific knowledge about what constitutes an anxiety and a pain response would permit effective treatment to be provided more efficiently.

Once researchers have determined if cry sounds are specific to emotional states, the clinical utility of using these acoustic characteristics needs to be addressed. Feasibility studies incorporating cry sounds into assessment procedures would be one such method. It is likely that, until technology advances to the stage where the equipment and time required to analyze cry sounds is both efficient and cost-effective, the value of acoustic and temporal analyses at the bedside will remain untested. However, subjective analyses can and need to be investigated as to their clinical applicability. The meaning of infant cries to adult listeners also deserves further attention. For example, Drummond *et al.* (1994) reported that mothers first view their newborn infant's cries as a rather annoying reflexive action that they endeavour to stop through trial and error attempts at soothing. With time, they come to see cry as the active communication of the infant's needs. They describe the parental role as a process of deciphering the information encoded in vocalizations and attending to the source of distress as promptly as possible.

Conclusion

Cry serves as an invaluable source of information concerning an infants' painful experiences for parents, clinicians and other concerned adults. It is a sensitive index of pain, even when the source is not immediately identifiable, and reflects the severity of distress. However, issues of specificity of the cry signal arise, and differentiating crying instigated by pain from crying initiated by hunger, fatigue, frustration or other aversive emotional states remains a challenge. The subjective judgments of attentive listeners and signal processing analyses of cry suggest qualitative differences between cry triggered by pain and other sources, but these qualities are not firmly established and their clinical or practical value has not been proven. Hence, concerned adults must consult other confirmatory sources of information. Nevertheless, it seems likely that more sophisticated approaches to signal processing and automated analysis of cry signals will come to yield these practical benefits. These developments will generate greater payoff if they recognize the needs, capabilities and limitations of listeners who must decode the cry signal and provide care for the child. The importance of refined measures of pain is reflected in the substantial risks to children for whom specific and effective analgesia is not provided.

ACKNOWLEDGEMENTS

Support for the preparation of this paper was provided to K.D. Craig by research grants from the Social Sciences and Humanities Research Council of Canada and the Medical Research Council of Canada; to C.A. Gilbert by the Social Sciences and Humanities Research Council of Canada; and to C.M. Lilley by the Medical Research Council of Canada.

REFERENCES

Abu-Saad, H.H. (1997) 'Sucrose analgesia.' *Pediatric Pain Letter*, **1**, 26–29.

—— Bours, C.J.J.W., Stevens, B., Hamers, J.P.H. (1998) 'Assessment of pain in the neonate.' *Seminars in Perinatology*, **22**, 402–416.

Alcock, J. (1993) *Animal Behavior: An Evolutionary Approach. 5th Edn.* Sunderland, MA: Sinauer.

Anand, K.J.S. (1997) 'Long-term effects of pain in neonates and infants.' *In:* Jensen, T.S., Turner, J.A., Wiesenfeld-Hallin, Z. (Eds.) *Proceedings of the VIIIth World Congress on Pain, Progress in Pain Research and Management. Vol. 8.* Seattle, WA: IASP Press, pp. 881–892.

Anand, K.J.S., McGrath, P.J. (1993) *Pain in Neonates.* Amsterdam: Elsevier.

Barr, R.G. (1992) 'Is this infant in pain?: Caveats from the clinical setting.' *APS Journal*, **1**, 187–190.

—— (1999) 'Infant crying behavior and colic: An interpretation in evolutionary perspective.' *In:* Trevathen, W., McKenna, J.J., Smith, E.O. (Eds.) *Evolutionary Medicine.* Oxford: Oxford University Press, pp. 27–51.

—— Rotman, A., Yaremko, J., Francouer, T.E. (1992) 'The crying of infants with colic: A controlled empirical description.' *Pediatrics*, **90**, 14–21.

—— Young, S.N., Wright, J.H., Cassidy, K.L., Hendricks, L., Bedard, Y., Yaremko, J., Leduc, J., Treherne, L.S. (1995) '"Sucrose analgesia" and diptheria–tetanus–pertussis immunizations at 2 and 4 months.' *Developmental and Behavioral Pediatrics*, **16**, 220–225.

Birns, B., Blank, M., Bridger, W.H. (1966) 'The effectiveness of various soothing techniques on human neonates.' *Psychosomatic Medicine*, **28**, 316–322.

Blass, E.M., Hoffmeyer, L.B. (1991) 'Sucrose as an analgesic for newborn infants.' *Pediatrics*, **87**, 215–218.

Brennan, M., Kirkland, J. (1982) 'Classification of infant cries using descriptive scales.' *Infant Behavior and Development*, **5**, 341–346.

—— —— (1983) 'Perceptual dimensions of infant cry signals: A semantic differential analysis.' *Perceptual and Motor Skills*, **57**, 575–581.

Brooks-Gunn, J., Lewis, M. (1982) 'Affective exchanges between normal and handicapped infants and their mothers.' *In:* Field, T., Fogel, A. (Eds.) *Emotion and Early Interaction.* Hillsdale, NJ: Erlbaum, pp. 161–188.

Cosmides, L., Tooby, J. (1989) 'Evolutionary psychology and the generation of culture. Part II.' *Ethology and Sociobiology*, **10**, 51–97.

Craig, K.D. (1998) 'The facial display of pain.' *In:* Finley, G.A., McGrath, P.J. (Eds.) *Measurement of Pain in Infants and Children.* Seattle: IASP Press, pp.103–122.

—— Grunau, R.V.E. (1993) 'Neonatal pain perception and behavioural measurement.' *In:* Anand, K.J.S., McGrath, P.J. (Eds.) *Pain in Neonates.* Amsterdam: Elsevier, pp. 67–105.

—— McMahon, R.S., Morison, J.D., Zaskow, C. (1984) 'Developmental changes in infant pain expression during immunization injections.' *Social Science and Medicine*, **19**, 1331–1337.

—— Prkachin, K.M., Grunau, R.V.E. (1992) 'The facial expression of pain.' *In:* Turk, D.C., Melzack, R. (Eds.) *Handbook of Pain Assessment.* New York: Guilford Press, pp. 225–274.

—— Whitfield, M.F., Grunau, R.V.E., Linton, J., Hadjistavropoulos, H.D. (1993) 'Pain in the preterm neonate: Behavioural and physiological indices.' *Pain*, **52**, 287–299.

—— Hadjistavropoulos, H.D., Grunau, R.V.E., Whitfield, M.F. (1994) 'A comparison of two measures of facial activity during pain in the newborn child.' *Journal of Pediatric Psychology*, **19**, 305–318.

—— Lilley, C.M., Gilbert, C.A. (1996) 'Social barriers to optimal pain management in infants and children.' *Clinical Journal of Pain*, **17**, 247–259.

Darwin, C.R. (1872) *Expression of Emotions in Man and Animals. (Republished* by Albermarle, London, 1976.)

Donovan, W.L., Leavitt, L.A., Walsh, R.O. (1997) 'Cognitive set and coping strategy affect mothers' sensitivity to infant cries: A signal detection approach.' *Child Development*, **68**, 760–772.

Drummond, J.E., Wiebe, C.F., Elliott, M.R. (1994) 'Maternal understanding of infant crying: What does a negative case tell us?' *Qualitative Health Research*, **4**, 208–223.

Ekman, P. (1985) *Telling Lies: Clues to Deceit in the Marketplace, Politics, and Marriage*. New York: Norton.

—— Friesen, W.J. (1978) *Investigators' Guide to the Facial Action Coding System*. Palo Alto, CA: Consulting Psychologist's Press.

Fogel, A., Reimers, M. (1989) 'On the psychobiology of emotions and their development.' *In:* Malatesta, C.Z., Culver, C., Tesman, J.R., Shephard, B. *The Development of Emotion Expression During the First Two Years of Life. Monographs of the Society for Research in Child Development, Serial No. 219, Vol. 54.* Chicago: Chicago University Press, pp. 105–113.

Franco, F. (1984) 'Differences in manner of phonation of infant cries: Relationship to communicative context.' *Language and Speech*, **27**, 59–78.

Fridlund, A.J. (1994) *Human Facial Expression: An Evolutionary View*. Academic Press.

Fuller, B.F. (1991) 'Acoustic discrimination of three types of infant cries.' *Nursing Research*, **40**, 156–160.

—— Horii, Y. (1988) 'Spectral energy distribution in four types of infant vocalizations.' *Journal of Communication Disorders*, **21**, 251–261,

Gladding, S.T. (1978) 'Empathy, gender, and training as factors in the identification of normal infant cry-signals.' *Perceptual and Motor Skills*, **47**, 267–270.

Gonzales, J.C., Routh, D.K., Saav, P.G., Armstrong, F.D., Shifman, L., Guerra, E., Fawcett, N. (1987) 'Effects of parental presence on children's reactions to injections: Behavioral, physiological, and subjective aspects.' *Journal of Pediatric Psychology*, **14**, 449–462.

Green, J.A., Jones, L.E., Gustafson, G.E. (1987) 'Perception of cries by parents and nonparents: Relation to cry acoustics.' *Developmental Psychology*, **23**, 370–382.

—— Gustafson, G.E., Irwin, J.R., Kalinowski, L.L., Wood, R.M. (1995) 'Infant crying: Acoustics, perception and communication.' *Early Development and Parenting*, **4**, 161–175.

Gross, A.M., Stern, R.M., Levin, R.B., Dale, J., Wajnilower, D.A. (1983) 'The effect of mother–child separation on the behavior of children experiencing a diagnostic medical procedure.' *Journal of Consulting and Clinical Psychology*, **51**, 783–785.

Gross, J.J., Fredrickson, B.L., Levenson, R.W. (1994) 'The psychophysiology of crying.' *Psychophysiology*, **31**, 460–468.

Grossman, R.G., Lawhon, G. (1993) 'Individualized supportive care to reduce pain and stress.' *In:* Anand, K.J.S., McGrath, P.J. (Eds.) *Pain in Neonates*. Amsterdam: Elsevier, pp. 233–250.

Grunau, R.V.E., Craig, K.D. (1987) 'Pain expression in neonates: Facial action and cry.' *Pain*, **28**, 395–410.

—— —— (1990) 'Facial activity as a measure of neonatal pain perception.' *In:* Tyler, D.C., Krane, E.J. (Eds.) *Advances in Pain Research and Therapy. Vol. 15. Pediatric Pain*. New York: Raven Press, pp. 147–155.

—— Johnston, C.C., Craig, K.D. (1990) 'Neonatal facial and cry responses to invasive and non-invasive procedures.' *Pain*, **42**, 295–305.

Gustafson, G.E., DeConti, K.A. (1990) 'Infant cries in the process of normal development.' *Early Child Development and Care*, **65**, 45–56.

—— Green, J.A. (1989) 'On the importance of fundamental frequency and other acoustic features in cry perception and infant development.' *Child Development*, **60**, 772–780.

—— —— (1991) 'Developmental coordination of cry sounds with visual regard and gestures.' *Infant Behavior and Development*, **14**, 51–57.

—— —— Cleland, J.W. (1994) 'Robustness of individual identity in the cries of human infants.' *Developmental Psychobiology*, **27**, 1–9.

Hadjistavropoulos, H.D., Craig, K.D., Grunau, R.V.E., Johnston, C.C. (1994) 'Judging pain in newborns: Facial and cry determinants.' *Journal of Pediatric Psychology*, **19**, 485–491.

—— —— —— Whitfield, M.F. (1997) 'Judging pain in infants: Behavioural, contextual, and developmental determinants.' *Pain*, **73**, 319–324.

Izard, C.E., Hembree, E.A., Dougherty, L.M., Spizzirri, C.C. (1983) 'Changes in facial expressions of 2- to 19-month-old infants following acute pain.' *Developmental Psychology*, **19**, 418–426.

—— Huebner, R.R. (1987) 'Infants' emotion expressions to acute pain: Developmental change and stability of individual differences.' *Developmental Psychology*, **23**, 105–113.

Jay, S.M., Ozolins, M., Elliott, C.H., Caldwell, S. (1983) 'Assessment of children's distress during painful medical procedures.' *Health Psychology*, **2**, 133–147.

Johnston, C.C., O'Shaughnessy, D.O. (1988) 'Acoustical attributes of infant pain cries: Discriminating features.'

In: Dubner, R., Gebhart, G.F., Bond, M.R. (Eds.) *Proceedings of the Vth World Congress on Pain.* Amsterdam: Elsevier, pp. 336–340.

—— Strada, M.E. (1986) 'Acute pain response in infants: A multidimensional description.' *Pain,* **24**, 373–382.

—— Stevens, B.J., Craig, K.D., Grunau, R.V.E. (1993) 'Developmental changes in pain expression in premature, full-term, two and four month old infants.' *Pain,* **52**, 201–208.

—— Stremler, R.L., Stevens, B.J., Horton, L.J. (1997) 'Effectiveness of oral sucrose and simulated rocking on pain response in preterm neonates.' *Pain,* **72**, 193–199.

Lawrence, J., Alcock, D., McGrath, P., Kay, J., MacMurray, S.B., Dulberg, C. (1993) 'The development of a tool to assess neonatal pain.' *Neonatal Network,* **12**, 59–66.

Lester, B.M. (1985) 'There's more to cry than meets the ear.' *In:* Lester, B.M., Boukydis, C.F.Z. (Eds.) *Infant Crying: Theoretical and Research Perspectives.* New York: Plenum, pp. 1–27.

Lewis, M., Michalson, L. (1983) *Children's Emotions and Moods: Developmental Theory and Measurement.* New York: Plenum.

Lilley, C.M., Craig, K.D., Grunau, R.V.E. (1997) 'The expression of pain in infants and toddlers: Developmental changes in facial action.' *Pain,* **72**, 161–170.

MacIntosh, N., Van Veen, L., Brameyer, H. (1993) 'The pain of heel prick and its measurement in preterm infants.' *Pain,* **52**, 71–74.

Malatesta, C.Z., Culver, C., Tesman, J.R., Shephard, B. (1989) *The Development of Emotion Expression During the First Two Years of Life. Monographs of the Society for Research in Child Development, Serial No. 219, Vol. 54.* Chicago: Chicago University Press.

Mangelsdorf, S.C., Shapiro, J.R., Marzolf, D. (1995) 'Developmental and temperamental differences in emotion regulation in infancy.' *Child Development,* **66**, 1817–1828.

McGrath, P.A. (1990) *Pain in Children: Nature, Assessment and Treatment.* New York: Guilford.

—— (1996) 'There is more to pain measurement in children than "ouch".' *Canadian Psychology,* **37**, 63–75.

Michelsson, K., Jarvenpaa, A-L., Rinne, A. (1983) 'Sound spectrographic analysis of pain cry in preterm infants.' *Early Human Development,* **8**, 141–149.

Murray, A.D. (1979) 'Infant crying as an elicitor of parental behavior: An examination of two models.' *Psychological Bulletin,* **86**, 191–215.

Porter, F.L., Miller, R.H., Marshall, R.E. (1986) 'Neonatal pain cries: Effects of circumcision on acoustic features and perceived urgency.' *Child Development,* **57**, 790–802.

—— Porges, S.W., Marshall, R.E. (1988) 'Newborn pain cries and vagal tone: Parallel change in response to circumcision.' *Child Development,* **59**, 495–505.

Raes, J., Dehaen, F., Despontin, M. (1990) 'Towards a standardized terminology and methodology for the measurement of durational pain cry characteristics.' *Early Child Development and Care,* **65**, 127–138.

Ramenghi, L.A., Wood, C.M., Griffith, G.C. Levene, M.I. (1996) 'Reduction of pain response in premature infants using intraoral sucrose.' *Archives of Disease in Childhood,* **74**, F126–F128.

Rinn, W.E. (1984) 'The neuropsychology of facial expression: A review of the neurological and psychological mechanisms for producing facial expression.' *Psychological Bulletin,* **95**, 52–77.

Scott, C.S., Riggs, K.W., Ling, E., Fitzgerald, C., Hill, M., Solimano, A., Grunau, R.V.E., Craig, K.D. (1999) 'Morphine pharmacokinetics and pain assessment in premature newborns.' *Journal of Pediatrics,* **135**, 423–429.

Solter, A. (1995) 'Why do babies cry?' *Pre- and Perinatal Psychology Journal,* **10**, 21–43.

Stevens, B.J., Johnston, C.C. (1991) 'Premature infants' response to pain: A pilot study.' *Nursing Quebec,* **11**, 90–95.

—— —— (1994) 'Physiological responses of premature infants to a painful stimulus.' *Nursing Research,* **43**, 226–231.

—— —— Horton, L. (1994) 'Factors that influence the behavioral responses of premature infants.' *Pain,* **59**, 101–109.

—— —— Petryshen, P., Taddio, A. (1996) 'Premature Infant Pain Profile: Development and early validation.' *Clinical Journal of Pain,* **12**, 13–22.

Taddio, A., Nulman, L., Goldbach, M., Ipp, M., Koren, G. (1994) 'Use of lidocaine–prilocaine cream for vaccination pain in infants.' *Journal of Pediatrics,* **124**, 643–648.

—— Goldbach, M., Ipp, M., Stevens, B., Koren, G. (1995a) 'Effect of neonatal circumcision on pain responses during vaccination in boys.' *Lancet,* **345**, 291–292.

—— Nulman, I., Koren, B.S., Stevens, B., Koren, G. (1995b) 'A revised measure of acute pain in infants.' *Journal of Pain and Symptom Management,* **10**, 456–463.

——— Stevens, B., Craig, K.D., Rastogi, P., Ben-David, S., Shennan, A., Mulligan, P., Koren, G. (1997) 'Efficacy and safety of lidocaine–prilocaine cream for pain during circumcision.' *New England Journal of Medicine*, **336**, 1197–1201.

Wasz-Höckert, O., Lind, J., Partanen, T., Valanne, E., Vuorenkoski, V. (1968) *The Infant Cry: A Spectrographic and Auditory Analysis. Clinics in Developmental Medicine No. 29*. London: Spastics International Medical Publications.

Worchel, F.F., Allen, M. (1997) 'Mothers' ability to discriminate cry types in low-birthweight premature and full-term infants.' *Children's Health Care*, **26**, 183–195.

Xie, Q., Ward, R.K., Laszlo, C.A. (1996) 'Automatic assessment of infant's levels of distress from the cry signals.' *IEEE Transactions on Speech and Audio Processing*, **4**, 253–265.

Zeskind, P.S., Lester, B.M. (1978) 'Acoustic features and auditory perceptions of newborns with prenatal and perinatal complications.' *Child Development*, **49**, 580–589.

——— Marshall, T.R. (1988) 'The relation between variation in pitch and maternal perceptions of infant crying.' *Child Development*, **59**, 193–196.

——— Sale, J., Maio, M.L., Huntington, L., Weiseman, J.R. (1985) 'Adult perceptions of pain and hunger cries: A synchrony of arousal.' *Child Development*, **56**, 549–554.

4
COLIC: THE 'TRANSIENT RESPONSIVITY' HYPOTHESIS

Ronald G. Barr and Megan Gunnar

Despite its salience in the early postnatal months, colic remains a mysterious and largely unexplained behavioral syndrome. This is perhaps surprising, since there has been a significant increase in clinical and empirical studies of early infant crying in recent years. These studies have served to support some, and to delimit other speculations about possible explanations of early excessive crying, particularly that which becomes clinically problematic. Clinical studies have provided evidence that some organic diseases can present as a colic-like syndrome (for reviews, see Barr 1996, Gormally and Barr 1997). These same studies also suggest that fewer diseases than expected present as colic syndrome, and that those that do account for only a small proportion (probably less than 5 per cent) of cases, depending upon the clinical setting (Gormally and Barr 1997, Sauls and Redfern 1997). Developmental studies of nonreferred samples have demonstrated that excessive crying equivalent to that seen with colic syndrome can occur in the context of emotionally normal families, optimal parenting and normal mother–infant interaction (St James-Roberts and Halil 1991, Miller *et al.* 1993, Barr 1998b, St James-Roberts *et al.* 1998). Consequently, it appears that neither organic nor pathological caretaking conditions are going to be sufficient to explain the majority of cases of colic syndrome.

In the absence of pathological explanations, the leading candidate for a nonpathological explanation is the hypothesis that colic is the earliest manifestation of a persistent 'difficult temperament' (Carey 1972, 1984; Weissbluth *et al.* 1984a; Weissbluth 1987). The hypothesis is understandable and reasonable. On the one hand, the concept of temperament has gained wide acceptance as a way of capturing individual behavioral differences considered to be primarily constitutional and biological in origin, present early in life, and relatively stable across time and situations, although expressed differently at different developmental stages and in different settings (Thomas *et al.* 1968, Goldsmith *et al.* 1987, Klevjord Rothbart 1989, Lewis 1989). Within the broader temperament construct, 'difficultness' is conceptualized as a dimension that includes a predisposition to negative affect, poor adaptability, greater intensity of reactions, and unpredictability. On the other hand, colic is a clinical syndrome in which the cardinal symptom is excessive crying, crying bouts are prolonged, and infants are less able to self-soothe or respond to soothing by caregivers (Barr *et al.* 1992; Stifter and Braungart 1992; St James-Roberts *et al.* 1993, 1995; Barr 1996). The crying is associated with increased facial activity and different cry acoustics, consistent with more vigorous and intense crying (Barr *et al.* 1992, Lester *et al.* 1992, Stifter and Braungart 1992, St James-Roberts *et al.* 1995, Zeskind and Barr 1997). The crying bouts are described as 'paroxysmal', implicating sudden onset, beginning and ending without warning, and unpredictability. Consequently, the behavioral characteristics of infants with colic syndrome closely 'map on to' the defining characteristics of temperamental 'difficultness'. Consistent with these parallels, infants with colic syndrome are usually rated as temperamentally difficult at the time they have colic (Carey 1972, 1984; Weissbluth *et al.* 1984a; Barr *et al.* 1992; Lester *et al.* 1992; White *et al.* 2000). However, colic crying tends to peak in the second month and resolve by the fourth, a pattern exactly paralleling crying patterns in normal infants (Barr 1990a,b, 1996; St James-Roberts and Halil 1991; St James-Roberts *et al.* 1995). Thus, the obvious exception to this mapping is that colic behavior is significantly reduced at 4 months, and seems to be at odds with the idea that 'difficult' temperament persists and is stable. However, this need not rule out the possibility that colic is a manifestation of early difficult temperament, since difficult temperament may be manifest differently at later ages.

In this chapter, we will argue that the hypothesis that colic is an early manifestation of difficult temperament is likely to be wrong despite its apparent reasonableness. As a more satisfactory hypothesis, we will suggest an alternative, referred to hereafter as the 'transient responsivity' hypothesis. This hypothesis takes the notion of *responsivity*—a core concept from the fields of temperament and emotion regulation—and uses it as the currency with which to formulate the hypothesis. We will suggest (1) that currently available evidence more strongly supports the transient responsivity than the temperament hypothesis, and (2) that the notion of responsivity permits us to generate empirically testable predictions to more directly test both hypotheses. We will come back to the notion of responsivity, but first we consider some of the evidence for and against the temperament hypothesis.

Evidence that colic is an early manifestation of difficult temperament

The first evidence was provided by Carey's report (1972) of the use of a 70-item questionnaire in 200 4- to 8-month-old infants in his practice. Maternal replies were correlated with office notes as to whether the infants had had colic when they were younger, as judged by modified Wessel's criteria (Wessel *et al.* 1954; see also Chapter 5). Carey reported a statistically significant correlation of colic history (n = 13/200) with the 'difficult' temperament cluster and with the one dimension of low sensory thresholds on the nine temperament dimensions.

In a subsequent study, Weissbluth *et al.* (1984a) asked parents (N = 37) of infants with previous 'Wessel's' colic by history to rate temperament by the Infant Temperament Questionnaire (Carey and McDevitt 1978) at 4 months of age following participation in a double-blind treatment trial with dicyclomine hydrochloride. They found that there were no significant differences in ratings on the nine dimensions of temperament, on the five temperament clusters, or on the general impression that the infant was 'easy', 'average' or 'difficult', between infants who did or did not improve with treatment. They also noted that the proportion of infants rated as 'difficult' was significantly higher than that reported for the normative sample for the Infant Temperament Questionnaire. Weissbluth *et al.* interpreted these results as support for the temperament hypothesis both because of the increased proportion of infants described as difficult and because the ratings of difficulty remained high despite successful treatment of the crying. There is a third, more indirect, argument

(Weissbluth 1987). Consistent with the suggestion that difficult temperament might manifest as colic earlier but something else later, there were no differences in sleep patterns within the group of colic infants that were or were not successfully treated, and sleep duration at 4 months (13.9 ± 2.2 hours) was similar to that previously reported for infants classified as 'difficult' (13.1 ± 1.8 hours) (Weissbluth 1981; see also Weissbluth and Lin 1983). In a separate report (Weissbluth *et al.* 1984b), night wakings and shorter total sleep duration were reported more commonly by parents of infants who had colic previously. Consequently, both earlier crying and later sleep patterns were consistently related to 'difficult' temperament ratings at 4 or 5 months by parents.

Finally, in a recent report seriously compromised by poor return rates in both colic (50 per cent) and control (33 per cent) subjects, as well as the fact that Wessel's colic status was determined by retrospective chart review, mothers of infants with colic were more likely to rate their infants higher on activity and negative mood dimensions, and these infants more often met cluster criteria for 'difficult' infants (Jacobson and Melvin 1995).

Support from these studies is actually weaker than at first sight for at least three reasons. First and most importantly, parent reports of temperament were all obtained soon after colic had resolved. Given that excessive crying is the cardinal symptom of colic syndrome, the risk that parent reports might still be affected by the earlier behavior would seem to be high. Second, there is an important 'measurement bias' in these studies. This is because crying and fussing are predominant behaviors both in the syndrome of colic and in the responses used to define the behavior clusters, especially those of the 'difficult' infant. Indeed, in the widely used Infant Charactcristics Questionnaire, the 'fussy–difficult' factor contributes almost 60 per cent of the variance to the 'difficult' infant dimension (Bates *et al.* 1979). Consequently, infants with colic are likely to be described as having difficult temperament 'by definition'. Finally, the studies do not appear to agree on which of the nine temperament dimensions is associated with colic, suggesting that the relationship of colic to any specific temperamental dimension is not very robust.

More recent *prospective* studies cast additional doubt on how closely colic and temperamental difficulty are related. A particularly important study in this regard was reported by Lehtonen *et al.* (1994). They asked parents for a general impression of their infants' overall temperament at 3 and 12 months, as well as their responses to a single question representing each of the nine temperament dimensions (activity, rhythmicity, adaptability, etc.) identified in the New York Longitudinal Study (Thomas *et al.* 1968). Each question was scored on a three-point scale. At 12 months, they also completed the revised Toddler Temperament Scale (Fullard *et al.* 1984). This questionnaire asks parents to rate specific behaviors, from which scores for each of the nine temperament dimensions are derived. In this sense, it provides a less impressionistic report of the behaviors presumed to reflect temperamental differences.

Consistent with previous findings, at 3 months the parents were more likely to perceive their previously colicky infants as having more intense reactions, and being more negative in mood, less persistent and more distractible. At 12 months, they were still perceived as being more active and less persistent. Furthermore, 23 per cent of infants with prior colic were perceived to be generally 'more difficult' than average, compared to 5 per cent of infants without prior colic. In stark contrast, however, there were no differences on any of the nine temperament dimensions derived from the 12 month Toddler Temperament Scale, based on actual behaviors of the infants. Consequently, while their parents retained a *generalized impression* of their infants' 'difficult' temperament, these general impressions were not supported by their more specific ratings of their childrens' behavior. Importantly, there were also no differences in sleep behaviors or patterns assessed at the ages of 8 and 12 months.

Two other prospective studies provide converging evidence that the relationship between early increased crying and temperament may be tenuous. The first suggests that temperament ratings taken prior to the development of colic may not predict crying at 6 weeks when colic is usually at its peak. Barr *et al.* (1988) asked mothers of 2-week-old infants to use a 17-item scale that provides a temperament score ranging from 'easy' to 'difficult' (Sostek and Anders 1977). Four weeks later, they completed a one-week diary that included crying and fussing behavior. The early temperament ratings did predict later duration and frequency of crying/fussing behavior, but the correlations were very modest (0.21 and 0.19 respectively), and only accounted for a small proportion of the variance (about 7 per cent) even after controlling for other possible confounders (such as breast- or formula-feeding). This translates into a very modest 17.0 minutes more crying and fussing per 24 hours for a 'difficult' infant (Barr *et al.* 1989). This was not a study of infants with 'colic'. However, it suggested that, even during the period of peak crying, those behaviors thought to be germane to the concept of 'difficult' temperament are far from explaining individual differences in crying, of which colic is the most extreme group. The second study suggested that having colic did not necessarily predict later temperament. Stifter and Braungart (1992) followed 100 normal infants from birth, of whom 10 met clinical criteria for colic. Prior to laboratory visits at 5 and 10 months, parents completed the Infant Behavior Questionnaire (Rothbart 1981) that measures six dimensions of temperament derived from ratings of specific infant behaviors. As in the Lehtonen *et al.* study, there were no differences in any of the six temperament dimensions at 5 or at 10 months.

In summary, the extent to which colic and difficult temperament are associated is more tenuous than might have been imagined. Infants with colic may be *perceived* to be more difficult infants later, but this is not congruent with reports based on specific behaviors, even when rated by the same parents. When colic (or crying) and temperament are measured prospectively, the association is weak or nonexistent. Neither is it clear that infants with colic have more difficulties with other regulatory functions (such as sleep) later. Because crying and fussing are predominant measures for parent reports both of colic and of difficult temperament, there is a measurement bias predisposing to them being associated. Compelling evidence that they are (or are not) related will require measures other than parent reports that are dependent on amounts of crying or fussing.

The notion of 'responsivity'
The notion of responsivity has emerged as a central concept in the fields of temperament and emotion regulation. The term 'responsivity' is usually used as a superordinate category that includes two subordinate dimensions, namely 'reactivity' and 'regulation' (Tables 4.1, 4.2). Conceptually, 'reactivity' refers to the excitability and/or arousability of responsive

TABLE 4.1

Aspects of the concept of 'responsivity', including 'type' and 'dynamics' of responses, indicating two subdimensions of responsivity dynamics: 'reactivity' and 'regulation'

Type:	Positive (*e.g.* smile) or Negative (*e.g.* cry)	
Dynamics:	Quality, intensity and timing of responses	
	System characteristics	*Parameters*
• *Reactivity*	Excitability/arousability	1. Threshold 2. Intensity 3. Onset time
• *Regulation*	Intrinsic/extrinsic modulation	1. Duration 2. Recovery rate

TABLE 4.2

Components of infant responses with examples of accessible, noninvasive measures for each system

Component	*System*	*Sample measures*
Subjective–experiential	Covert subjective	Verbal report (not available in infants)
Behavioral	Overt behavior	Vocalizations Facial activity Motor activity
Physiological	Covert	
	Autonomic	Heart period Vagal tone
	Hypothalamic pituitary adrenal	Cortisol

behavioral and physiological systems; 'regulation' refers to the processes (intrinsic or extrinsic) that may modulate this reactivity (for reviews, see Rothbart and Derryberry 1981, Thompson 1994). As a rubric for describing individual differences, it is assumed that, in response to the same stimulus, individuals can differ in both the *type* and the *dynamics* of their response. In infants, 'type' usually refers to whether the response has a negative or positive valence. Thus, for example, one infant may cry while another infant may smile in response to the same stimulus (say, a tickle or a stranger's face). The 'dynamics' of a response refers to the *intensity* or *temporal course* of the response. Thus, for example, while two infants may cry in response to the same stimulus, one may cry very loudly very quickly, while another may only fuss after a considerable delay.

There are a number of advantages to employing these as core concepts in studies of temperament and emotion regulation. First, they capture well the sense of the temperament construct. To use the metaphor suggested by Thompson (1994), dynamics refers not to the tune, but to the ways the tune is played by different individuals. Thomas and Chess (1977) referred to this as the "how" of behavior, or the "behavioral style". Considering response

45

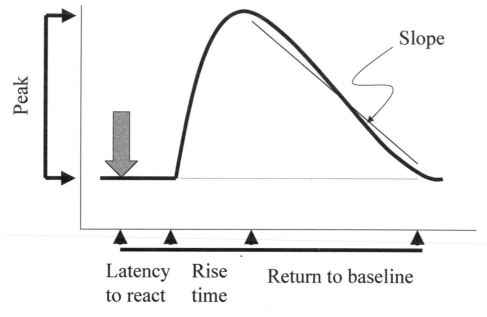

Fig. 4.1. Graphical illustration of measures of dynamic parameters of responsivity (reactivity and regulation). The grey arrow represents the time of application of a discrete stimulus to a system. Reactivity can be measured by peak height, latency to react and rise time. Regulation can be measured by the slope of the return to baseline and time to return to baseline.

dynamics highlights the important principle that, to be biologically adaptive, responses must be able to be flexible (rather than stereotypic), situationally responsive, and adaptable to a wide variety of conditions (Hofer 1994, Thompson 1994).

Second, the responsivity concepts provide an approach to distinguishing, conceptually and to some extent empirically, the dynamics of reactivity from the dynamics of response regulation (Lewis 1989, Worobey and Lewis 1989, Thompson 1994, Lewis and Ramsay 1995b, Braungart-Ricker and Stifter 1996). Assuming a starting state, responses are initiated by a stimulus, rise in intensity, come to a peak, and then subside over time (Fig. 4.1). In principle at least, this permits a number of parameters of reactivity and regulation to be operationalized. *Reactivity* measures of response 'intensity' can be captured by determining the *threshold* (or sensitivity) of the system to reacting as a function of the intensity of the stimulation required to provoke a reaction (Rothbart and Derryberry 1981, Lewis 1989) The *peak height* of the response (to a standard stimulus) can provide another measure of the intensity of the system's reactivity. 'Temporal' reactivity measures include the *latency to react*, and the *rise time* from initiation of the reaction to its peak. *Regulation* can be captured in principle by measures of recovery. This could include the *slope* of the recovery and/or the *time to return* to baseline. It should be noted that these are descriptions of the response process, not direct measures of the mechanisms that may be implicated in the process.

The third advantage of reactivity and regulation concepts is that they can be applied at a number of levels of description, including subjective–experiential, behavioral and physiological components (Rothbart and Derryberry 1981, Lewis 1989). This facilitates investigation of temperament as an essentially psychobiological construct implicating the biological structures integrally involved with manifest behavior (Rothbart and Derryberry 1981, Goldsmith *et al.* 1987, Lewis 1989, Plomin 1989). The subjective-experiential, behavioral and physiological systems are integrally related in complex ways, and their reactivity and regulation properties are not necessarily isomorphic (Fox 1989, Stansbury and Gunnar 1994). In animals and human infants, the subjective–experiential components are available only by inference. However, the type and dynamics of behavioral and some physiological systems (heart rate, vagal tone, hypothalamic–pituitary–adrenal [HPA] axis) are measureable in noninvasive ways (for review, see Fox 1994a). In the context of the present argument, this is particularly important. Measurement of responsivity characteristics in temperament-relevant behavioral and physiological systems may permit us to empirically test competing hypotheses concerning putative relationships between difficult temperament and colic.

LIMITATIONS TO THE RESPONSIVITY CONCEPT

Despite these advantages, there are a number of conceptual, empirical and measurement limitations to the concept of responsivity, five of which are germane to the argument to be pursued here. The first is the conceptual assumption that reactivity and regulation dimensions of the response are independent. On the basis of some definitions, there is some empirical support for this distinction. For example, Lewis and Ramsay reported no age change in "maximum" behavioral crying responses (reactivity) to innoculation (possibly because of ceiling effects), while quieting (regulation) occurred more rapidly with age (Ramsay and Lewis 1994, Lewis and Ramsay 1995b). However, the measures may represent only a 'first approximation' of reactive and regulatory processes. It is not at all clear, for example, that regulatory processes come into play only once the system has reached its peak response. Indeed, it is more likely that regulatory processes are implicated from the start. If so, the 'peak' measure of intensity (and other 'reactivity' measures) represents some *combination* of reactive and regulatory properties of the system (Rothbart and Derryberry 1981). A second limitation is that it is not always clear which of the various potential indices of 'reactivity' or 'regulation' are most appropriate. As an illustration, both latency of return to baseline and slope are used as indices of regulation. However, latencies of return to baseline may be the same for both responses, while the slopes are different, and dependent on the peak attained (Fig. 4.2). In such cases, it is not clear *a priori* whether it should be concluded that 'regulation' is the same or different. The third limitation relates to the availability of measures. The operational distinction between reactivity and regulation depends on continuous, or at least frequent, sampling of the phasic response. However, logistic or feasibility limitations often constrain the numbers of samples available. Consequently, studies of responsivity are often limited to differences between one baseline and one post-stimulus response sample. Indeed, for all studies of cortisol responsivity in infants, we know of only a few that have sampled post-stimulus cortisol more than once. With so few post-stimulus measurements, it is unclear whether the pre- to post-stressor response indexes

47

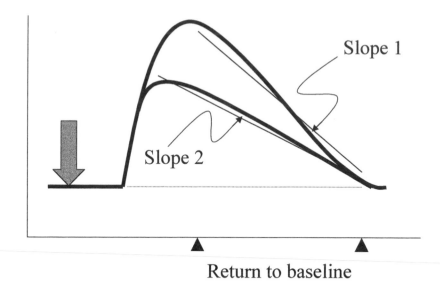

Fig. 4.2. Graphical illustration of different results obtained from two measures of 'regulation'. For two different responses to a stimulus, Slope 1 is different from Slope 2, but the time to return to baseline is the same.

reactivity, regulation, or some combination of both. Fourth, it is not clear whether the dynamics of multiple behavioral and physiological responses are related in lawful ways despite their different temporal courses. Fox and Calkins (1993) have argued that they should be, but this has yet to be demonstrated. Finally, it is unlikely that responsivity represents a unitary dimension of general arousal that applies across response systems. More likely, responses will vary across response systems of an individual, as well as amongst individuals (Lacey 1967, Rothbart and Derryberry 1981). If infants with colic and with difficult temperament are different, it may be the patterns of responsivity amongst systems that distinguish them.

These limitations need not vitiate the value of the responsivity, reactivity and regulation constructs, nor of the intensity and temporal measures of these response systems. Indeed, many of these concerns would be diminished if and when the determinants and/or the mechanisms underlying different parts of the phasic responses were known. However, they are a reminder that the results of studies of responsivity must be carefully described and interpreted to prevent misleading conclusions. Keeping these caveats in mind, we turn now to see whether these concepts may be useful as a strategy for approaching the problem of infant colic and whether colic is related to difficult temperament.

Colic: the 'transient responsivity' hypothesis
In the first instance, we employ the responsivity, reactivity and regulation constructs to provide a conceptual statement of the hypothesis that infants with colic will manifest a 'transient increased responsivity' relative to non-colic infants. Then, using the same constructs, we

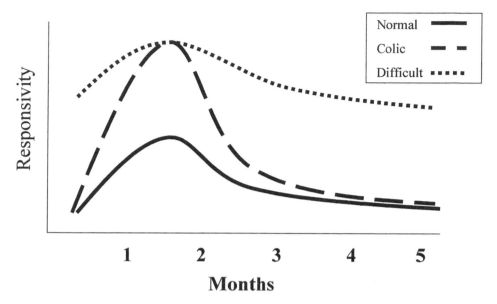

Fig. 4.3. Graphical illustration of age-related course of responsivity measures that might be expected according to the transient responsivity hypothesis of infant colic *(long broken lines)*, compared to the persistent difficult temperament hypothesis *(short broken lines)*, and to infants without colic *(solid line)*.

can compare what might be expected on the assumption that colic is an early manifestation of an infant with 'difficult' temperament. Finally, we propose a variation on the original, indicating that there may be both a 'weak' and a 'strong' version of the hypothesis.

The simplest and most general statement of the hypothesis is that, on appropriate responsivity measures, infants with colic compared to those without will manifest increased levels of responsivity during the first three months of life, but that this increased responsiveness will be transient, not persistent. Because of the behavioral phenomenology of infant colic in which the increased crying follows an 'n-shaped' curve over the first three months, we predict that the responsivity will be greater sometime during the second month (6 weeks, say). However, because it is transient (rather than persistent), it should be the same as in infants without colic at birth and after the colic has resolved (at 5 months, say). This is illustrated graphically in Figure 4.3. Note that the mean responsivity of normal infants also shows an increase and a decrease in responsivity during the first three months, but that this pattern is exaggerated in infants with colic. This reflects the current evidence that essentially all of the features associated with the crying of infants with colic (peak pattern, evening clustering, unsoothable crying bouts, pain facies, acoustic properties of the cries, post-feed crying) are also found in infants without colic but that they are less intense, less prolonged, or less frequent (Barr 2000). Note also that there would be no colic/normal differences in responsivity either at birth or at 5 months.

By contrast, when the hypothesis that colic is an early manifestation of difficult temperament is formulated in terms of the responsivity concept, it is also predicted that infants with colic will manifest increased levels of responsivity during the first three months, but that these levels of responsivity will be persistent, rather than transient (Fig. 4.3). In this case, the n-shaped curve would be present for infants both with and without colic, but the curve for colic would be higher than, and run 'parallel' to, the curve for normals. Note that, if responsivity was measured only at 2 months, there would be no means of distinguishing between the transient responsivity and difficult temperament hypotheses, as is currently the case with parent report measures of difficult temperament. However, if measures of responsivity were taken soon after birth and at 5 months, they would provide two tests for distinguishing between the transient responsivity and persistent difficult temperament hypotheses.

As indicated earlier, responsivity is the more general superordinate concept that includes the two components of reactivity and regulation. Because they are conceptualized to be independent of each other, the behavioral manifestations of colic may be understood in terms of either one or both components of responsivity. Consequently, if we incorporate the two subdimensions of reactivity and regulation, then the transient responsivity hypothesis can be stated in terms of three slightly more complex, but also more specific, versions of the hypothesis. The first version is that infants with colic will have *both* increased reactivity *and* decreased regulation at 2 months compared to infants without colic, but there will be no differences at birth or at 5 months. In this case, the 'curves' of reactivity and regulation for infants with and without colic will be the same as those for 'responsivity' in Figure 4.3.

The second version of the hypothesis (which can be called the 'transient *reactivity*' hypothesis) is that infants with colic *differ in reactivity*, but have the *same regulatory* capacities as normal infants. In this case, infants with colic will have increased reactivity at 2 months compared to infants without colic, no reactivity differences at birth or at 5 months, and no differences in regulation at any age. Since 'reactivity' is expected to account for the behavioral phenomenology, the n-shaped curve (and colic/normal differences) would be reflected only in the values for the reactivity measures. It is not clear what shape the curve for regulatory measures would have, but consistent with most developmental assumptions, it would probably improve, and in any case would not be different for infants with and without colic.

The third version of the hypothesis (which can be called the 'transient *regulatory*' hypothesis) is that infants with colic have *decreased regulatory* capacities, but the same reactivity as infants without. In this case, infants with colic will have decreased regulation at 2 months (that is, their responses to stimuli will be greater in the absence of regulation), no regulatory differences at birth and at 5 months, and no differences in reactivity at any age (Fig. 4.4). Of these three versions of the transient responsivity hypothesis, there are reasons to think that the evidence is most consistent with the transient regulatory hypothesis. We will review the evidence favouring this version of the hypothesis shortly.

Although seldom explicitly stated, it is most likely that infants with difficult temperament would be those with a combination of increased reactivity *and* decreased regulation (Rothbart and Derryberry 1981, Lewis 1989). Furthermore, both increased reactivity and decreased regulation would be present at birth (reflecting the fact that temperament is largely constitutional and genetic, and assuming that these responsivity properties were expressed

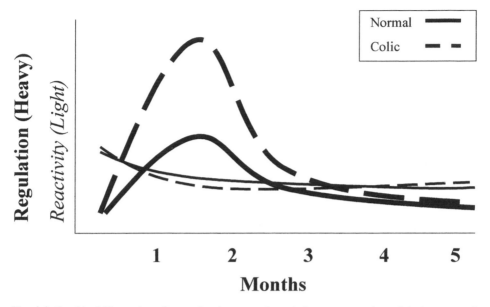

Fig. 4.4. Graphical illustration of age-related course of regulation measures that might be expected according to the more specific transient regulation hypothesis if infants with colic were different from infants without colic on measures of regulation (*bold broken lines and bold solid lines*, respectively), but not on measures of reactivity (*thin broken lines* and *solid lines*, respectively).

at birth) and persistent (reflecting the fact that temperament is relatively stable). If infants with colic were infants with difficult temperament, then both their reactivity and regulation scores would be higher and parallel to those of infants without colic (Fig. 4.5). Note that there are now many potential points at which to test the persistent temperament hypothesis against one or other of the versions of the transient responsivity hypothesis.

Strong and weak versions of the transient responsivity hypothesis

Although rarely systematically studied, there are an increasing number of observations in the literature that suggest that (1) increased responsivity does not necessarily have the same 'meaning' at different ages, and (2) early increased responsivity may be related to later lower responsivity (or better regulation) on a variety of measures. In an early observation, Bell *et al.* (1971) reported that infants who had intense motor reactions to removal of a nipple as newborns had less intense motor reactions to presentation of a barrier in the preschool period. More recently, using pre- to post-pain stimulus cortisol differences, a number of authors have reported that an elevated 'stress' response is associated with more optimal functioning in the newborn period (Gunnar *et al.* 1987, 1995; Magnano *et al.* 1992; Spangler and Scheubeck 1993; Ramsay and Lewis 1995) but with less optimal functioning in later infancy (Spangler *et al.* 1994, Gunnar *et al.* 1995, Ramsay and Lewis 1995). Furthermore, elevated stress responses early may be associated with reduced stress responses later (Gunnar *et al.* 1995, Lewis and Ramsay 1995b). Thus, for example, Gunnar *et al.* (1995) found that

51

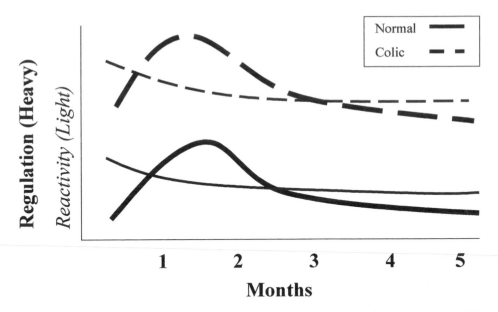

Fig. 4.5. Graphical illustration of age-related courses of reactivity and regulation measures that might be expected according to the persistent difficult temperament hypothesis, in which infants with colic would have higher scores on both measures before, during and after the period in which colic occurs than would infants without colic.

infants who cry more and have higher cortisol responses to heel stick stimuli at birth cry less and have lower cortisol responses when immunized at 6 months, and their parents rate them as having less 'distress to limitations' on the Infant Behavior Questionnaire. Ramsay and Lewis (1995) reported that an optimal birth condition was associated with a high cortisol response to immunization at 2 months but a low cortisol response at 6 months. Similar findings have also been reported for vagal tone, a different physiological response system likely to be integral to emotional expression and regulation (Porges *et al.* 1994). Newborn infants with high vagal tone—a parasympathetic measure of responsivity—manifest more irritability and difficulty in self-soothing. However, 3-month-old infants with high vagal tone require less soothing and score high on the 'soothability' dimension of the Infant Behavior Questionnaire (Huffman *et al.* 1998). Finally, newborns who take longer to soothe to pacifier become more rhythmic, approachful of new situations, adaptable and pleasant by 9 months of age (Riese 1995).

These interesting 'inversions' in reactivity and/or regulatory measures of responsivity in normal infants raise another possible version of the transient responsivity hypothesis. The core assumption of the transient responsivity hypothesis is that infants with colic are otherwise normal, but as a group represent the upper end of the spectrum of normal behavioral and emotional development. Assuming these individual differences can be captured by measures of responsivity, then the form of the hypothesis that we have been describing until now might be called the *'weak'* form of the hypothesis; namely, that infants with colic

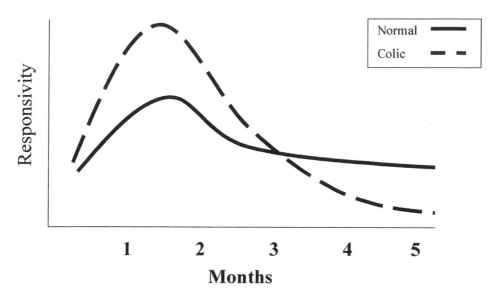

Fig. 4.6. Graphical illustration of the strong form of the transient responsivity hypothesis, in which infants with colic would have higher scores than infants without colic on responsivity measures during the time they had colic, but lower scores after colic resolved.

compared to those without will have increased responsivity early, but will be *the same* as other infants by 5 months. However, if increased responsivity early becomes lower responsivity later, then the *'strong'* form of the hypothesis would be that infants with higher responsivity earlier (*i.e.* infants with colic) will actually be *less responsive* (*i.e.* less reactive and/or better regulated) than infants without colic at 5 months (Fig. 4.6). If this were shown to be true, it would be even stronger evidence against the hypothesis that colic is an early manifestation of persistent difficult temperament.

Evidence supporting the 'transient responsivity' hypothesis of infant colic
A number of observations provide partial support for the weak—and even the strong—forms of the transient responsivity hypothesis of infant colic. In some cases, they also challenge the difficult temperament hypothesis. None of these studies were carried out specifically to test either hypothesis, so the evidence remains tentative at best. As will be seen, whether some of the measures reported are good indices of general responsivity or more specifically reactivity and/or regulation is not always clear (see Limitations to the responsivity concept, above). Nevertheless, the evidence does tend to support the potential usefulness of considering colic syndrome in the light of these constructs.

THE 'BIOBEHAVIORAL SHIFT'
The first argument is a very general one; namely, that many behavioral and physiological functions—including but not limited to crying—manifest developmental n- (or u-) shaped curves during the first three months. For crying behavior, the evidence is increasingly

strong. The n-shaped curve for crying has been described not only for normally developing infants in Western caregiving settings (Brazelton 1962, Hunziker and Barr 1986, Barr 1990a, St James-Roberts and Halil 1991, St James-Roberts *et al.* 1995, Alvarez and St James-Roberts 1996) but also in !Kung San hunter-gatherers (Barr *et al.* 1991a) and, at least partially, in Manali infants (St James-Roberts *et al.* 1994) in whom caregiving practice is radically different. It is also present in age-corrected preterm infants despite an additional eight weeks of extrauterine experience (Barr *et al.* 1996, Malone 1997). Consequently, the overall pattern of a decrease in crying behavior is quite marked. This is consistent with the behavior pattern that might be expected for the transient responsivity hypothesis. One of the possible reasons for this apparent discontinuity is that crying does not stay the same over this period; rather, fairly dramatic shifts in crying quality begin to occur at about 3 months. Crying becomes more modulated, context-dependent, intentional and 'communicative' (Bell and Ainsworth 1972, Gekoski *et al.* 1983, Franco 1984, Hopkins and von Wulfften Palthe 1987, Barr 1990a). However, such changes do not rule out the possibility that individual differences in crying persist throughout this period (consistent with the persistent difficult temperament hypothesis).

The evidence for individual stability in crying is mixed. In one report, individual differences in crying were stable only for the first three months, but not after. For fussing, they were not stable until after 6 weeks (St James-Roberts and Plewis 1996). In another, infant 'distress' (crying plus fussing plus 'colic' crying) was reduced by more than 50 per cent at 5 months of age in three groups of infants (defined as 'persistent', 'evening' and 'moderate' criers at 6 weeks), but individual differences were moderately stable (r = 0.54, p<0.001) (St James-Roberts *et al.* 1998). It remains unclear whether this individual difference persists beyond 5 months, and to what extent this might be accounted for by caregiving style, since the mothers of persistent criers had a lower inclination to respond to crying at 5 months (St James-Roberts *et al.* 1998). Similar developmental curves have been described in whole or in part for many other infant parameters, ranging from changes in sleep patterns (Parmelee and Stern 1972, Anders *et al.* 1992), nutrient intakes (Fomon 1974), incomplete absorption of lactose carbohydrate (Douwes *et al.* 1980, Barr *et al.* 1984, Miller *et al.* 1992), and measures of attention and habituation for visual stimuli (Bornstein *et al.* 1996, Hood *et al.* 1996, Johnson 1996, Slater *et al.* 1996) to cortisol response to handling during pain and stress procedures.

Developmental changes in cortisol response are of particular interest in regard to colic, because of the assumption that infants with colic may be experiencing increased 'stress'. The necessity for relatively standard immunizations at 2, 4 and 6 months has provided an opportunity to study salivary cortisol responses longitudinally. There is a developmental 'dampening' of cortisol responsivity between 2–4 and 6 months of age, with a further decrease in responsivity by 15–18 months (Gunnar *et al.* 1989, 1996; Ramsay and Lewis 1994; Lewis and Ramsay 1995a,b; Larson *et al.* 1998). In addition, individual stability in cortisol responses become apparent only between 4 months and later, but not between 2 and 4 or 6 months (Lewis and Ramsay 1995a,b).

These and other findings have been interpreted as suggesting that there is a 'biobehavioral shift' (Emde *et al.* 1976) occurring at 2–3 months that is expressed in many aspects of the infant's functioning. Further, the relatively weak, and often absent, stabilities across this developmental period for many of these parameters, including those traditionally used in studies of temperament and emotional regulation, compared to the stronger stabilities later in the first year suggest that early individual differences may be more transient than stable (Rothbart 1981, St James-Roberts and Wolke 1988, Worobey and Lewis 1989, Izard and Porges 1991, Kagan and Snidman 1991, Fox 1994b, Snidman *et al.* 1995). Exactly what this biobehavioral shift consists of, what its determinants are, and how it is organized remain matters of considerable debate (Emde *et al.* 1976, Prechtl 1984, Barr 1998a). However, if infants with colic are otherwise normal infants, it seems at least reasonably likely that their increased crying could be but one manifestation of individual differences that are transient rather than persistent, as is true for these other functions.

DURATION-FREQUENCY DISSOCIATION IN CRYING
The second line of argument stems from an interesting feature of the phenomenological descriptions of crying in infants with and without colic. Descriptions of crying in everyday contexts have often been limited to measures of crying duration (total duration per day, or per period of observation), with little attention to parameters such as frequency and bout length. However, in studies of caregiving effects on the crying of normal infants, duration appears to be susceptible to modification but frequency is much less so (Barr 1990b). Thus, for example, in a randomized controlled trial of increased carrying and holding by parents, crying and fussing duration was reduced by 43 per cent at 6 weeks of age in the group receiving 'supplemental carrying', but there was no difference in the frequency of crying/fussing bouts (Hunziker and Barr 1986, Barr 1989). Caregiving of infants of the !Kung San hunter-gatherers is usually characterized as 'indulgent', and features constant holding, carrying in a sling, upright posture, 'continuous' breast-feeding (about four times an hour for one to two minutes per feed), and virtually immediate responsivity to cries and frets. Despite the radical differences in caregiving style from that typical of Dutch and American infants, cry/fret frequency is the same, but duration of crying and fretting is only about half as long (Barr *et al.* 1991a). These observations suggest that parameters such as frequency and duration of crying bouts are dissociable and may be subject to different determinants. Of course, this might be accounted for simply by the fact that caregivers are more likely to respond to crying, thereby shortening the crying bouts. However, many of the elements of !Kung San caregiving (including carrying) are constant (rather than responsive), and the crying differences in the carrying study were due to increased carrying that was not associated with crying (Barr 1990b). Thus, caregiving strategies may not affect whether an infant cries, but could modify whether or not crying persists. Furthermore, this dissociation could be cast in terms of the reactivity and regulation components of responsivity. It may be suggesting that caregiving components are modifiers of cry/fuss regulation, but have little or no effect on reactivity.

Applied to the behavioral phenomenology of colic, a number of observations provide interesting support for the possibility that decreased *regulation* is an important, and perhaps specific, feature of the crying of infants with colic. Other than crying, resistance to soothing (decreased regulation) is the most frequently cited clinical characteristic (Barr 1991). When the crying of infants meeting modified Wessel's criteria (Wessel *et al.* 1954) for colic was compared to that of normal infants and clinically problematic infants who did not meet Wessel's criteria, the frequency of crying bouts was the same in all three groups; however, bout length was longer only in infants with Wessel's colic (Barr *et al.* 1992). In contrast to the situation in normal infants, increased carrying is ineffective as a treatment for increased crying in infants meeting modified Wessel's criteria, implying that difficulty in regulation of crying (at least by caregiving techniques) is characteristic of infants with colic (Barr *et al.* 1991b). Finally, in a controlled comparison by St. James-Roberts *et al.* (1995), the crying bouts of 'persistent criers' were more likely to be resistant to soothing and to require a greater variety of soothing maneouvers. Together, these findings imply that it is the inability to arrest crying once started, rather than the presence of crying itself, that is specific to infants with colic. If presence or absence of crying reflects reactivity, and duration (or bout length) of crying reflects regulation, then the responsivity dimension most important for understanding infants with colic may be decreased regulation rather than increased reactivity (the transient regulation hypothesis). However, since most of these studies do not independently measure crying intensity (a reactivity measure), this only suggests, but does not demonstrate, specific differences in capacities to regulate crying.

REACTIVITY AND REGULATION IN COLIC STUDIES
The third line of argument derives from controlled studies of infants with and without colic which used measures that could be seen as measuring reactive and/or regulatory dimensions of responsiveness in infants. In the first of these (the previously mentioned study of Stifter and Braungart 1992), 10 of 100 infants followed prospectively from birth were identified as meeting clinical criteria for colic in the second month of life. At birth, 5 and 10 months (but unfortunately not while they manifested colic symptoms), they were administered age-appropriate stimuli designed to elicit negative 'reactivity' (crying responses). However, since the presence or absence of crying as well as intensity and duration measures were used, it is probably more appropriate to interpret this as a study of negative reactivity *and* regulation, *i.e.* 'responsivity'. At birth, alert inactive infants were administered a pacifier withdrawal task (repeated withdrawals after one minute of sucking) and a rubber band snap to the heel. At 5 months, the infants underwent the arm restraint procedure, in which their mothers held their infants' arms at their sides (and maintained a neutral composure) until the infant cried for 20 seconds. At 10 months, the infants were exposed to toy removal. Mothers moved a toy that the infant had been playing with for 90 seconds out of reach but within sight of the infant until the infant cried for 20 seconds. In each case, duration and intensity of crying was recorded. Importantly for the purposes of our argument, the infants with or without prior colic showed no differences in the presence or absence, intensity or duration of crying for any of the tasks at any age. In a later replication, infants with prior colic (n = 11) did cry more than infants without colic to arm restraint at 5 months, but there were no differences in crying response at 10 months (Stifter 1997).

Although these are small samples, these studies are important in the present context for two reasons. First, since the studies were specifically designed to elicit temperamental differences in 'negative reactivity', the absence of differences was quite striking, and quite incompatible with a persistent 'difficult infant' hypothesis. Since equivalent measures were not taken when the infants were manifesting colic symptoms, it remains unclear as to whether these infants ever had differences in responsivity. Consequently, if infants with colic do have differences in responsivity, they are likely to be transient (not present before or after colic) rather than persistent. The second reason is that, perhaps surprisingly, the infants with colic actually cried only about 70 per cent as long as their matched control group during the arm restraint and toy removal tasks at 5 and 10 months respectively (Stifter and Braungart 1992). Because of the small sample sizes, it is theoretically possible that differences in responsivity were missed in this study. However, the fact that crying tended to be less in infants with colic at 5 and 10 months reduces the likelihood that significant *increases* in negative responsivity predicted by the persistent temperament hypothesis were missed despite the small sample sizes. If anything, it is suggestive that the 'strong' form of the transient responsivity hypothesis is more likely to be correct.

To date, only two controlled studies have measured putative indices of responsivity during the time infants manifested colic. White *et al.* (2000) used an analogue to a 'real life' setting by having infants with and without colic undergo a mock physical examination consisting of four phases: (1) Baseline; (2) a Measurement phase consisting of undressing the infant and taking temperature, weight, height and head circumference measures; (3) Rest; and (4) a Physical Exam including ears, mouth, eyes, heart and respiration, followed by a Denver II Developmental Screen. From the videotape, behavioral measures of aggregate crying duration, intensity and consolability were extracted. In addition, heart rate and vagal tone were calculated for each phase, and three salivary cortisol samples were taken (Baseline, post-Measurement, post-Physical Exam). Since the stimuli were not discrete and the measures were aggregated within phases, these are best thought of as behavioral and physiological measures of responsivity, rather than measures of reactivity and regulation. In addition, parents completed 24-hour diaries of infant behavior (Hunziker and Barr 1986, Barr *et al.* 1988) for three days to confirm that infants met modified Wessel's criteria for colic.

With respect to our argument, there were two main findings. The first was that infants with colic were behaviorally more negatively responsive. Overall, infants with colic had about twice the amount of negative vocalizations as infants without, and a greater proportion of these vocalizations were rated as moderate or intense. Consolability was scored only in those infants who had moderate or intense cries. Of these, half of the infants with colic, but none of the infants without, were 'inconsolable', and consolability scores were significantly poorer for infants with colic. This might be taken to index regulation since crying intensity is partially controlled for by considering only moderate or intense cries. However, since there were more intense cries amongst infants with colic (*i.e.* cry intensity was not controlled), it is probably more conservatively considered as evidence of increased responsivity in infants with colic. The second main finding was the absence of important differences on physiological measures of heart rate, vagal tone and salivary cortisol secretion, despite clear evidence of expected responses to the exam stress. At least in this stimulus setting, the increased responsivity appeared to be specific to behavioral, but not physiological, systems.

Three additional findings deserve mention. First, all three measures of behavioral responsivity were moderately strongly and significantly correlated with diary measures of total daily crying (all r = 0.44–0.57), suggesting that the laboratory behavioral measures of responsivity are relevant to at least one behavioral feature of colic. Second, there were no significant correlations between any baseline physiological measures and negative behavior during the examination. However, for most measures during the Measurement and Physical Exam periods, physiological–behavioral correlations were significant and of the same order of magnitude in infants with and without colic. This implies that, from the point of view of the organization of their physiological–behavioral systems, infants with colic were otherwise normal despite the differences in behavioral responsivity. In addition, it appears that the greater crying of infants with colic can be supported with otherwise similar activation of relevant physiological systems. Third, as found in previous studies, infants with colic were rated as having more 'distress to limitations', the core of the difficult temperament dimension on the Infant Behavior Questionnaire. This supports the expectation that infants with colic are not easily distinguishable from infants with difficult temperament at the time when colic is manifest.

The final study complements the two previous studies but is more specifically focused on assessing *regulation* of crying behavior during the period when infants manifest colic. In previous studies of normal infants, the taste of sucrose (or, more accurately, sweet taste— Barr *et al.* 1999a) applied to the anterior tongue produces dramatic calming in already crying newborns, an effect that persists for minutes after the taste stimulus is gone (Blass *et al.* 1989; Smith *et al.* 1990; Blass and Smith 1992; Barr *et al.* 1994, 1999a; Graillon *et al.* 1997). In nonhuman species, sucrose tastes are equally effective at blocking distress vocalizations in response to maternal separation. This effect requires a functioning central opioid-dependent system, since sucrose has the same effect as morphine injections, and both sucrose and morphine effects are blocked by opioid antagonists (Panksepp *et al.* 1978; Kehoe and Blass 1986a,b; Blass *et al.* 1987, 1989, 1990; Smith *et al.* 1990). Furthermore, of the central transmitter systems, the opioid system has the most specific and powerful effect on distress vocalization reduction (Panksepp *et al.* 1980). Sucrose induced orogustatory calming is functionally distinct from pacifier (or contact) induced orotactile calming, and pacifier induced calming is not opioid-dependent. Pacifier calming is stimulus-bound (*i.e.* effective only while the pacifier is in the mouth—Wolff 1987, Smith *et al.* 1990), whereas sucrose calming persists for minutes after the taste stimulus is over. In animals, contact calming is not blocked by opioid antagonists (Blass *et al.* 1990, 1995). In human infants, orogustatory but not pacifier calming is disturbed in infants of methadone-dependent mothers and infants with postmature syndrome, consistent with differential involvement of opioid systems in these two types of calming (Smith *et al.* 1992, Blass and Ciaramitaro 1994). Interestingly, sucrose taste effects are also able to be elicited at 6 weeks of age—the age when crying and colic peak—but, as would be expected if this system were relevant to crying regulation, are much diminished in magnitude (Barr *et al.* 1994, Zeifman *et al.* 1996). These findings suggest that sucrose taste may be useful as a biobehavioral probe of a relatively specific central, opioid-dependent calming system possibly implicated in distress regulation, and of the pattern of early infant crying, including colic.

In a review of orogustatory calming effects, Barr and Young (1999) argued that the sucrose taste calming response is actually a biphasic response. The early phase (marked by increased mouthing) is due to the presence of the liquid tastes in the mouth, its magnitude is dependent on salience of the taste, and it is probably not opioid-dependent. The late phase is not dependent on the continuing presence of the stimulus, its magnitude is dependent on the sweetness (or positive hedonic value) of the stimulus, and it probably is opioid-dependent. This makes the sucrose taste response a potentially interesting probe of crying regulation for two reasons. First, by starting with equivalently crying infants, the taste response isolates the extent to which the implicated mechanisms *regulate* negative responsiveness. Second, to the extent that the two phases of the taste response can be distinguished, it provides indices of two putative regulatory mechanisms, one probably related to an opioid-dependent central system, and one not. Consequently, differential early and late phase responses might index relatively specific central mechanisms contributing to regulation of negative responsivity characteristics of infants.

If, as previously suggested, the crying of infants with colic is a manifestation of individual differences in the regulatory component of its responsive systems, then it would be predicted that infants with and without colic would differ on one or both phases of the sucrose taste response. To test this prediction (Barr *et al.* 1999b), infants with and without colic were observed prior to a feed until they established at least 15 seconds of continuous crying, at which time they were provided with three 250μl tastes of 50 per cent sucrose solution 30 seconds apart to the anterior tongue. Prior to another feed, they received three water tastes. Both percentage time crying per minute and percentage time mouthing per minute were calculated for each subject for four minutes following each tastant. As expected, in normal infants, the calming response to sucrose was greater than for water throughout the four minutes post-administration (Fig. 4.7). After the first minute, water effectively produced no calming, whereas crying was stably reduced to about 65 per cent during minutes 3 and 4. In infants with colic, the response to water was the same as in the normal infants. In addition, sucrose reduced crying about the same amount in infants with colic as with normals during the first minute (to about 55 per cent). However, by three minutes post-taste completion, crying had increased to more than 90 per cent of the time in infants with colic. For mouthing (not shown in Fig. 4.7), sucrose produced a greater response than water in infants with and without colic, the mouthing response peaked in the first minute and dropped sharply in the second, and there was no difference between groups. This implies that the salience of the sucrose taste was the same for both.

For the purposes of our argument, these results are important for a number of reasons. The first is that they are the second demonstration that infants with colic differ on a measure of responsivity during the time they manifest colic behavior. The second is that, because initial crying state is equivalent, they specifically implicate regulation of negative responsivity, independent of reactivity to the inciting stimulus. Third, if the biphasic hypothesis concerning orogustatory responses (Barr and Young 1999) holds, the results implicate differences specifically in regard to one modality of regulation (sweet taste), but not another (taste contact). Fourth, there is reasonable evidence for a putative and quite specific opioid-based mechanism for this regulatory process. In this instance, taste tests may implicate determinants of the manifest regulatory processes previously defined only in temporal terms.

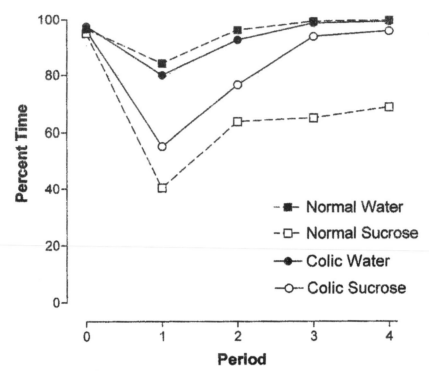

Fig. 4.7. Percentage time crying following water *(closed symbols)* and sucrose *(open symbols)* in infants with *(circles)* and without *(squares)* colic before taste administration (period 0) and in each minute following stimulus administration (periods 1 through 4) when tastes are administered to crying infants before a feeding. (Reprinted by permission from Barr *et al.* 1999b.)

Summary and conclusions

The transient responsivity hypothesis uses the concepts of responsivity, reactivity and regulation developed in the fields of temperament and emotion regulation as a framework to capture potentially defining functional characteristics of the clinical syndrome of infant colic. Beginning with well-established clinical features, it posits that, given appropriate measures, infants with colic will manifest increased responsivity during the period when colic syndrome is manifest, but that this increased responsivity will be transient (that is, not present before or following colic syndrome-like behavior). The predictions that follow from this hypothesis are different to those that follow from the leading alternative hypothesis; namely, that colic is an early behavioral manifestation of infants with difficult temperament. If so, they should show increased responsivity when colic is manifest, but this will be persistent (present before and after colic), not transient. Because responsivity will be a manifestation of some interplay between its two putatively independent components of reactivity and regulation, more specific hypotheses (and predictions) using these constructs can be generated.

No current study systematically addresses the predictions of the transient responsivity hypothesis. This would require a prospective study from birth in which appropriate measures of reactivity and regulation were taken before, during and after the period when colic is manifest, and in which reliable measures of colic behavior were used to classify infants with and without colic. However, we have argued that findings from three available studies converge in support of the transient responsivity hypothesis, and are inconsistent with the persistent temperament hypothesis. The longitudinal studies of Stifter and colleagues (Stifter and Braungart 1992, Stifter 1997) suggest that infants with and without colic have similar responsivity characteristics (for emotional negativity, or crying) before and after the colic period. These results support the 'transient' prediction, and are counter to the persistent difficult temperament prediction. The mock physical examination study of White *et al.* (2000) is the first to document increased behavioral responsivity during the colic period, and shows no difference in three physiologically responsive systems. This suggests that responsivity differences may not be generalized across all subsystems, and that the *pattern* of responsivity differences may contribute to understanding clinical crying syndromes. The sucrose taste response study of Barr *et al.* (1999b) focused specifically on the regulatory component of negative responsivity. Consistent with predictions, it documented diminished regulatory functioning which, intriguingly, may be specific to only one of two possible distress regulatory systems available to infants at this age. Along with the phenomenological evidence that infants with colic do not cry more often, but cry for longer once started, these findings heighten interest in the 'transient regulation' variant of the transient responsivity hypothesis. To date, there is no specific direct evidence for or against the possible role of increased reactivity.

Given almost 20 years of study of individual differences in temperament in terms of responsivity, reactivity and regulation in normal infants, and the remarkably close mapping between the phenomenological behaviors typical of infants with difficult temperament and colic, it is surprising that there have been so few attempts to apply these normative developmental constructs to understanding clinical crying syndromes. Perhaps this is due to an *a priori* assumption that colic behavior is a symptom or a sign of a distinct clinical syndrome due to organic or, even more specifically, gastrointestinal pathophysiological processes. Despite generating different predictions, both the transient responsivity and persistent difficult temperament hypotheses start from the assumption that colic is a manifestation of individual differences in otherwise normal infants. It also shifts the focus of interest from the gastrointestinal tract to the central nervous system. In light of the accumulating evidence that pathophysiological processes will not account for most cases of colic syndrome, and the extent to which current, though still incomplete, evidence appears to support this approach, careful examination of responsivity, reactivity and regulation properties may yet contribute to making the clinical colic syndrome less mysterious to concerned parents and clinicians.

ACKNOWLEDGEMENTS

Ronald Barr was supported by an Academic Award from the Montreal Children's Hospital Foundation and Project Support from the Hospital for Sick Children's Foundation (XG-96-003). Megan Gunnar was supported by a National Institutes of Mental Health Research Scientist Award (MH 00946)

REFERENCES

Alvarez, M., St James-Roberts, I. (1996) 'Infant fussing and crying patterns in the first year in an urban community in Denmark.' *Acta Paediatrica*, **85**, 463–466.

Anders, T.F., Halpern, L.F, Hua, J. (1992) 'Sleeping through the night: A developmental perspective.' *Pediatrics*, **90**, 554–560.

Barr, R.G. (1989) 'Recasting a clinical enigma: The problem of early infant crying.' *In:* Zelazo, P.H., Barr, R.G. (Eds.) *Challenges to Developmental Paradigms.* New York: Lawrence Erlbaum, pp. 43–64

—— (1990a) 'The normal crying curve: what do we really know?' *Developmental Medicine and Child Neurology*, **32**, 356–362.

—— (1990b) 'The early crying paradox: a modest proposal.' *Human Nature*, **1**, 355–389.

—— (1991) 'Colic and gas.' *In:* Walker, W.A., Durie, P.R., Hamilton, J.R., Walker-Smith, J.A., Watkins, J.G. (Eds.) *Pediatric Gastrointestinal Disease: Pathophysiology, Diagnosis and Management.* Burlington, VT: Decker, B.C., pp. 55–61.

—— (1996) 'Colic.' *In:* Walker, W.A., Durie, P.R., Hamilton, J.R., Walker-Smith, J.A., Watkins, J.B. (Eds.) *Pediatric Gastrointestinal Disease: Pathophysiology, Diagnosis and Management. 2nd Edn.* St. Louis: Mosby, pp. 241–250.

—— (1998a) 'Reflections on n-shaped curves in early infancy: Regulater or re-organized development?' Program of the International Conference on Infant Studies 35 (Abstract).

—— (1998b) 'Crying in the first year of life: good news in the midst of distress.' *Child: Care, Health and Development*, **24**, 425–439.

—— (2000) 'Excessive crying.' *In:* Lewis, M., Sameroff, A.J. (Eds.) *Handbook of Developmental Psychopathology. 2nd Edn.* New York: Plenum Press. *(In press.)*

—— Young, S.N. (1999) 'A two phase model of the soothing taste response: Implications for a taste probe of temperament and emotion regulation.' *In:* Lewis, M., Ramsay, D. (Eds.) *Soothing and Stress.* Mahwah, NJ: Lawrence Erlbaum, pp. 109–137.

—— Hanley, J., Patterson, D.K., Wooldridge, J.A. (1984) 'Breath hydrogen excretion of normal newborn infants in response to usual feeding patterns: evidence for "functional lactase insufficiency" beyond the first month of life.' *Journal of Pediatrics*, **104**, 527–533.

—— Kramer, M.S., Leduc, D.G., Boisjoly, C., McVey-White, L., Pless, I.B. (1988) 'Parental diary of infant cry and fuss behaviour.' *Archives of Disease in Childhood*, **63**, 380–387.

—— —— Pless, I.B., Boisjoly, C., Leduc, D. (1989) 'Feeding and temperament as determinants of early infant cry/fuss behaviour.' *Pediatrics*, **84**, 514–521.

—— Konner, M., Bakeman, R., Adamson, L. (1991a) 'Crying in !Kung San infants: a test of the cultural specificity hypothesis.' *Developmental Medicine and Child Neurology*, **33**, 601–610.

—— McMullan, S.J., Spiess, H., Leduc, D.J., Yaremko, J., Barfield, R., Francoeur, T.E., Hunziker, U.A. (1991b) 'Carrying as colic "therapy": a randomized controlled trial.' *Pediatrics*, **87**, 623–630.

—— Rotman, A., Yaremko, J., Leduc, D., Francoeur, T.E. (1992) 'The crying of infants with colic: a controlled empirical description.' *Pediatrics*, **90**, 14–21.

—— Quek, V., Cousineau, D., Oberlander, T.F., Brian, J.A., Young, S.N. (1994) 'Effects of intraoral sucrose on crying, mouthing and hand–mouth contact in newborn and six-week-old infants.' *Developmental Medicine and Child Neurology*, **36**, 608–618.

—— Chen, S., Hopkins, B., Westra, T. (1996) 'Crying patterns in preterm infants.' *Developmental Medicine and Child Neurology*, **38**, 345–355.

—— Pantel, M.S., Young, S.N., Wright, J.H., Hendricks, L.A., Gravel, R.G. (1999a) 'The response of crying newborns to sucrose: Is it a "sweetness" effect?' *Physiology and Behavior*, **66**, 409–417.

—— Young, S.N., Wright, J.H., Gravel, R., Alkawaf, R. (1999b) 'Differential calming response to sucrose taste in crying infants with and without colic.' *Pediatrics*, **103**, 1–9. (www.pediatrics.org/cgi/content/full/103/5/e68)

Bates, J.E., Freeland, C.A., Lounsbury, M.L. (1979) 'Measurement of infant difficultness.' *Child Development*, **50**, 794–803.

Bell, R.Q., Weller, G.M., Waldrop, M.F. (1971) *Newborn and Preschooler: Organization of Behavior and Relations Between Periods. Monographs of the Society for Research in Child Development, Serial No. 142, Vol. 36, No. 1.* Chicago: Chicago University Press.

Bell, S.M., Ainsworth, D.S. (1972) 'Infant crying and maternal responsiveness.' *Child Development*, **43**, 1171–1190.

Blass, E.M., Ciaramitaro, V. (1994) *A New Look at Some Old Mechanisms in Human Newborns: Taste and Tactile Determinants of State, Affect and Action. Monographs of the Society for Research in Child Development, Serial No. 239, Vol. 59.* Chicago: Chicago University Press.

—— Smith, B.A. (1992) 'Differential effects of sucrose, fructose, glucose, and lactose on crying in 1- to 3-day-old human infants: Qualitative and quantitative considerations.' *Developmental Psychology*, **28**, 804–810.

—— Fitzgerald, E., Kehoe, P. (1987) 'Interactions between sucrose, pain and isolation distress.' *Pharmacology, Biochemistry and Behavior*, **26**, 483–489.

—— Fillion, T.J., Rochat, P., Hoffmeyer, L.B., Metzher, M.A. (1989) 'Sensorimotor and motivational determinants of hand–mouth coordination in 1–3-day-old human infants.' *Developmental Psychology*, **25**, 963–975.

—— —— Weller, A., Brunson, L. (1990) 'Separation of opioid from nonopioid mediation of affect in neonatal rats: nonopioid mechanisms mediate maternal contact influences.' *Behavioral Neuroscience*, **104**, 625–636.

—— Shide, D.J., Zaw-Mon, C., Sorrentino, J. (1995) 'Mother as shield: Differential effects of contact and nursing on pain responsivity in infant rats – evidence for nonopioid mediation.' *Behavioral Neuroscience*, **109**, 342–353.

Bornstein, M.H., Brown, E., Slater, A. (1996) 'Patterns of stability and continuity in attention across early infancy.' *Journal of Reproductive Infant Psychology*, **14**, 195–206.

Braungart-Ricker, J., Stifter, C. (1996) 'Infants' responses to frustrating situations: Continuity and change in reactivity and regulation.' *Child Development*, **67**, 1767–1779.

Brazelton, T.B. (1962) 'Crying in infancy.' *Pediatrics*, **29**, 579–588.

Carey, W.B. (1972) 'Clinical applications of infant temperament measures.' *Behavioral Pediatrics*, **81**, 823–828.

—— (1984) '"Colic" – Primary excessive crying as an infant–environment interaction.' *Pediatric Clinics of North America*, **31**, 993–1005.

Carey, W.B., McDevitt, S.C. (1978) 'Revision of the Infant Temperament Questionnaire.' *Pediatrics*, **61**, 735–739.

Douwes, A.C., Oosterkamp, R.F., Fernandes, J., Los, T., Jongbloed, A.A. (1980) 'Sugar malabsorption in healthy neonates estimated by breath hydrogen.' *Archives of Disease in Childhood*, **55**, 512–515.

Emde, R.N., Gaensbauer, T.J., Harmon, R.J. (1976) *Emotional Expression in Infancy: A Biobehavioral Study.* New York: International University Press.

Fomon, S.J. (1974) *Infant Nutrition. 2nd Edn.* Philadelphia: W.B. Saunders.

Fox, N.A. (1989) 'Psychophysiological correlates of emotional reactivity during the first year of life.' *Developmental Psychology*, **25**, 364–372.

—— (Ed.) (1994a) *The Development of Emotion Regulation: Biological and Behavioral Considerations.* Chicago: University of Chicago Press.

—— (1994b) 'Dynamic cerebral processes underlying emotion regulation.' *In:* Fox, N.A. (Ed.) *The Development of Emotion Regulation: Biological and Behavioral Considerations.* Chicago: University of Chicago Press, pp. 152–166

Franco, F. (1984) 'Differences in manner of phonation of infant cries: relationship to communicative context.' *Language and Speech*, **27**, 59–78.

Fullard, W., McDevitt, S.C., Carey, W.B. (1984) 'Assessing temperament in one- to three-year old children.' *Journal of Pediatric Psychology*, **9**, 205–217.

Gekoski, M.J., Rovee-Collier, C.K., Carulli-Rabinowitz, V. (1983) 'A longitudinal analysis of inhibition of vocal distress: The origins of social expectations?' *Infant Behavioral Development*, **6**, 339–351.

Goldsmith, H.H., Buss, A.H., Plomin, R., Rothbart, M.K., Thomas, A., Hinde, R.A., McCall, R.B. (1987) 'Roundtable: What is temperament? Four approaches.' *Child Development*, **58**, 505–529.

Gormally, S.M., Barr, R.G. (1997) 'Of clinical pies and clinical clues: proposal for a clinical approach to complaints of early crying and colic.' *Ambulatory Child Health*, **3**, 137–153.

Graillon, A., Barr, R.G., Young, S.N., Wright, J.H., Hendricks, L.A. (1997) 'Differential response to oral sucrose, quinine and corn oil in crying human newborns.' *Physiology and Behavior*, **62**, 317–325.

Gunnar, M.R., Isensee, J., Fust, S. (1987) 'Adrenocortical activity and the Brazelton Neonatal Assesment Scale: moderating effects of the newborn biomedical status.' *Child Development*, **58**, 1448–1458.

—— Mangelsdorf, S., Larson, M., Hertsgaard, L. (1989) 'Attachment, temperament, and adrenocortical activity in infancy: A study of psychoendocrine regulation.' *Developmental Psychology*, **25**, 355–363.

—— Porter, F.L., Wolf, C.M., Rigatuso, J., Larson, M.C. (1995) 'Neonatal stress reactivity: Predictions to later emotional temperament.' *Child Development*, **66**, 1–13.

63

—— Broderson, L., Krueger, K., Rigatuso, J. (1996) 'Dampening of adrenocortical responses during infancy: Normative changes and individual differences.' *Child Development*, **67**, 877–889.

Hofer, M.A. (1994) 'Hidden regulators in attachment, separation and loss.' *In:* Fox, N.A. (Ed.) *The Development of Emotion Regulation: Biological and Behavioral Considerations.* Chicago: University of Chicago Press, pp. 192–207

Hood, B.M., Murray, L., King, F., Hooper, R., Atkinson, J., Braddick, O. (1996) 'Habituation changes in early infancy: Longitudinal measures from birth to 6 months.' *Journal of Reproductive Infant Psychology*, **14**, 177–185.

Hopkins, B., von Wulfften Palthe, T. (1987) 'The development of the crying state during early infancy.' *Developmental Psychobiology*, **20**, 165–175.

Huffman, L.C., Bryan, Y.E., del Carmen, R., Pedersen, F.A., Porges, S.W., Doussard-Roosevelt, J.A. (1998) 'Infant temperament and cardiac vagal tone:assesment at twelve weeks of age.' *Child Development*, **69**, 624–635.

Hunziker, U.A., Barr, R.G. (1986) 'Increased carrying reduces infant crying: A randomized controlled trial.' *Pediatrics*, **77**, 641–648.

Izard, C.E., Porges, S.W. (1991) 'Infant cardiac activity: Developmental changes and relations with attachment.' *Developmental Psychology*, **27**, 432–439.

Jacobson, D., Melvin, N. (1995) 'A comparison of temperament and maternal bother in infants with and without colic.' *Journal of Pediatric Nursing*, **10**, 181–188.

Johnson, S.P. (1996) 'Habituation patterns and object perception in young infants.' *Journal of Reproductive Infant Psychology*, **14**, 207–218.

Kagan, J., Snidman, N. (1991) 'Infant predictors of inhibited and uninhibited profiles.' *Psychological Science*, **2**, 40–44.

Kehoe, P., Blass, E.M. (1986a) 'Opioid-mediation of separation distress in 10-day-old rats: reversal of stress with maternal stimuli.' *Developmental Psychobiology*, **19**, 385–398.

—— —— (1986b) 'Behaviorally functional opioid systems in infant rats: II. Evidence for pharmacological, physiological, and psychological mediation of pain and stress.' *Behavioral Neuroscience*, **100**, 624–630.

Klevjord Rothbart, M. (1989) 'Biological processes in temperament.' *In:* Kohnstamm, G.A., Bates, J.E., Klevjord Rothbart, M. (Eds.) *Temperament in Childhood.* New York: John Wiley, pp. 77–110.

Lacey, J.I. (1967) 'Somatic response patterning and stress: Some revisions of activation theory.' *In:* Appley, M.H., Trumbull, R. (Eds.) *Psychological Stress: Issues in Research.* New York: Appleton-Century-Crofts, pp. 14–42.

Larson, M.C., Prudhome-White, B., Cochran, A., Donzella, B., Gunnar, M. (1998) 'Dampening of the cortisol response to handling at 3-months in human infants and its relation to sleep, circadian cortisol activity, and behavioral distress.' *Developmental Psychobiology*, **33**, 327–337.

Lehtonen, L., Korhonen, T., Korvenranta, H. (1994) 'Temperament and sleeping pattern in infantile colic during the first year of life.' *Journal of Development and Behavioural Pediatrics*, **15**, 416–420.

Lester, B.M., Boukydis, C.F.Z., Garcia-Coll, C.T., Hole, W.T, Peucker, M. (1992) 'Infantile colic: Acoustic cry characteristics, maternal perception of cry, and temperament.' *Infant Behavior and Development*, **15**, 15–26.

Lewis, M. (1989) 'Culture and biology: The role of temperament.' *In:* Zelazo, P.R., Barr, R.G. (Eds.) *Challenges to Developmental Paradigms: Implications for Theory, Assessment and Treatment.* Hillsdale, NJ: Lawrence Erlbaum, pp. 203–226.

—— Ramsay, D.S. (1995a) 'Developmental change in infants' responses to stress.' *Child Development*, **66**, 657–670.

—— —— (1995b) 'Stability and change in cortisol and behavioral response to stress during the first 18 months of life.' *Developmental Psychobiology*, **28**, 419–428.

Magnano, C.L., Gardner, J.M., Karmel, B.Z. (1992) 'Differences in salivary cortisol levels in cocaine-exposed and noncocaine-exposed NICU infants.' *Developmental Psychobiology*, **25**, 93–103.

Malone, A. (1997) 'The crying pattern of preterm infants.' *Paper presented at the 6th International Workshop on Infant Cry Research, Bowness-on-Windermere, July 4, 1997.*

Miller, A.R., Barr, R.G., Eaton, W.O. (1993) 'Crying and motor behavior of six-week-old infants and postpartum maternal mood.' *Pediatrics*, **92**, 551–558.

Miller, J.B., Bokdam, M., McVeagh, P., Miller, J.J. (1992) 'Variability of breath hydrogen excretion in breast-fed infants during the first three months of life.' *Journal of Pediatrics*, **121**, 410–413.

Panksepp, J., Vilberg, T., Bean, N.J., Coy, D.H., Kastin, A.J. (1978) 'Reduction of distress vocalization in chicks by opiate-like peptides.' *Brain Research Bulletin*, **3**, 663–667.

—— Meeker, R., Bean, N.J. (1980) 'The neurochemical control of crying.' *Pharmacology, Biochemistry and Behavior*, **12**, 437–443.

Parmelee, A.H., Stern, E. (1972) 'Development of states in infants.' *In:* Clemente, C.D., Purpura, D.P., Mayer, F.E. (Eds.) *Sleep and the Maturing Nervous System*. New York: Academic Press, pp. 199–215

Plomin, R. (1989) 'Environment and genes: determinants of behavior.' *American Psychologist*, 44, 105–111.

Porges, S.W., Doussard-Roosevelt, J.A., Maiti, A.K. (1994) 'Vagal tone and the physiological regulation of emotion.' *In:* Fox, N.A. (Ed.) *The Development of Emotion Regulation: Biological and Behavioral Considerations*. Chicago: University of Chicago Press, pp. 167–191.

Prechtl, H.F.R. (Ed.) (1984) *Continuity of Neural Functions from Prenatal to Postnatal Life. Clinics in Developmental Medicine No. 94*. London: Spastics International Medical Publications.

Ramsay, D.S., Lewis, M. (1994) 'Developmental change in infant cortisol and behavioral response to inoculation.' *Child Development*, **65**, 1491–1502.

—— —— (1995) 'The effects of birth condition on infants' cortisol response to stress.' *Pediatrics*, **95**, 546–549.

Riese, M.L. (1995) 'Mothers' ratings of infant temperament: Relation to neonatal latency to soothe by pacifier.' *Journal of Genetic Psychology*, **156**, 23–31.

Rothbart, M.K. (1981) 'Measurement of infant temperament.' *Child Development*, **52**, 569–578.

—— Derryberry, D. (1981) 'Development of individual differences in temperament.' *In:* Brown, A.L., Lamb, M.E. (Eds.) *Advances in Developmental Psychology*. Hillsdale, NJ: Lawarence Erlbaum, pp. 37–86.

Sauls, H.S., Redfern, D.E. (1997) *Colic and Excessive Crying*. Columbus, OH: Ross Products Division Abbott Laboratories.

Slater, A., Brown, E., Mattock, A., Bornstein, M.H. (1996) 'Continuity and change in habituation in the first 4 months from birth.' *J Reproductive Infant Psychol*, **14**, 187–194.

Smith, B.A., Fillion, T.J., Blass, E.M. (1990) 'Orally mediated sources of calming in 1 to 3-day old human infants.' *Developmental Psychology*, **26**, 731–737.

—— Stevens, K., Torgerson, W.S., Kim, J.H. (1992) 'Diminished reactivity of postmature human infants to sucrose compared with term infants.' *Developmental Psychology*, **28**, 811–820.

Snidman, N., Kagan, J., Riordan, L., Shannon, D.C. (1995) 'Cardiac function and behavioral reactivity during infancy.' *Psychophysiology*, **32**, 199–207.

Sostek, A.M., Anders, T.F. (1977) 'Relationship among the Brazelton Neonatal Scale, Bayley Infant Scales, and early temperament.' *Child Development*, **48**, 320–323.

Spangler, G., Scheubeck, R. (1993) 'Behavioral organization in newborns and its relation to adrenocortical and cardiac activity.' *Child Development*, **64**, 622–633.

—— Schieche, M., Ilg, U., Maier, U., Ackermann, C. (1994) 'Maternal sensitivity as an external organizer for biobehavioral regulation in infancy.' *Developmental Psychobiology*, **27**, 425–437.

St James-Roberts, I., Halil, T. (1991) 'Infant crying patterns in the first year: Normal community and clinical findings.' *Journal of Child Psychology and Psychiatry*, **32**, 951–968.

—— Plewis, I. (1996) 'Individual differences, daily fluctuations, and developmental changes in amounts of infant waking, fussing, crying, feeding and sleeping.' *Child Development*, **67**, 1–36.

—— Wolke, D. (1988) 'Convergences and discrepancies among mothers' and professionals' assessments of difficult neonatal behaviour.' *Journal of Child Psychology and Psychiatry*, **29**, 21–42.

—— Hurry, J., Bowyer, J. (1993) 'Objective confirmation of crying durations in infants referred for excessive crying.' *Archives of Disease in Childhood*, **68**, 82–84.

—— Bowyer, J., Varghese, S., Sawdon, J. (1994) 'Infant crying patterns in Manali and London.' *Child: Care, Health and Development*, **20**, 323–337.

—— Conroy, S., Wilsher, K. (1995) 'Clinical, developmental and social aspects of infant crying and colic.' *Early Development and Parenting*, **4**, 177–189.

—— —— —— (1998) 'Links between maternal care and persistent infant crying in the early months.' *Child: Care, Health and Development*, **24**, 353–376.

Stansbury, K., Gunnar, M. (1994) 'Adrenocortical activity and emotion regulation.' *In:* Fox, N.A. (Ed.) *The Development of Emotion Regulation: Biological and Behavioral Considerations*. Chicago: University of Chicago Press, pp. 108–134.

Stifter, C.A., Braungart, J. (1992) 'Infant colic: A transient condition with no apparent effects.' *Journal of Applied Developmental Psychology*, **13**, 447–462.

Thomas, A., Chess, S., Birch, H. (1968) *Temperament and Behavior Disorders in Children*. New York: New York University Press.

Thompson, R.A. (1994) 'Emotion regulation: A theme in search of definition.' *In:* Fox, N.A. (Ed.) *The Development of Emotion Regulation: Biological and Behavioral Considerations.* Chicago: University of Chicago Press, pp. 25–52.

Weissbluth, M. (1981) 'Sleep duration and infant temperament.' *Journal of Pediatrics*, **99**, 817–819.

—— (1987) 'Sleep and the colicky infant.' *In:* Guilleminault, C. (Ed.) *Sleep and Its Disorders in Children.* New York: Raven Press, pp. 129–140.

—— Lin, K. (1983) 'Sleep patterns, attention spans and infant temperament.' *Journal of Development and Behavioral Pediatrics*, **4**, 34–36.

—— Christoffel, K.K., Davis, T. (1984a) 'Treatment of infantile colic with dicyclomine hydrochloride.' *Journal of Pediatrics*, **104**, 951–955.

—— Davis, T, Poncher, J. (1984b) 'Night waking in 4–8 month old infants.' *Journal of Pediatrics*, **104**, 477–480.

Wessel, M.A., Cobb, J.C., Jackson, E.B., Harris, G.S., Detwiler, A.C. (1954) 'Paroxysmal fussing in infancy, sometimes called "colic".' *Pediatrics*, **14**, 421–434.

White, B.P., Gunnar, M.R., Larson, M.C., Donzella, B., Barr, R.G. (2000) 'Physiological reactivity and daily rhythms in infants with and without colic.' *Child Development. (In press.)*

Wolff, P.H. (1987) *The Development of Behavioral States and the Expression of Emotions in Early Infancy: New Proposals for Investigation.* Chicago: University of Chicago Press.

Worobey, J., Lewis, M. (1989) 'Individual differences in the reactivity of young infants.' *Developmental Psychology*, **25**, 663–667.

Zeifman, D., Delaney, S., Blass, E.M. (1996) 'Sweet taste, looking, and calm in 2- and 4-week-old infants: The eyes have it.' *Developmental Psychology*, **32**, 1090–1099.

Zeskind, P.S., Barr, R.G. (1997) 'Acoustic characteristics of naturally occurring cries of infants with "colic".' *Child Development*, **68**, 394–403.

5
'CLINICAL PIES' FOR ETIOLOGY AND OUTCOME IN INFANTS PRESENTING WITH EARLY INCREASED CRYING

Liisa Lehtonen, Siobhan Gormally and Ronald G. Barr

More often than we think, newspapers and journals report the abuse or even the death of infants whose crying is persistent and inconsolable (O'Neill 1993, Duncan *et al.* 1996). In one such case reported in *Life* magazine in September 1996, a 2-month-old was shaken by his 18-year-old father because "I just wanted him to stop crying." The shaking was so severe that he subsequently died of brain injuries (Duncan *et al.* 1996). Death of an infant as a sequel of excessive crying is relatively rare, even if it should be nonexistent. The crying is unlikely to be the 'only' causal factor: although the anecdotes are rarely sufficiently inciteful on this score, the excessive crying is probably only the trigger in an already fragile family system.

These reports stand in stark contrast to the standard description of excessive crying in many pediatric textbooks. They usually present the clinical problem of excessive crying in terms of the behavioral syndrome of colic, and typically describe it as benign and self-limited. To make matters more confusing, there is also anecdotal evidence that the outcome of colic can be quite positive. A parent of one of our study subjects with colic wrote that "Catherine is now mobile (crawling) and has been for a month. She has a monster appetite and has eight teeth! She has a very even temper and adjusted to the babysitter beautifully when I went back to work." A short surf on the internet with the keyword 'colic' will unearth dozens of similar testimonials from parents of colic 'graduates' reassuring others whose infants with colic are still 'in school' that they will indeed outgrow it and become wonderful, responsive 1-year-olds. Thus, the textbooks are correct most of the time; colic syndrome is relatively benign and self-limited, but not always.

For the clinician, these discrepant descriptions provide an important reminder and some significant challenges. The reminder is that the typical description of colic syndrome as benign is at least incomplete and arguably seriously deficient. Even though mortality is low, morbidity may be much more common. The question is how clinicians can be helpful to frustrated parents in the face of these outcomes. One challenge is to be aware of what is known regarding three of their essential clinical responsibilities, namely: (1) the etiology of colic syndrome; (2) in particular, what organic diseases account for the syndrome; and (3) what the prognosis is. A second and more difficult challenge for the clinician—and the one that is of interest to parents—is to know, not just that colic syndrome could have this or that etiology or outcome, but whether *this specific infant* has a specific etiology or is at risk for a specific outcome.

Meeting these challenges is often difficult in the clinical setting for many complaints even when the etiologies, pathogeneses and alternative treatment modalities have been well studied. It is even more difficult for early crying complaints. Only recently has the problem of colic been subject to controlled comparisons, treatment trials and longitudinal studies. Furthermore, the results are widely distributed in clinical, developmental and nursing journals, making integration difficult for the clinician. Even if they are read together, it is unclear that the authors of different studies are talking about the same phenomenon. The word 'colic' has been variably used to refer to a presumably distinct type of crying (or crying bout), to a presumably distinct behavioral crying syndrome, and sometimes to a clinical complaint about crying. To make matters worse, some authors limit the term to crying that is due to organic, or even more specifically gastrointestinal, causes (a diagnosis of inclusion) and others, paradoxically, to crying in infants in whom organic disease has been ruled out or who are 'otherwise well' (a diagnosis of exclusion). Such problems exacerbate rather than facilitate the clinician's job when faced with a complaint of persistent, excessive crying in an infant.

Because of these problems, we set out to investigate whether the available literature could be brought together in a way that could be at once conceptually coherent and helpful to these challenges facing the clinician. In an initial report (Gormally and Barr 1997), we proposed a 'clinical pie' (pie chart) as an heuristic device with which to organize the literature and more adequately guide a clinical approach to crying complaints in the first three months. It was clear that this approach would be more meaningful and clinically useful if it could be interpreted in the light of known outcomes of early colic syndrome. Longitudinal and outcome studies are becoming more plentiful, although there are significant limitations in those that are available. Consequently, in this chapter, we do three things: (1) describe a diagnostic pie for crying complaints and, in relation to the pie, (2) summarize the evidence for organic diseases and clinical clues that might indicate their presence in a specific infant; and (3) review available longitudinal studies and develop a prognostic pie to describe probable outcomes for infants with colic. The results are encouraging in that some general principles of potential value to the clinician for both diagnosis and counselling regarding outcome are emerging, and they highlight a number of important questions that remain to be answered.

Background

Although far from consistent or universally accepted, most clinical descriptions of colic syndrome take crying behavior that is considered excessive and/or persistent as the cardinal presenting symptom (Barr 1991). More specific details about what characteristics the crying must have to consititute colic remain controversial. However, the full-fledged syndrome is usually qualitatively described in terms of three dimensions. First, the pattern of crying has age-dependent and diurnal features. The total duration of daily crying usually begins to increase about two weeks after birth, reaches its zenith during the second month, and declines to more stable but lower levels by the fourth month. Within the day, it tends to cluster during the later afternoon and evening hours. Second, there are a number of associated behavioral features, some of which are common and some of which are more variable. The most common and well-replicated features are that the crying bouts are prolonged (and sometimes referred to as 'colic bouts'), and that they are resistant to soothing (Barr 1990a, Stifter and Braungart 1992, St James-Roberts *et al.* 1996, St James-Roberts 2000). More variable features include the infant clenching its fists, flexing its legs over the abdomen, arching its back, having an active and grimacing face, and being flushed. While it remains an open question as to whether this specifically represents 'pain' as compared to more vigorous crying, this configuration contributes to the caregiver's concern that the infant is in pain when it cries (Geertsma and Hyams 1989, Barr and Geertsma 1993). The abdomen is sometimes described as hard and/or distended. The crying bout may be associated with regurgitation and the passing of gas per rectum, contributing to the presumed localization of pain in the intestine. The third dimension refers to the unpredictability of crying, usually captured in the term 'paroxysmal' crying. This refers variously to cry bouts that have a rapid onset, begin and end without warning, and/or are unrelated to other events (such as soothing efforts) in the environment.

Capturing these qualitative dimensions in a definition that is useful clinically has not been an easy task. By far and away the most widely *used* definition has come to be known as 'Wessel's rule of threes'; namely, that an infant has colic (or is a 'serious paroxysmal fusser' in Wessel *et al.*'s original description) if it cries for more than three hours a day for more than three days a week for more than three weeks (Wessel *et al.* 1954). It helpfully focuses on quantifiable measures of crying duration, and has been a useful 'benchmark' for comparing studies and trying to determine whether populations of crying infants are comparable. For clinical purposes, however, it has a number of recognized limitations. One of these is that few parents or clinicians are willing to wait for three weeks to see if the increased crying will persist in order to 'meet' criteria for colic, so the third criterion is often dropped. This produces what might reasonably be considered a broader 'modified Wessel's criteria' (crying for more than three hours a day for more than three days a week). Because of its wide acceptance and use, we have retained modified Wessel's criteria in our proposed diagnostic pie (see below). However, readers should be aware that even this modification is used differently (Barr 1995a). For example, in some studies 'crying' is interpreted as including fussing (*e.g.* Barr *et al.* 1992), whereas in others, fussing is excluded or not recorded. Clearly, what is included in the term 'crying' is going to affect which infants meet even modified Wessel's criteria.

Another limitation has prompted a revision in the opposite direction, one that narrows the definition. Because Wessel *et al.*'s rules use only crying duration measures, other investigators have required that infants also meet additional criteria in an attempt to capture and quantify some of the other dimensions of the typical 'syndrome'. This produces what might be referred to as 'Wessel's plus' modifications. By subdividing crying into 'crying' and 'colicky crying' (the latter being that which was 'pain sounding' and difficult to soothe), Lehtonen *et al.* (1994) separated out infants with 'severe colic' as those whose parents recorded at least three hours per day of 'colic crying' for at least three days a week. These could be considered as one kind of 'Wessel's plus' infants. The most formal attempt has

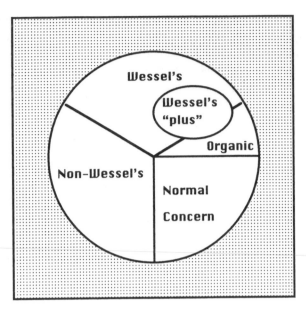

Fig. 5.1. The 'Gormally and Barr' diagnostic pie for crying complaints. The stippled background represents all crying infants, and the circle represents those that present to the clinician with a complaint about crying. The pie slices represent different presentations of crying complaints based on phenomenology rather than etiology. In only one slice (organic) is etiology suggested, and it is represented as accounting for 5–10 per cent of cases. (Reprinted by permission from Gormally and Barr 1997.)

been proposed by Lester *et al.* (1990, see their Appendix) in which they limit their studies to infants who meet Wessel's criteria as a minimum, but whose parents also specifically report paroxysmal or sudden onsets, a perceived high pitch or 'pain' quality, behavioral characteristics of hypertonia, and inconsolability. Another kind of 'Wessel's plus' infants occur when authors (especially in diet trial studies) report on infants who, in addition to crying, also presented with increased vomiting, diarrhea, weight loss, other symptoms implicating (but not demonstrating) possible organic disease, and high prevalences of atopic manifestations in their families (Lester *et al.* 1990, Wolke and Meyer 1995). Finally, some authors report on infants who, prior to entry into the study, have already been seen in other (often many other) settings and/or failed other (often many other) treatments. These too are likely to be 'more severe' than infants who simply meet modified Wessel's criteria and are derived from nonreferred community samples. To situate these infants in relation to early crying complaints, the 'diagnostic pie' incorporates the notion of 'Wessel's plus' infants as well.

There is a third recognized limitation to the usefulness of Wessel's criteria, however modified for clinical purposes. This has to do with the fact that they do not take into account the caregiving context in which the crying occurs. Presumably, evolution did not 'design' the crying of infants to be reported as a symptom or observed as a sign for infants to be diagnosed as having 'colic'. More probably, it functions as a signal, and the extent to which it functions in the best interests of the infant is importantly dependent on how the caregiver interprets and responds to the signal (Barr 1998b, 1999, 2000). As a result, it is unlikely to be the case that there will be a one-to-one correspondence between a specific amount or intensity of crying and an 'abnormal' amount of crying.

In the evaluation of crying complaints, this significantly limits the clinical usefulness of any criteria based solely on duration of crying, in a number of ways. One is that other, possibly qualitative, features of crying are likely to contribute, either uniquely or in addition to durational indices, to caregiver concern (Barr 1990b, Barr et al. 1992). Second, the definition takes no account of the effort of the caregiver in reducing crying. Infants might well cry less than the cut-off (and be classified as 'non-colic') because their mothers have been 'working overtime' carrying, soothing and attending to their infants, whereas other infants whose mothers leave them to 'cry out' meet the definition. A third example is that the same amount of crying may not be problematic in an infant whose mother is psychologically healthy, but will be if the mother has postpartum depression (Barr and Geertsma 1993, Miller et al. 1993). Finally, durational definitions are arbitrary. It is not at all apparent why a frustrated mother whose infant cries 175 minutes/day for 3 days/week should be told her baby does not have a problem while another mother whose infant cries 185 minutes/day for 3 days/week should be told her baby does have a problem. In all of these cases, knowing that the amount of crying is quantitatively 'normal' may be reassuring, but the crying remains palpably real, and parents' concerns about its presence and characteristics need to be addressed. For these and other reasons, the concept of a 'normal' amount of crying is difficult to define, conceptually problematic, and possibly clinically useless (Barr 1993). To address considerations such as these, the diagnostic pie is constructed to include crying concerns brought to clinicians that do not meet modified Wessel's durational criteria.

The diagnostic pie for crying complaints

In light of these considerations, there are two important organizational principles incorporated in the proposed diagnostic pie (Fig. 5.1). The first is that the background square represents all infants regardless of the amount of crying they do. The circle represents *crying complaints* brought to the clinician, not infants whose crying meets any particular definition for colic syndrome. Consequently, what determines whether an infant is inside or outside the circle is not solely dependent on what the infant does, but also on factors such as the level of the concern of the caregiver, cultural predispositions to consider crying a clinical problem, available health facilities, and so on. This means that there will be infants both 'inside' and 'outside' the circle whose crying is otherwise the same. This is consistent with a number of studies comparing crying in referred and non-referred samples. While, on average, referred infants do in fact cry more than nonreferred infants, there is also a significant overlap between the two groups (St James-Roberts and Halil 1991; Barr et al. 1992; Hill et al. 1992; St James-Roberts et al. 1993, 1995).

The second principle is that, with the exception of the organic segment, the slices are based on the phenomenology of crying, not on its etiology. This respects the growing evidence that the behavioral syndrome we think of as 'colic' is, in most cases, the upper end of the spectrum of a continuum of otherwise developmentally appropriate behavior (Barr

1998b, 1999; Gormally and Barr 1997). It has two further advantages. On the one hand, it does not inappropriately and narrowly limit discussion of colic to crying with an 'organic' cause. On the other hand, it similarly does not assume that colic crying is due to psychogenic, caregiving or familial etiologies. It is, after all, completely appropriate for caregivers to be concerned about crying that is persistent, difficult to soothe and gives the appearance that the infant is in pain. Indeed, we would probably be concerned if caregivers were not worried about such behavior. Further, although less well-studied, it is increasingly apparent that colic may occur despite optimal caregiving (St James-Roberts *et al.* 1998, Barr 2000). As with organic diseases, whether caregiver factors cause, exacerbate or maintain persistent, unsoothable crying should be an empirical question in each case, rather than being (often inappropriately) assumed to be etiologic.

CLINICAL 'SLICES'
Crying due to organic disease
This refers to infants whose crying meets at least modified Wessel's criteria and in whom definitive signs and symptoms confirm the presence of an organic disease process. This is the only slice in which knowledge of the etiology is implicated in its description. Defining which children should be included in this slice is an important responsibility for clinicians, and the available 'clinical clues' for so doing will be discussed subsequently. In the absence of a definitive community-based study in which the sample is uncontaminated by referral bias and a consistent evaluation for organic etiologies has been applied to all infants, a good estimate of the incidence of colic due to organic disease is difficult to come by. However, on the basis of recent reviews, it seems likely that organic disease is implicated in about 5 per cent or less of cases (Miller and Barr 1991, Treem 1994, Barr 1996, Gormally and Barr 1997, Sauls and Redfern 1997).

Wessel's crying
This slice refers to infants who have an increased quantity of crying as represented by them meeting modified Wessel's criteria for amounts of crying and fussing. In addition, the crying follows the typical pattern (peak during the second month, and evening clustering), and the child has a normal physical examination. These infants may also manifest the typical behavioral features, although two of these (crying after a feed and abdominal distension) are not likely to be diagnostically helpful (Barr *et al.* 1992). They may manifest more facial activity (or more 'pain facies') when they cry, may be reported as having more 'sick sounding' cries, and their cries may have more dysphonation or a higher dominant frequency compared to cries of normal infants. (For a description of dysphonation and dominant frequency, see Chapter 9.) However, none of these features are specific to infants with Wessel's colic (Barr *et al.* 1992, Zeskind and Barr 1997). It is estimated that infants who meet modified Wessel's criteria account for about one-third of crying complaints brought to the clinician, but this figure is based on a single study (Barr *et al.* 1992) and might well be different in other settings. In sum, these infants meet modified Wessel's criteria for *quantities* of crying and fussing, but also have exaggerated but not unique *behavioral* and *qualitative* characteristics to their crying.

Non-Wessel's crying

Another one-third or so of infants are referred to as non-Wessel's crying infants. The essential difference with these infants is that they have the exaggerated behavioral and qualitative characteristics seen with Wessel's infants, but do not meet criteria for increased duration of crying. Their physical examinations are also normal, and the crying pattern shows the typical peak and evening clustering. This slice recognizes that aspects of crying other than duration may well be a cause of concern (Barr 1990b, St James-Roberts *et al.* 1996). Clearly, this is the group about which we know the least. In one study, mothers of infants who complained of their crying even though it was quantitatively the same as that of control infants rated their after-feed cries as more sick-sounding (Barr *et al.* 1992). A second study revealed more dysphonation in their after-feed cries on acoustic analysis; this was due to an increase in the amount of dysphonation from prefeed levels, whereas normal infants decreased the amount of dysphonation post-feed (Zeskind and Barr 1997). Consequently, the concerns of these parents cannot simply be dismissed as being due to biased reporting due to heightened anxiety. This slice would also include those infants whose crying fails to meet quantitative Wessel's criteria because their mothers are 'working overtime' trying to reduce the crying behavior.

Normal concern

This slice includes those infants in whom the duration, pattern and quality of crying, associated behavioral characteristics and physical examination are normal, but the parents are simply concerned about what the typical pattern of increased crying in the first few weeks of life might mean. Although first- and later-born infants cry the same amounts (St James-Roberts and Halil 1991), parents are more likely to take their first-borns to clinicians with crying complaints. Often they simply will not have heard that crying typically increases in the first two months (Brazelton 1962, Barr 1990b), and are frustrated that this is occurring despite their best efforts at optimal caregiving.

Wessel's 'plus' crying

These are infants whose crying and fussing duration meets modified Wessel's criteria as a minimum, but who must meet other criteria as well to be considered to have 'colic'. Unfortunately, as previously discussed, there is no uniform practice as to what these extra criteria should be. The only thing they all are likely to have in common is that they are the most severe criers, have more frequent atypical behavioral features, and more indicators of organic disease that are, nevertheless, nonspecific and nondiagnostic. Furthermore, most studies of such infants do not report the 'denominator' from which these infants are selected, so it is very difficult to know what percentage of crying complaints these infants represent. For these reasons, these infants are represented as a circle (rather than a slice) on the border between Wessel's infants and those with organic disease. It remains unclear whether such infants in whom organic disease is never diagnosed represent a distinct subgroup who may have other crying syndromes beyond the first three months (DeGangi *et al.* 1991; van den Boom and Hacksma 1994; Papousek and von Hofacker 1995, 1998; Barr 2000) or are simply the extreme of infants with increased amounts of crying.

Etiology

One of the reasons parents bring their crying infants to clinicians is their concern that the crying represents a disease process. Making that determination is an important responsibility of clinicians. Even if disease is relatively rare (less than 5 per cent), the responsibility is no less, and arguably the challenge of being able to detect those with disease is greater. To address this problem, we reviewed 48 original articles and 13 major reviews from the pediatric literature published during the last 31 years. Papers were ascertained by a Medline search from 1966 through 1998 using the keywords 'crying' and 'colic' for infants under 1 year of age. The articles were reviewed to determine the answers to two questions: (1) which organic entities can present as colic syndrome, and (2) what clinical clues could be derived from the presentations to identify whether a *specific* infant with colic syndrome has an organic disease?

There were a number of problems in attempting to answer these questions. First, because almost any disease can present with crying in infants, many organic entities are listed as being causal of colic. However, we wanted to determine whether crying having the behavioral characteristics of *colic syndrome* as previously described could be caused by specific organic diseases. Consequently, we did not include febrile infants with increased crying, usually of recent or acute onset. Nor did we include nonfebrile infants with increased crying, also usually of recent onset, but who were older than 4 months. Infants with these presentations are also diagnostically difficult cases, but they have a different set of possible etiologies (see Chapter 6; and Poole 1991, De Lorenzo and Fisher 1995, Trocinski and Pearigen 1998, Barr 2000).The second problem was that the descriptions of the crying phenomenology were often incomplete, so that we had to make clinical judgments as to whether the reported cases fell within the 'colic' group. Third, the kinds of evidence provided by these reports was quite variable both in type and quality. The articles included qualitative descriptions, case reports and clinical treatment trials. Some provided compelling evidence that a particular disease could present as colic syndrome, whereas in others the evidence was weaker because of lack of description, methodological weaknesses, the possibility of alternative interpretations, or often, overinterpretation of the results. On the basis of these qualitative dimensions, we categorized the evidence for each specific etiology as strong, moderate or weak. Finally, we extracted 'clinical clues' that characterized infants whose crying syndrome was associated with organic disease from those in whom it was not. We were interested both in clues that might be specific to a particular disease, and in those that were not specific but that might increase the likelihood of organic disease being present.

ORGANIC ENTITIES THAT CAN PRESENT AS COLIC SYNDROME (TABLE 5.1)

Organic diseases for which we consider the evidence to be *strong* include cow's milk protein intolerance, isolated fructose intolerance, maternal drug effects (especially fluoxetine hydrochloride [Prozac]), infantile migraine, and anomalous left coronary artery. Each is important for different reasons, but they have in common the possibility of a specific treatment. Cow's milk protein intolerance is important because it is almost certainly the most common of the organic entities that can present as colic-like syndrome. It has been the subject of at least 14 clinical trials (Jakobsson and Lindberg 1978, 1983; Evans *et al.*

TABLE 5.1
Organic etiologies for colic syndrome

Strong	Moderate	Weak
Cow's milk protein intolerance	Reflux esophagitis	Lactose intolerance
Isolated fructose intolerance	Infant abuse	Glaucoma
Fluoxetine hydrochloride (Prozac)		CNS abnormalities (Chiari type I)
Infantile migraine		Urinary tract infection
Anomalous left coronary artery		

1981; Kahn *et al.* 1985; Stahlberg and Savilahti 1986; Thomas *et al.* 1987; Taubman 1988; Campbell 1989; Forsyth 1989; Lothe and Lindberg 1989; Iacono *et al.* 1991; Schrander *et al.* 1993; Oggero *et al.* 1994; Hill *et al.* 1995) and has been extensively reviewed (Geertsma and Hyams 1989, Miller and Barr 1991, Wolke 1993, Treem 1994, Wolke and Meyer 1995, Barr 1996, Sauls and Redfern 1997). There is good evidence that cow's milk protein allergens can be passed by breast milk and that crying can be affected in selected cases (Barr 1996). The methodologically most rigorous diet trial is that of Forsyth (1989). He reported a decrease in crying following a change to casein hydrolysate formula, but the beneficial effects decreased over time, were small in magnitude, and were clinically meaningful for only two of the 17 highly selected infants. Although increased crying occurs in 20–40 per cent of infants with cow's milk protein intolerance, only four of 65 (6 per cent) who had crying as the main symptom were intolerant to cow's milk in a prospective epidemiological study (Schrander *et al.* 1993). In a recent prospective double-blind study of referred (probably Wessel's plus) infants with colic, a statistically significant and clinically meaningful reduction in crying (>25 per cent) was reported for breast or formula-fed infants placed on a low allergen diet, but the improvements were most apparent (though not statistically significant) for the subgroup of breast-fed infants younger than 6 weeks (Hill *et al.* 1995). Together, these and other studies suggest that cow's milk protein is probably a real, but infrequent, cause of colic syndrome.

Evidence for the other four causes comes from detailed case studies. Wales *et al.* (1989) report a fairly convincing case of a crying infant given daily fennel or blackcurrant drinks from 1 week of age, whose crying was associated with 'wind' and abdominal distension and post-feed 'screaming'. Isolated fructose intolerance was documented when she was older by breath hydrogen and blood tests following fructose challenge.

Lester *et al.* (1993) reported a very convincing case study of colic syndrome in a breast-fed infant whose mother was taking fluoxetine hydrochloride (Prozac). Symptoms disappeared when the baby was bottle-fed and reappeared when breast-feeding was restarted, and elevated concentrations of fluoxetine were documented in the infant's serum.

Diagnosing migraine in infants is always difficult. Katerji and Painter (1994) describe a crying syndrome that early on sounded like a colic syndrome, but progressed by 4 months to daily 1.5–4 hour bouts of inconsolable crying associated with face-scratching, back arching, vomiting and a staring expression with upper lid retraction (Collier's sign). Symptoms disappeared within a week following treatment with cyproheptadine, a serotonergic

5-HT2 receptor antagonist. Finally, Mahle (1998) reported an infant whose increased crying began at 2 weeks and was predictably postprandial, was diagnosed as having 'colic' by three physicians, and was treated unsuccessfully with an antispasmodic–sedative combination (Donnatol), glycerin suppositories, and two formula changes (to soy-based and elemental formulae respectively). At 12 weeks, the increased crying had persisted and difficult breathing developed. Physical examination revealed subcostal retractions, end expiratory wheezes, and hepatomegaly. Imaging studies revealed cardiomegaly, pulmonary edema and an anomalous left coronary artery. Symptoms resolved completely with surgical repair.

Organic diseases for which there is *moderately* convincing evidence that they can present with colic include reflux esophagitis and shaken baby syndrome. Evidence for the former is limited to two retrospective studies (Berezin *et al.* 1995, Heine *et al.* 1995). Both report on referred and probably highly selected samples, with limited descriptions of the crying characteristics. From both studies, five of 42 infants under 3 months of age had significant gastroesophageal reflux or endoscopic histologic evidence of esophagitis. All had associated increased frequency of regurgitation or vomiting. (For a good review of possible mechanisms, see Hyman 1994.)

Despite the limitations of the anecdotal evidence, infant abuse can almost certainly present as a colic-like syndrome. Crying is widely cited as a precipitating event in fatal cases (Weston 1968, Kadushin and Martin 1981, Duncan *et al.* 1996), and is also the chief presenting complaint in infants who have had repetitive and violent shaking (Ludwig 1984, Singer and Rosenberg 1992).

Weaker evidence exists for the possibility that lactose intolerance, eye pathology, central nervous system abnormalities and urinary tract infection may cause colic. Of these, lactose intolerance has had the most attention, because the time courses of crying symptoms and incomplete lactose absorption (as indexed by breath hydrogen excretion) are roughly similar, both in the first few months of life and within the day (Douwes *et al.* 1980, Barr *et al.* 1984, Miller *et al.* 1992). However, clinical studies have significant methodological problems and have provided only mixed support at best (Barr 1996, Gormally and Barr 1997). Treatment trials to date have been consistently ineffective (Danielsson and Hwang 1985, Stahlberg and Savilahti 1986, Miller *et al.* 1990, Metcalf *et al.* 1994).

With regard to eye pathology, the best evidence, despite an incomplete description, is a case of congenital glaucoma (Talbot *et al.* 1992). Most eye pathologies listed as causes of colic have very acute onset, and therefore are not relevant to colic syndrome.

Central nervous systems abnormalities might also be expected to be more commonly represented, but few cases have been documented. The best is an infant with a Chiari type 1 malformation whose retrospective history is consistent with colic syndrome (Listernick and Tomita 1991).

Urinary tract infection also might be expected to present as colic syndrome. However, to date the two case series (Du 1976, Browne and Lillystone 1991) provide only weak support at best, and the urinary infections may have been coincident rather than causal (Gormally and Barr 1997).

In summary, on the basis of current evidence, the number of organic diseases that have been documented to present as colic syndrome are fewer than might be expected. Those in which organic diseases are causal (as with, for example, cow's milk protein intolerance) constitute a smaller proportion of all cases of colic syndrome than usually assumed. The important caveat is that there may be more cases than those for which we have evidence. However, although it is possible that the estimates are significantly compromised by lack of evidence, it is unlikely that organic disease will account for most, or even a large number of cases.

CLINICAL CLUES OF ORGANIC DISEASE

The second question was whether there were clinical clues in the phenomenology of crying, the history or the physical examination that helped differentiate which infants had an organic disease causing their colic syndrome. Specific clues were rare indeed, unless one counts diagnostic tests such as urinalysis for urinary tract infection, or esophagoscopy for esophagitis. However, some nonspecific clues were suggested, if not established, by the cases. First, concerning behavioral clues, an organic etiology appears to be more likely in infants whose cries are high-pitched, who regularly arch their backs when they cry, or whose crying does not manifest a diurnal pattern. Second, there may be a useful general principle concerning the presentation of organic disease as colic syndrome; namely, that colic syndrome is not due to organic disease in the absence of additional signs and symptoms. At least in the cases reviewed, there was always some other positive symptom or sign in the history or physical examination that made the presentation of colic 'atypical'. Of these, increased frequency of regurgitation, vomiting or diarrhea were the most common, probably because of the prevalence of reports of cow's milk protein intolerance. Others, such as Collier's sign in the case of the infant with migraine, were only reported once. Finding other symptoms and signs is in part a function of how carefully they are sought. However, the principle underlines the importance of the completeness of the history and physical examination. Third, in regard to cow's milk protein intolerance, timing of symptoms may be relevant. Breast-fed infants who responded to maternal dietary intervention tended to be younger (<6 weeks— Hill *et al.* 1995), while a late onset of increased crying in the third month, especially following a switch from breast to formula feeding, may raise the likelihood of protein intolerance in others (Schrander *et al.* 1993). Finally, and not surprisingly, it was very common for infants with unusual and excessive crying due to organic disease to have the crying persist beyond 4 months. This feature is of little help at the time of presentation and is not diagnostic. However, it emphasizes the importance of monitoring these infants until the symptoms resolve.

The fact that organic disease presents relatively rarely as colic syndrome heightens the importance of being able to identify those in whom it is present. Unfortunately, none of these clinical clues is diagnostic, and all simply raise the probability that there may be an organic disease in any particular infant. Clearly, the task of identification remains a challenge, and clinicians could benefit from a more complete data base on which to base these judgments.

Prognosis

A second parental motivation for bringing infants with excessive crying to clinicians is concern about what the outcome will be for their child. This is no less important for the clinician, who must decide which infants to follow closely and whether there is an increased risk for subsequent disease and/or dysfunction. Although there is only a modest literature concerning organic etiology, follow-up studies of colic outcome are rarer still. Furthermore, those that do exist have many of the same limitations as the etiologic studies. In much the same way that interest has focused on gastrointestinal pathophysiology in regard to etiology, longitudinal studies have tended to focus on temperament on the assumption that colic is an early manifestation of relatively stable temperamental traits that manifest later as the 'difficult child'. Such biases, while understandable, risk overlooking other more important, if less immediately obvious, outcomes.

Despite its limitations, this is an important literature for clinicians faced with the problem of infant colic. To address these problems, we reviewed 55 articles addressing the long-term outcome of infants with colic published during the last 44 years. Papers were ascertained by a search of Medline (1996–1997) and PsychInfo (1967–1997) databases using the keywords 'infantile colic', 'crying infant', and 'irritable infant'. This produced 768 studies. We also included four studies that were 'in press' at the time of the review. In trying to determine which studies to include, a number of additional limitations were readily apparent. One is that the method of determining whether an infant has (or had) colic syndrome varies widely from direct behavioral observation or diary records at the time colic was occurring to asking a single question of a parent months after the colic had resolved. A second is that many studies are retrospective and/or only begin to record or observe infants after 3 months, the age by which 'typical' colic has resolved. A third limitation is that only two studies had parental measures prior to the onset of colic or the crying complaint. Consequently, it is often impossible to know whether parental characteristics present after the infant had colic were 'caused' by the colic or were also present before. Finally, some longitudinal studies discuss infants with 'irritability', persistent mother–infant distress syndrome, the 'difficult' infant or 'dysregulated' infants, rather than crying behavior or colic syndrome *per se*. Whether these infants are the same as infants with colic is not self-evident. Some of the issues concerning the continuity or discontinuity of colic syndrome and these later presentations of crying concerns are discussed elsewhere (Barr 2000).

In light of these constraints, we chose to limit this review to studies that (a) explicitly studied infants with the behavioral syndrome of colic and (b) were prospective from the time that colic status was obtained (whether by observation, diary or history). Within this group, we ascertained six cohorts of infants with colic (a total of 178 infants) in which the diagnosis was made *during* the period of excessive crying ('concurrent' diagnosis) and cases were followed prospectively. There were an additional five cohorts in which colic status was ascertained *following* the colic period ('recall' diagnosis) and cases were followed prospectively. The latter studies are more likely to represent parental *perceptions* of infant behavior than the behavior itself. Consequently, the results of the studies in which colic status is determined when it is happening are likely to be 'stronger' evidence of outcome than those in which colic status is determined after the fact. The time lines for determining 'colic case status' and follow-up contacts for all 11 cohorts are illustrated in Figure 5.2. The overall results by 'domain' of outcome are represented in Table 5.2.

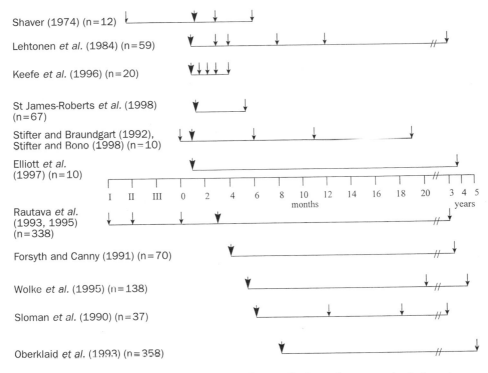

Fig. 5.2. Studies and timelines of longitudinal samples contributing to the prognostic pie for outcomes of infants with colic. Authors are listed at left; number of subjects are listed in brackets. The 'time axis' in the middle of the figure represents months of age of the infants (to the right of 0, or birth) and trimester of pregancy (I, II or III to the left of 0, or birth). Studies listed above the 'time axis' represent studies in which colic status was determined during the age when colic occurred. For studies below the time axis, colic status was obtained only by recall. Large arrowheads indicate the age (in months) at which colic status was ascertained. Small arrowheads indicate the age at which outcome variables were assessed.

Outcomes from Studies in Which Colic Status Was Determined at the Time It Was Happening

In the earliest study, Shaver (1974) reported outcomes determined by interview of 12 mothers of infants with 'diagnosed colic' (undefined) and 45 mothers of infants without colic. Interviews occurred when the infants were 6 weeks, 3 and 6 months old. They were compared on 54 'items' concerning maternal characteristics and mother–infant interaction. Most of the outcomes were not significantly different. There were no differences in maternal characteristics of sensitivity, responsiveness or affection, psychological adaptation to the infants, personality, or number of stress events. Mothers of infants with colic reported a decline in confidence in coping and being less accepting of their infants at 3 months, but these differences had resolved by 6 months. The infants with colic were still described as having 'increased irritability', 'increased tenseness', 'more feeding problems' and 'lower overall functioning' (undefined) at 6 months. Given the potential for biased recall and that

TABLE 5.2
Outcome of colic syndrome by domain.

| | Diagnosis obtained | |
	During colic	By recall
INFANT		
Health		
Weight gain delay	Transient?	
Allergy, eczema, asthma	None	None
Developmental delay	None	Transient or none
Crying	Much reduced	
Behavior disturbances	None	Increased
Difficult temperament	No	Yes/no
Sleep problems	None	Increased
Negative reactivity	None	
PARENT (MOTHER)		
Self-confidence (efficacy)	At risk	
Depression	At risk	
Personality differences	None	
Stress increased	None	
INFANT–CAREGIVER INTERACTION		
Responsiveness (sensitivity) affected	No	Yes
Caregiving flexibility differences	No	
Attachment non-secure	No	
Perception of infant as 'problematic'	Yes	Yes
FAMILY		
Stress increased	Transient	
Interaction difficulties	Transient	
Marital adjustment problems	No	
Family functioning affected	No	Yes

at least two differences (of 54) might be expected by chance, this small study suggests that the outcome may be fairly good.

A Finnish study followed 59 infants with colic and 58 age-matched controls (Lehtonen 1994). Colic status was determined by parental diary records. Mothers of infants with colic reported a mean of 2 hours/day of 'colicky' (painful sounding, difficult to soothe) crying and 4 hours/day of total crying (that is, they met at least modified Wessel's colic criteria). A subgroup of 36 infants were designated as having 'severe' colic, defined as at least 3 hours/day of 'colicky' crying for three days a week (a version of 'Wessel's plus' colic).

There were a wide variety of outcome measures in a number of domains. Concerning physical health, weight gain was slightly less in colic infants during the first 16 weeks, but no different thereafter. Otherwise, there were no differences in health as assessed by parental report of infections, allergies or presence of eczema and by physical examinations at 4, 8 and 12 months. Concerning development, no differences were found on tests of gross motor, fine motor, language or social development as assessed by a screening scale from

Helsinki University Hospital at 4 and 8 months or a Gesell Scale examination at 12 months. In light of the assumption that colic is an early manifestation of temperament, the findings regarding temperament assessment are particularly interesting. No group differences were found on any of the nine temperament dimensions of the Toddler Temperament Scale (Fullard *et al.* 1984) at 12 or 36 months. However, when choosing optional responses to the statement, "In general, the temperament of your child is (a) about average, (b) more difficult than average, (c) easier than average", the mothers whose infants had previously had colic were more likely to report their infants as 'more difficult' at 3 months (24 *vs* 4 per cent), 12 months (23 *vs* 5 per cent) and 36 months (29 *vs* 16 per cent) (Lehtonen *et al.* 1994). In regard to other infant behaviors, no differences were reported for duration of sleep during the night or during the day, nor for percentage of infants who woke at least once every night at any age.

Family psychological characteristics were assessed by family interview when the infants had colic and at 12 months of age (Raiha *et al.* 1996, 1997). Families of infants with colic reported expectable differences in domains of family affect, functioning and structure when the infants had colic. For example, there was a more negative family atmosphere when the infant cried, less flexibility, and more unresolved conflicts in families with infants with colic. At 12 months, all families scored within the normal range on all measures, but statistically significant differences were found for fewer positive responses in domains of family communication, function and affect. At 36 months, there were trends toward less optimal scores on the McMaster Family Assessment Device (Epstein *et al.* 1983) in the families whose infants had previously 'severe' colic, but they were not statistically reliable (Raiha *et al.* 1997).

Importantly, this relatively unselected cohort more objectively defined colic status, assessed both infant and family outcomes, and followed the families longer. In general, outcome was remarkably positive in most areas once colic resolved, including infant health and development, temperamentally relevant behaviors, and family functioning. The discrepancy between the lack of difference on all temperament subscales and the overall maternal impression of 'difficultness' suggests that early colic may have lasting effects on maternal *perception* of infant difficultness even in the face of equivalent infant behaviors.

Keefe *et al.* (1996) reported a short-term longitudinal study of a convenience sample of 20 Caucasian middle and upper middle class infants with colic ('irritable infants'), defined as greater than 2.5 hours of 'crying'/day over the past week on the Fussiness Rating Scale with cry duration and intensity indices above the median, compared to 20 infants without colic. Mother–infant interaction was assessed by observation of feedings with the Nursing Child Assessment Feeding Scale (NCAFS—Barnard *et al.* 1989). On testing when the infants were 7 weeks old, the mothers of those with colic scored lower on one of four subscales (maternal growth fostering) and on the overall 'maternal scale', and the infants scored lower on one of two subscales (responsiveness) and on the overall 'infant scale'. However, at 12 weeks, there were no mother or infant differences on this interaction measure, and no differences in crying or sleep behavior in the infants. Although limited in its outcome measures, the study does provide direct behavioral observations of infant and mother–infant interaction. In this relatively low-risk sample, the outcome appears equivalent for infants with and without colic.

St. James-Roberts *et al.* (1998) reported groups selected from an unreferred community sample of infants to represent 'persistent' criers (roughly equivalent to modified Wessel's colic; n = 68), 'evening' criers (did not meet Wessel's criteria, but cried or fussed at least one hour in the evenings; n = 38), and 'moderate' criers (non-colic; n = 55). The infants were followed from 6 weeks to 5 months of age. Crying amounts were documented by audio recordings (at 6 weeks) and diaries (at 6 weeks and 5 months). In addition to crying, outcome measures included diary measures of caregiving, direct behavioral observations (including maternal sensitivity and intrusiveness during a play session) and counts of maternal and infant behaviors, and questionnaires for maternal depression (the Edinburgh Depression Scale—Cox 1987), maternal responsiveness and attitudes to spoiling (Crockenberg and Smith 1982), flexibility of maternal caregiving style (Schedule-Demand Inventory—Power 1990), infant temperament (Infant Characteristics Questionnaire—Bates *et al.* 1979), and (at 5 months only) maternal satisfaction, adjustment and daily hassles. This represents the most complete description of behavioral outcome, and particularly observed outcome, to date.

Differences in infant distress (fussing + crying + 'colic' crying) were significant by design at 6 weeks. At 5 months, overall distress behavior was reduced by more than half in all groups but, importantly, was still significantly different between groups and moderately stable across the two ages (r = 0.54, p<0.001). Despite the earlier and continuing differences in distress behavior, there were no differences in caregiving behaviors by diary or direct observation except, not surprisingly, increased time spent carrying and soothing, especially while they were crying. There were no differences in global ratings from direct observation of maternal sensitivity and affection, nor for sensitivity and intrusiveness in the play situation. On questionnaire measures, neither flexibility of caregiving (scheduled *vs* infant demand approaches) nor marital adjustment were different among groups. There were four differences. The mothers of 'persistent' criers were a little less likely to respond to crying than the mothers of non-colic ('moderate') criers, were more likely to consider them 'difficult' on temperament scales, and reported more daily hassles. Finally, the maternal depression scores were still higher, and a higher percentage of mothers with persistent or evening criers had scores above the clinical cut-off (9 and 16 per cent respectively) than in the control group (0 per cent). However, these percentages were much reduced compared to the same scores at 6 weeks (23, 27 and 2 per cent respectively).

Given the number of measures, domains of behavior, and infant and maternal characteristics that were measured, these outcomes might be considered quite encouraging. In particular, direct observation of maternal–infant interaction was intact, at least on these measures. Of the differences that did persist, most (attitude concerning response to crying, reported difficult temperament, and more daily hassles) might be expected, especially since crying differences, while reduced, were still present at 5 months. The differences in self-report of maternal depression were potentially the most important. However, these too became less in association with the decline in crying amounts relative to the rates reported at 6 weeks. Furthermore, it is not known what the rates of depressive symptoms were prior to the onset of colic. It is possible that they were the same, or that a prior vulnerability to depression interacted with the increased crying to make the depression manifest. Whether this is a transient or persistent outcome remains an open question.

Stifter and Braungart reported on 10 unreferred infants who met interview-ascertained Wessel's criteria for colic, identified prospectively from a cohort of 100 infants followed from birth and seen at 5, 10 (Stifter and Braungart 1992) and 18 months (Stifter and Bono 1998). Although a small sample, it is important because they had both infant reactivity measures (crying response to pacifier withdrawal and rubber band snap to the heel) and maternal personality measures (neuroticism and extraversion scales of the NEO-AC Personality Inventory [Costa and McCrae], and maternal responsiveness on the Crockenberg and Smith [1982] scale) *prior to* the onset of colic. At 5 and 10 months, they assessed infant temperament (by the Infant Behavior Questionnaire—Rothbart 1981), maternal responsiveness during a five-minute play session, infant development (with the Bayley Mental Scale—Bayley 1969), infant negative reactivity to arm restraint (at 5 months) and toy removal procedures (at 10 months), and maternal self-efficacy and separation anxiety. At 18 months, they assessed attachment classification.

The results were remarkably consistent across the domains measured. Importantly, there were no differences at birth on either the infant responsivity measures or the maternal personality and responsivity measures. Similarly, at 5 and 10 months, there were no differences concerning infant mental development, maternal perceptions of infant temperament (all subscales), or directly observed maternal responsiveness. There were also no differences in observed negative reactivity of infants; indeed, if anything, those with previous colic cried less in response to the mildly aversive stimuli. At 18 months, only two infants had insecure/resistant attachments, and, generally, infants with prior colic had attachment classifications that were similar to those for infants without colic. There were 'statistically significant' differences on perceived maternal self-efficacy at 5 months, but this was due to the scores of two of the 10 mothers (Stifter and Bono 1998, Barr 1998a). Interestingly, the insecurely attached infants were those of the mothers with lower earlier perceived self-efficacy. These findings are obviously questionable statistically because of the small sample size. However, they are remarkably consistent with those from other studies, and add confidence to the overall findings because of the measures taken prior to the onset of colic, and the direct behavioral observations taken afterwards.

In the final study with concurrently measured colic, Elliott *et al.* (1997) report another small convenience sample of 10 infants with colic based on questionnaire responses to three questions regarding crying episodes in their infants that, the authors state, is equivalent to meeting Wessel's criteria. When the infants were between 2 and 4 years of age, they had no differences on measures of child behavior (the Child Behavior Checklist for 2- to 3-year-olds—Achenbach and Edelbrock 1986), family function, parent or infant measures from direct observation of parent–infant interaction (Nursing Child Assessment Feeding Scale—Barnard *et al.* 1989), questions about child health, or a general question about infant temperament. The only reported difference was in response to a question about major family disruptions, on which families of infants with prior colic reported more.

LONGITUDINAL STUDIES IN WHICH COLIC STATUS WAS DETERMINED AFTER INCREASED CRYING RESOLVED

Five longitudinal studies were found in which the determination of whether the infants had

colic was made after the increased crying had resolved. The time of assessment by questionnaire or interview ranged from 3 months (Rautava *et al.* 1993) to 8 months (Oberklaid *et
al.* 1993). Only two (Sloman *et al.* 1990, Wolke *et al.* 1995) specified the amount of crying
in the question. Because such determinations were retrospective, more subject to recall bias,
and without other more 'objective' confirmation of crying amounts, it is more appropriate
to consider these infants to have a 'perceived crying problem' rather than 'colic'. In terms
of the diagnostic pie (Fig. 5.1, p. 70), these infants met criteria for being inside the circle
rather than being inside any particular slice of the pie. There is an additional important
constraint to interpretation. Since the parent is the reporter of both the colic status and the
later concerns, it is difficult to know whether the reported outcomes are actually due to prior
colic, or to the perception of otherwise typical increases in crying as problematic. While
associations of perceptions are important, they may or may not reflect real differences in
behavior of the infant or the caregiver.

Of these studies, the one with the earliest assessment of colic was that of Rautava *et
al.* (1993, 1995). They reported a cohort of 1443 Finnish families who were recruited during
the first trimester and then followed to three years postpartum. Colic status was determined
at three months postpartum, by parental responses to a question as to whether their infant
had 'quite a lot of colic' (18 per cent) or 'a lot of colic' (10 per cent) on a five-point scale.
On a confidential *prepartum* questionnaire of more than 60 questions, colic was more likely
to be reported later if there was dissatisfaction with marital life (*e.g.* perceived worsening
of the sexual relationship), more stress experiences (*e.g.* social isolation) or stress symptoms
(*e.g.* work distressing during pregnancy), and more symptoms of illness (*e.g.* sickness
during pregnancy, sick leave). Disappointment with the delivery (*e.g.* with appearance or
health of the baby) was reported by greater numbers of both mothers and fathers who later
reported colic. Importantly, there was no association of later colic with any sociodemographic
or educational variable. Although it is a little unclear how many of these significant responses
might have occurred by chance, the associations make sense, and suggest that perceived
prenatal and perinatal difficulties might well be associated with later perceptions that
increased crying was a problem.

At three years postpartum, 865 mothers (and 753 fathers) completed questionnaires
concerning family and infant functioning. Families that had earlier perceived their infant's
crying as colic continued to be more likely to report dissatisfaction in daily family life (*e.g.*
unequal responsibility for household activities, fewer shared leisure activities) and their infants
were reported to have more frequent problems falling asleep and more temper tantrums.
However, there were no reported differences for behavior problems other than sleep (Child
Behavior Checklist—Achenbach and Edelbrock 1986), for development (Denver Developmental Screening Test—Frankenburg *et al.* 1971), or for suspected or verified allergens or
special diets.

Forsyth and colleagues (Forsyth *et al.* 1985, Forsyth and Canny 1991) reported a
longitudinal study in which infants from pediatric practices were reported by interview at
4 months to have moderate or severe excessive crying, spitting, colic or feeding problems.
Thirty-five per cent had at least one of these problems. Of these, 65 per cent were described
as having excessive crying and 31 per cent as having colic, but symptom overlap was not

reported. Infants with previous crying and/or feeding problems were more likely to be seen as 'vulnerable' (20 *vs* 11 per cent) and to have more behavioral problems (19 *vs* 11 per cent) at 3.5 years of age. Differences in reported prevalence of asthma (1.7 *vs* 4.4 per cent) and eczema (8.8 *vs* 5.4 per cent) were nonsignificant.

In another large community sample in Germany, Wolke *et al.* (1995) followed 432 infants from 5 to 56 months of age. This study is limited to questionnaire responses, but is unique in systematically asking parents to describe separately their infant's behaviors, characteristics of these behaviors that might be problematic, and their own distress associated with these behaviors. At 5 months, 32 per cent of the infants were defined as *still having* a crying problem or as having had a crying problem *before* that age. Parents of these infants reported more night wakenings at 20 months (30 *vs* 17 per cent) and more frequent cosleeping at 56 months (36 *vs* 23 per cent). However, the more remarkable finding was the general lack of significant associations among crying, feeding and sleeping behaviors as well as among problematic characteristics of these behaviors (Barr 1995b, Wolke *et al.* 1995). With few exceptions, neither normative behaviors nor problem behaviors tended to be predictive of later problems, but expressed *distress* concerning the problem behaviors did. Although limited to questionnaire responses, this study is particularly important in emphasizing the importance of perceived concern as a factor in subsequent outcome.

As part of a larger study of low-level lead exposure in White, middle- to upper-middle-class families, Sloman *et al.* (1990) interviewed mothers of 6-month-old infants by asking whether they considered that their child had colic, and the duration (number of hours a day?), pattern (three days a week?), and persistence (at least one month?) of crying. Infants who were reported to have cried at least one hour per day, whose crying was unsoothable, and who answered affirmatively to the pattern and persistence questions were considered to have had 'colic' (17 per cent). There was no relation between cord blood lead at birth or capillary blood lead at 6 months and colic status. The positive findings were lower scores on the mental and motor indices of the Bayley Scales of Infant Development (Bayley 1969) at 6 months, and this difference was statistically independent of a number of possible confounding factors. Importantly, however, there were no differences at 12, 18 and 24 months. The infants with a colic history were also rated as less responsive, unhappier during testing, less persistent, and less able to maintain optimal functioning during the test on the associated Infant Behavior Record (Bayley 1969), an examiner rating of behavior during the testing procedure. At 6 months, mothers rated them as more withdrawing, intense and negative in mood on the Infant Temperament Questionnaire (Fullard *et al.* 1984), but there was no significant difference in the proportions of infants classified as 'difficult' (10.8 *vs* 9.2 per cent). Apparently, temperament was not assessed at later ages. Parents of infants with colic also scored lower on two scales (emotional and verbal responsivity of the mother and opportunities for variety in daily routine) of the Home Observation for Measurement of the Environment (HOME—B. Caldwell, unpublished).

Despite the retrospective determination of colic status, this study is important because of the determination of developmental outcome by direct testing. The results were interpreted by the authors as evidence for a 'transient developmental lag', possibly secondary to reduced interaction between the difficult infant and reduced stimulation. The associated examiner and parent ratings at 6 months could have meant that the differences were due to testability, rather than differences in cognitive function. However, at least in this relatively advantaged sample, these differences did not persist, suggesting that if developmental lags do occur, they are reversible in sufficiently supportive contexts.

Oberklaid *et al.* (1993) reported on a cohort of infants (N = 1583) that was a stratified random population sample first assessed between 4 and 8 months and again during the preschool period (4–5 years). This was primarily a study of temperament, but infants were ranked separately on a three-item rating (four-point scale: none to severe) concerning colic, sleeping problems and excessive crying. Infants in the top 25 per cent of the sample on the summed score were considered to have infant behavior problems. About 8 per cent more of these than control infants were likely to score high for preschool behavior problems on the Preschool Behavior Questionnaire (Behar and Springfield 1979). Importantly, however, the authors interpret these (and other) results to reflect parental *perception* of difficulties, consistent with the findings in the study by Wolke *et al.* (1995). Among other sources of evidence, global parental perception of 'difficultness' during infancy and of infant behavior problems predicted preschool behavior problems, but maternal *ratings* of infant behavior (on the Revised Infant Temperament Questionnaire—Carey and McDevitt 1978) did not.

SUMMARY OF FOLLOW-UP STUDIES

The results of prospective studies in which colic status was determined at the time of the increased crying are remarkably similar. For the most part, the infants with colic included in these samples met at least modified Wessel's criteria for colic, and some met 'Wessel's plus' criteria. Of the cohorts described, at least three—including the two largest (Lehtonen *et al.* 1994, St James-Roberts *et al.* 1998)—consisted of non-referred infants, thereby removing a number of referral biases that might have complicated the outcome picture. The results suggest that infants with colic will be as healthy as controls, and not distinguishable behaviorally. Importantly, there were no apparent lasting disruptions of mother–infant interaction, at least as assessed by direct observations of relatively short interaction sessions. This might be qualified by the possibility that an infant with prior colic in a family with a 'vulnerable' parent (with, for example, low perceived self-efficacy) might be at increased risk for a poor interactive outcome later. Furthermore, there is some indication that, despite lack of evidence for behavioral or sleeping differences, infants with previous colic may be *perceived* to be more difficult and as having more sleeping problems even up to three years later. There is evidence for at least transient reductions in coping confidence and depressive symptoms in mothers.There is also the possibility of residual differences in the family interactions of infants with prior colic. An important, unresolved question is whether these differences were present prior to, were caused by, or were moderated by the experience of having an infant with colic.

The results from the studies in which the determination of whether infants had colic was made *after* increased crying had resolved are also remarkably similar. Infants in these samples were those in whom increased crying had been seen as a problem. In terms of the clinical pie, these included infants who would have met Wessel's criteria, but also those who did not. Applied to a community setting (when the subjects are not referred), the subjects in these studies would all be 'inside' the circle. In a clinical setting, fewer subjects would be inside the circle because of the additional motivation that would be required for them to come to the clinic to raise crying as a concern.

Again, however, the results are remarkably positive, consistent, and indeed similar to those found previously. First, on the basis of the admittedly limited available health measures, infants with colic were as healthy as controls. Second, evidence for developmental delay was mixed (Sloman *et al.* 1990, Rautava *et al.* 1995), but if present, it was transient. This is qualified by the caveat that this is true in a relatively low-risk, middle-class sample. Whether such a delay might be more persistent in the presence of additional risk factors remains unknown. Third, the strongest associations reported were to *perceived* subsequent behavior problems in these as in the previous studies. Since the determination of colic status was retrospective, that might be expected for the latter group of studies. However, these studies reinforce the importance of the perception of problematic increased crying as a predictor of persistent differences in perception of behavior, if not of actual behavior itself. Finally, there is additional evidence that some difficulties in later family function are also predicted by earlier perceived excessive crying. However, the study by Rautava *et al.* suggests, although it does not yet demonstrate, that some of these difficulties may have been present prior to the onset of colic.

A prognostic pie for infants with colic

There are a number of limitations to constructing a 'prognostic pie' analogous to the 'diagnostic pie' for infants with crying complaints. The first is that the duration of follow-up is different, so that it is not clear whether some outcomes that are present early (*e.g.* maternal depressive symptoms) are transient or persistent. The second is that rare or difficult-to-ascertain outcomes (such as child abuse) are unlikely to be reported. A third is that the degree of overlap of outcomes, both within and especially amongst studies, is not known. A fourth is that there is still little evidence of parental attitudes and characteristics prior to the onset of colic. Consequently, some sequelae may be due to pre-colic difficulties, rather than to colic itself. Finally, some studies report significant associations, but not the numbers of infants or families so affected, making estimation of the 'size' of an outcome slice difficult.

In light of these constraints, only a very preliminary 'worst case' scenario prognostic pie is presented (Fig. 5.3). The organizational principles incorporated in this pie are similar to those in the diagnostic pie. As before, the circle represents crying complaints. However, in this pie it is not necessarily the case that these infants were brought to the clinician, but rather that they met criteria for colic when approached in the community. The slices are outcomes reported (to date) derived from those studies in which it is possible to estimate the *differential* prevalence of these problems in infants with colic (*i.e.* the percentage of infants with colic with these problems in follow-up minus the percentage of infants without colic with these problems). No adjustment is made for likely possible overlap of problems (*e.g.* 'perceived vulnerability' of the infant might coexist with 'family problems'). This is a 'worst case' prognostic pie in the sense that the outcomes are not adjusted for any of the constraints in the available data that will tend to inflate the estimates of slice size (differences in follow-up duration, overlap of outcomes, pre-colic status). Furthermore, we have not

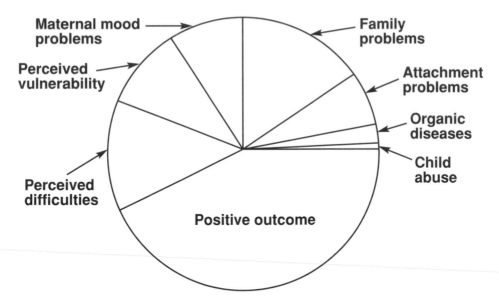

Fig. 5.3. A clinical prognostic pie for colic. This represents a 'worst case' scenario for prognosis, since it does not account for probable overlap in some of the outcomes (see text). The size of slices is estimated from differences in the rates of these outcomes in infants with and without colic. Organic disease and child abuse slices are included, but there are no studies that compare rates of occurrence for these important, but relatively rare, outcomes.

distinguished the results of studies of perceived colic (ascertained after colic resolved) from those of concurrently documented colic. Finally, we have included reference to abuse (prevalence unknown) as an outcome and to organic disease (prevalence also unknown). The justification for the latter is that, in the review for literature describing organic etiologies, crying secondary to organic disease so often persisted beyond 3 months.

Despite these limitations, the prognostic pie does capture many important features of the overall pattern of results suggested by the longitudinal studies. First, the physical, health, and behavioral outcomes for infants are remarkably good. Other than the very small but extremely important group of infants whose crying persists because of underlying organic disease or who suffer abuse, evidence of illness after colic is resolved is so far non-existent. Second, the most common outcome *for infants* is that they are *perceived* to be more vulnerable and/or difficult in about 25 per cent (or less) of the cases. Whether this has any as yet undefined negative effects on the infant is, so far, not clear. At least on available evidence, it does not seem to have affected infant–caregiver interaction on the basis of direct observations. Third, the most common outcome *for caregivers* is that maternal mood (self-perception, depression) may be affected, at least transiently, and family relationships may be problematic for quite a long time. Fourth, a possible outcome *for caregiver–infant interaction* is insecure or resistant attachments. The evidence for this is the weakest, since this prevalence was no different than that found in the control sample (Stifter and Bono

1998). However, we included this because it was found in the infants whose mothers had compromised self-esteem, presumably due to well-documented excessive crying.

Summary and implications

The diagnostic and prognostic pies are one way of providing a concise heuristic framework for summarizing the available literature for two of the important challenges facing clinicians dealing with crying complaints in nonfebrile infants in the first three months of life. By understanding the principles on which they are organized, they can be adjusted accordingly if applied to different settings, or in the face of new data. For example, since the bulk of the follow-up studies are from community samples, it is possible that the type or size of outcomes in the prognostic pie would be different if new studies using different measures became available or if only 'referred' or 'clinical' samples were studied. Even in this form, however, there are a number of implications for both research and practice that these pies highlight.

The first implication applies equally to the diagnostic and prognostic pies. In both cases, the number of infants with colic is relatively large compared to the number that (in the diagnostic pie) have an organic disease underlying their behavioral syndrome or (in the prognostic pie) a poor prognosis for the infant or the family. The encouraging implication is that outcome is good for infant and family in most cases, and should provide much needed reassurance for harried parents and clinicians. The discouraging implication is that it accentuates the difficulty for the clinician of being able to decide *which* infant with colic has underlying organic disease and/or is at risk for a problematic outcome. The clinician can assume neither that colic syndrome is benign nor that there is a uniformly good outcome. However, the data base for 'clinical clues' for organic disease and 'prognostic clues' is, as we have seen, remarkably weak. On the basis of available studies, we have proposed some possible clinical clues, but these have yet to be systematically and prospectively evaluated. There is clearly some important work that can be done to define these clues and improve clinical decision-making.

A second implication concerns a challenge highlighted by an important limitation in the prognostic pie. Because the outcomes were drawn from different studies, we have no idea whether the families with problems were also the families who perceived that their infants were difficult. On the one hand, it is possible that *all* of the poor outcomes for the infants, for the caregivers and for infant–caregiver attachment occurred in very few families. If this was so, and if these infant–caregiver dyads could be identified at or prior to presentation, then it might be very advantageous to concentrate clinical efforts on these families. On the other hand, it is also possible that poor outcomes are expressed differently in different families. The consequences of having an infant with colic might be expressed as maternal depressive mood in one family but as perceived vulnerability of the infant in another. In the Finnish cohort (Lehtonen 1994), a subanalysis suggested that there was little overlap between the families with problems and the families who perceived their infants as difficult. However, the only way we will know with certainty is if all of the potentially negative outcomes are assessed in the same prospective cohort to determine whether they cluster together in a few families or are differentially expressed in many families.

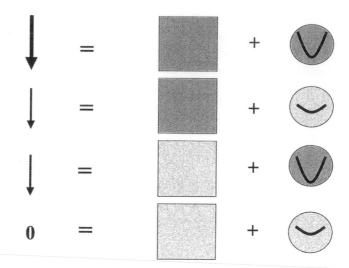

Fig. 5.4. Diagrammatic representation of the 'double hit' hypothesis for negative prognostic outcome in infants with colic. Circles represent infants; squares represent family environments. Gray circles (with an increased crying curve) represent infants with colic (one 'hit'); gray squares represent stressed, or at-risk, family environments (a second 'hit'). The right column represents chance of increased risk of poor outcome.

A third implication is highlighted by another important limitation in the prognostic pie; namely, the absence of sufficient understanding of parental attitudes and characteristics prior to the onset of colic. The one study with prepartum measures (Rautava *et al*. 1993) did report familial differences in those who later said their infants had had colic, and also reported increased family functioning difficulties later, but it is not known whether those with prepartum and postpartum differences were the same families. The measures at birth in the cohort of Stifter and Braungart (1992) showed no maternal differences, but the sample of infants with colic was very small (N = 10) so that important differences may have been missed.

However, exactly this kind of information might be the most important missing link for integrating a number of findings into what might be called the 'double hit' hypothesis (Fig. 5.4). This is the proposal that negative outcomes for colic are the consequence, not of colic (or increased crying) *per se*, but of the interaction between an infant with colic (one 'hit') and an 'at risk' contextual factor (a second 'hit'). The presence of colic by itself in an otherwise intact family context would not typically increase the likelihood of a poor outcome, while a fragile family context in the absence of colic also would not typically have a poor outcome. However, an increased incidence of poor outcomes would occur in fragile families that also had an infant with colic.

There is at least a suggestion of this in the study of Stifter and Bono (1998), where the insecure/resistant attachments occurred in the two families in which the infants had colic and the mothers experienced low self-efficacy. This is also indirectly supported by findings in other studies that did not meet selection criteria for inclusion in this review, but contribute to the impression that the outcome for families with an infant with colic is much worse than this review would suggest. For example, Papousek and von Hofacker (1995, 1998) describe a clinical sample of families who might be considered to have 'persistent mother–infant distress' syndrome (Barr 1998a). Most presented after the early crying peak at 2 months, but showed no decline in crying amounts that remained at the level of infants with Wessel's colic. In addition, however, these infants had increased rates of feeding and/or sleeping disturbances, mild developmental delay and organic risk factors, and their parents more often reported prior psychosocial risk factors, prenatal emotional distress, a high rate of maternal psychopathology and postnatal parental conflicts. Since this is not a prospective longitudinal study, it is difficult to know whether the colic or the 'at risk' family characteristics came first. However, both the infants and the parents in this sample were much more troubled than our review of follow-up studies would predict. At least by history, the density of 'at risk' parental, infant and familial characteristics preceding and concurrent with the onset of colic was much greater than that found in their own control subjects or in the samples reviewed here. Clearly, these families were coping with more than just the single 'hit' of an infant with colic.

If the double hit hypothesis holds, it suggests that the relatively good outcomes seen in the studies used to construct the prognostic pie may not hold for families in which prior risks were also present. Furthermore, such families may be more concentrated in clinical settings, especially referral ones. If it could be demonstrated to be true, however, then presence of a second significant risk factor might be the best prognostic indicator for a poor outcome following colic. This would be particularly important in clinical settings that were able to provide continuous care and anticipatory guidance.

Finally, both the diagnostic and prognostic pies provide some guidance for deciding what, and which infants, should be monitored beyond the colic period. The diagnostic pie clearly indicates that infants whose colic does not resolve must be followed, since this was one of the most frequent behavioral characteristics of infants shown subsequently to have organic disease. Persistent crying beyond 3 or 4 months should not simply be 'dismissed' as colic. The prognostic pie indicates that appropriate care in the families of infants with prior colic should include a check of how parents perceive their infants now and whether there is evidence of disturbance of maternal mood, self-perception or familial disharmony. In many cases, relatively simple counselling may be effective in ameliorating these sequelae (van den Boom 1994, 1995).

The recent increase in careful clinical reports of infants with colic, and especially in controlled observational and, in some cases, experimental studies has begun to improve our understanding of this confusing crying syndrome. Together, they suggest that organic disease is rare, and that most infants have very good outcomes, but catastrophic outcomes are also possible. Deciding which infants have organic disease or whose families are at risk for poor outcomes remains an important, and at least a somewhat more focused, challenge.

ACKNOWLEDGEMENTS

The authors gratefully acknowledge financial support for this work as follows: Liisa Lehtonen by the Finnish Academy of Science (#36772) and by a McGill University–Montreal Children's Hospital Fellowship; Siobhan

Gormally by the Allen Ross Memorial Fellowship from the Montreal Children's Hospital; and Ronald Barr by the Louis Sessenwein Trust Academic Award and the Medical Research Council of Canada.

REFERENCES

Achenbach, T., Edelbrock, C. (1986) *Manual for the Child Behavior Check List and Revised Child Behavior Profile.* Burlington, VT: Dept of Psychiatry, University of Vermont.

Barnard, K.E., Hammond, M.A., Booth, C., Bee, H., Mitchell, S.K., Spieker, S.J. (1989) 'Measurement and meaning of parent–child interaction.' *In:* Morrison, F.J., Lord, C.I., Keating, D.P. (Eds.) *Applied Developmental Psychology, Vol. 3.* San Diego: Academic Press, pp. 39–80.

Barr, R.G. (1990a) 'The "colic" enigma: prolonged episodes of a normal predisposition to cry.' *Infant Mental Health Journal,* **11**, 340–348.

—— (1990b) 'The normal crying curve: what do we really know?' *Developmental Medicine and Child Neurology,* **32**, 356–362.

—— (1991) 'Colic and gas.' *In:* Walker, W.A., Durie, P.R., Hamilton, J.R., Walker-Smith, J.A., Watkins, J.G. (Eds.) *Pediatric Gastrointestinal Disease: Pathophysiology, Diagnosis and Management.* Burlington, VT: Decker, B.C., pp. 55–61

—— (1993) 'Normality: a clinically useless concept; the case of infant crying and colic.' *Journal of Developmental and Behavioral Pediatrics,* **14**, 264–270.

—— (1995a) 'Infant crying and colic: it's a family affair: invited commentary.' *Infant Mental Health Journal,* **16**, 218–220.

—— (1995c) 'The enigma of infant crying: the emergence of defining dimensions.' *Early Development and Parenting,* **4**, 225–232.

—— (1996) 'Colic.' *In:* Walker, W.A., Durie, P.R., Hamilton, J.R., Walker-Smith, J.A., Watkins, J.B. (Eds.) *Pediatric Gastrointestinal Disease: Pathophysiology, Diagnosis and Management. 2nd Edn.* St. Louis: Mosby, pp. 241–250.

—— (1998a) 'Crying in the first year of life: good news in the midst of distress.' *Child: Care, Health and Development,* **24**, 425–439.

—— (1998b) 'Reflections on measuring pain in infants: dissociation in responsive systems and "honest signalling".' *Archives of Disease in Childhood,* **79**, F152–F156.

—— (1999) 'Infant cry behaviour and colic: An interpretation in evolutionary perspective.' *In:* Trevathen, W., Smith, E.O., McKenna, J.J. (Eds.) *Evolutionary Medicine.* New York: Oxford University Press, pp. 27–51.

—— (2000) 'Excessive crying.' *In:* Lewis, M., Sameroff, A.J. (Eds.) *Handbook of Developmental Psychopathology. 2nd. Edn.* New York: Plenum Press. *(In press.)*

—— Geertsma, M.A. (1993) 'Colic: The pain perplex.' *In:* Schechter, N.L., Berde, C.B., Yaster, M. (Eds.) *Pain in Infants, Children, and Adolescents.* Philadelphia: Williams & Wilkins, pp. 587–596

—— Hanley, J., Patterson, D.K., Wooldridge, J.A. (1984) 'Breath hydrogen excretion of normal newborn infants in response to usual feeding patterns: evidence for "functional lactase insufficiency" beyond the first month of life.' *Journal of Pediatrics,* **104**, 527–533.

—— Rotman, A., Yaremko, J., Leduc, D., Francoeur, T.E. (1992) 'The crying of infants with colic: a controlled empirical description.' *Pediatrics,* **90**, 14–21.

Bates, J.E., Freeland, C.A., Lounsbury, M.L. (1979) 'Measurement of infant difficultness.' *Child Development,* **50**, 794–803.

Bayley, N. (1969) *Bayley Scales of Mental Development.* New York: Psychological Corporation.

Behar, L., Springfield, S. (1974) 'A behavioral rating scale for the preschool child.' *Developmental Psychology,* **10**, 601–610.

Berezin, S., Glassman, M.S., Bostwick, H., Halata, M. (1995) 'Esophagitis as a cause of infant colic.' *Clinical Pediatrics,* **34**, 158–159.

Brazelton, T.B. (1962) 'Crying in infancy.' *Pediatrics,* **29**, 579–588.

Browne, G., Lillystone, D. (1991) 'Renal disease presenting as severe unremitting colic.' *Medical Journal of Australia,* **154**, 93–94.

Carey, W.B., McDevitt, S.C. (1978) 'Revision of the Infant Temperament Questionnaire.' *Pediatrics,* **68**, 735–739.

Campbell, J.P.M. (1989) 'Dietary treatment of infant colic: a double-blind study.' *Journal of the Royal College of General Practitioners,* **39**, 11–14.

Cox, J.L. (1987) 'Detection of postnatal depression: development of the 10-item Edinburgh Postnatal Depression Scale.' *British Journal of Psychiatry,* **150**, 782–786.

Crockenberg, S., Smith, P. (1982) 'Antecedents of mother–infant interaction and infant irritability in the first three months of life.' *Infant Behavior and Development*, **5**, 105–119.

Danielsson, B., Hwang, C.P. (1985) 'Treatment of infantile colic with surface active substance (Simethicone).' *Acta Paediatrica Scandinavica*, **74**, 446–450.

De Lorenzo, R.A., Fisher, R. (1995) 'Infant with crying and fever.' *Annals of Emergency Medicine*, **25**, 699–705.

DeGangi, G.A., DiPietro, J.A., Greenspan, S.I., Porges, S.W. (1991) 'Psychophysiological characteristics of the regulatory disordered infant.' *Infant Behavior and Development*, **14**, 37–50.

Douwes, A.C., Oosterkamp, R.F., Fernandes, J., Los, T., Jongbloed, A.A. (1980) 'Sugar malabsorption in healthy neonates estimated by breath hydrogen.' *Archives of Disease in Childhood*, **55**, 512–515.

Du, J.N.H. (1976) 'Colic as the sole symptom of urinary tract infection in infants.' *Canadian Medical Association Journal*, **115**, 334–337.

Duncan, D.E., Briggs, J., Bensimhon, M. (1996) 'One deadly week.' *Life*, 52–58.

Elliott, M.R., Pedersen, E.L., Mogan, J. (1997) 'Early infant crying: Child and family follow-up at three years.' *Canadian Journal of Nursing Research*, **29** (2), 47–67.

Epstein, N.B., Baldwin, L.M., Bishop, D.S. (1983) 'The McMaster Family Assessment Device.' *Jornal of Marital and Family Therapy*, **9**, 171–180.

Evans, R.W., Fergusson, D.M., Allardyce, R.A., Taylor, B. (1981) 'Maternal diet and infantile colic in breast-fed infants.' *Lancet*, **i**, 1340–1342.

Forsyth, B.W.C. (1989) 'Colic and the effect of changing formulas: a double-blind, multiple-crossover study.' *Journal of Pediatrics*, **115**, 521–526.

—— Canny, P.F. (1991) 'Perceptions of vulnerability 3¹/₂ years after problems of feeding and crying behavior in early infancy.' *Pediatrics*, **88**, 757–763.

—— Leventhal, J.M., McCarthy, P.L. (1985) 'Mothers' perceptions of problems of feeding and crying behaviours.' *American Journal of Diseases of Children*, **139**, 269–272.

Frankenburg, W.K., Goldstein, A.D., Camp, B.W. (1971) 'The revised Denver Developmental Screening Test: Its accuracy as a screening instrument.' *Journal of Pediatrics*, **79**, 988 995.

Fullard, W., McDevitt, S.C., Carey, W.B. (1984) 'Assessing temperament in one- to three-year-old children.' *Journal of Pediatric Psychology*, **9**, 205–217.

Geertsma, M.A., Hyams, J.S. (1989) 'Colic—a pain syndrome of infancy?' *Pediatric Clinics of North America*, **36**, 905–919.

Gormally, S.M., Barr, R.G. (1997) 'Of clinical pies and clinical clues: proposal for a clinical approach to complaints of early crying and colic.' *Ambulatory Child Health*, **3**, 137–153.

Heine, R.G., Jaquiery, A., Lubitz, L., Cameron, D.J.S., Catto-Smith, A.G. (1995) 'Role of gastro-oesophageal reflux in infant irritability.' *Archives of Disease in Childhood*, **73**, 121–125.

Hill, D.J., Menahem, S., Hudson, I., Sheffield, L., Oberklaid, F., Hosking, C.S. (1992) 'Charting infant distress: An aid to defining colic.' *Journal of Pediatrics*, **121**, 755–758.

—— Hudson, I.L., Sheffield, L.J., Shelton, M.J., Menahem, S., Hosking, C.S. (1995) 'A low allergen diet is a significant intervention in infantile colic: Results of a community-based study.' *Journal of Allergy and Clinical Immunology*, **96**, 886–892.

Hyman, P.E. (1994) 'Gastroesophageal reflux: one reason why baby won't eat.' *Journal of Pediatrics*, **125**, S103–S109.

Iacono, G., Carroccio, A., Montalto, G., Cavataio, F., Bragion, E., Lorello, D., Balsamo, V., Notarbartoll, A. (1991) 'Severe infantile colic and food intolerance: A long-term prospective study.' *Journal of Pediatric Gastroenterology and Nutrition*, **12**, 332–335.

Jakobsson, I., Lindberg, T. (1978) 'Cow's milk as a cause of infantile colic in breast-fed infants.' *Lancet*, **ii**, 437–439.

Jakobsson, I., Lindberg, T. (1983) 'Cow's milk proteins cause infantile colic in breast-fed infants: A double-blind crossover study.' *Pediatrics*, **71**, 268–271.

Kadushin, A., Martin, J.A. (1981) *Child Abuse: An Interactional Event.* New York: Columbia University Press.

Kahn, A., Mozin, M.J., Casimir, G., Montauk, L., Blum, D. (1985) 'Insomnia and cow's milk allergy in infants.' *Pediatrics*, **76**, 880–884.

Katerji, M., Painter, M. (1994) 'Infantile migraine presenting as colic.' *Journal of Child Neurology*, **8**, 336–337.

Keefe, M.R., Kotzer, A.M., Froese-Fretz, A., Curtin, M. (1996) 'A longitudinal comparison of irritable and nonirritable infants.' *Nursing Research*, **45**, 4–9.

Lehtonen, L. (1994) 'Infantile colic.' PhD thesis, University of Türkü.

93

—— Korhonen, T., Korvenranta, H. (1994) 'Temperament and sleeping pattern in infantile colic during the first year of life.' *Journal of Developmental and Behavioral Pediatrics*, **15**, 416–420.

Lester, B.M., Boukydis, C.F.Z., Garcia-Coll, C.T., Hole, W.T. (1990) 'Symposium on infantile colic: Introduction.' *Infant Mental Health Journal*, **11**, 320–333.

—— Cucca, J., Andreozzi, L., Flanagan, P., Oh, W. (1993) 'Possible association between fluoxetine hydrochloride and colic in an infant.' *Journal of the American Academy of Child and Adolescent Psychiatry*, **32**, 1253–1255.

Listernick, R., Tomita, T. (1991) 'Persistent crying in infancy as a presentation of Chiari type I malformation.' *Journal of Pediatrics*, **118**, 567–569.

Lothe, L., Lindberg, T. (1989) 'Cow's milk whey protein elicits symptoms of infantile colic in colicky formula-fed infants: A double-blind crossover study.' *Pediatrics*, **83**, 262–266.

Ludwig, S. (1984) 'Shaken baby syndrome: a review of 20 cases.' *Annals of Emergency Medicine*, **13**, 104–107.

Mahle, W.T. (1998) 'A dangerous case of colic: anomalous left coronary artery presenting with paroxysms of irritability.' *Pediatric Emergency Care*, **14**, 24–27.

Metcalf, T.J., Irons, T.G., Sher, L.D., Young, P.C. (1994) 'Simiethicone in the treatment of infant colic: A randomized placebo-controlled, multicenter trial.' *Pediatrics*, **94**, 29–34.

Miller, A.R., Barr, R.G. (1991) 'Infantile colic: Is it a gut issue?' *Pediatric Clinics of North America*, **38**, 1407–1423.

—— —— Eaton, W.O. (1993) 'Crying and motor behavior of six-week-old infants and postpartum maternal mood.' *Pediatrics*, **92**, 551–558.

Miller, J.B., Bokdam, M., McVeagh, P., Miller, J.J. (1992) 'Variability of breath hydrogen excretion in breast-fed infants during the first three months of life.' *Journal of Pediatrics*, **121**, 410–413.

Miller, J.J., McVeagh, P., Fleet, G.H., Petocz, P., Brand, J.C. (1990) 'Effect of yeast lactase enzyme on "colic" in infants fed human milk.' *Journal of Pediatrics*, **117**, 261–263.

Oberklaid, F., Sanson, A., Pedlow, R., Prior, M. (1993) 'Predicting school behavior problems from temperament and other variables in infancy.' *Pediatrics*, **91**, 113–120.

Oggero, R., Garbo, G., Savino, F., Mostert, M. (1994) 'Dietary modifications versus dicyclomine hydrochloride in the treatment of severe colics.' *Acta Paediatrica*, **83**, 222–225.

Papousek, M., von Hofacker, N. (1995) 'Persistent crying and parenting: Search for a butterfly in a dynamic system.' *Early Development and Parenting*, **4**, 209–224.

—— —— (1998) 'Persistent crying in early infancy: a non-trivial condition of risk for the developing mother–infant relationship.' *Child: Care, Health and Development*, **24**, 395–424.

Poole, S.R. (1991) 'The infant with acute, unexplained, excessive crying.' *Pediatrics*, **88**, 450–455.

Power, T.G. (1990) 'Maternal perceptions of infant difficultness: The influence of maternal attitudes and attributions.' *Infant Behavior and Development*, **13**, 421–437.

Raiha, H., Lehtonen, L., Korhonen, T., Korvenranta, H. (1996) 'Family life one year after infantile colic.' *Archives of Pediatric and Adolescent Medicine*, **150**, 1032–1036.

—— —— —— —— (1997) 'Family functioning three years after infantile colic.' *Journal of Developmental and Behavioral Pediatrics*, **18**, 290–294.

Rautava, P., Helenius, H., Lehtonen, L. (1993) 'Psychosocial predisposing factors for infantile colic.' *British Medical Journal*, **307**, 600–604.

—— Lehtonen, L., Helenius, H., Silanpaa, M. (1995) 'Infantile colic: child and family three years later.' *Pediatrics*, **96**, 43–47.

Rothbart, M.K. (1981) 'Measurement of infant temperament.' *Child Development*, **52**, 569–578.

Sauls, H.S., Redfern, D.E. (1997) *Colic and Excessive Crying*. Columbus, OH: Ross Products Division Abbott Laboratories.

Schrander, J.J.P., van den Bogart, J.P.H., Forget, P.P., Schrander-Stumpel, C.T.R.M., Kuijten, R.H., Kester, A.D.M. (1993) 'Cow's milk protein intolerance in infants under 1 year of age: a prospective epidemiological study.' *European Journal of Pediatrics*, **152**, 640–644.

Shaver, B.A. (1974) 'Maternal personality and early adaptation as related to infantile colic.' *In:* Shereshefsky, P.M., Yarrow, L.J. (Eds.) *Psychological Aspects of a First Pregnancy and Early Postnatal Adaptation.* New York: Raven Press, pp. 209–215.

Singer, J.I., Rosenberg, N.M. (1992) 'A fatal case of colic.' *Pediatric Emergency Care*, **8**, 171–172.

Sloman, J., Bellinger, D.C., Krentzel, C.P. (1990) 'Infantile colic and transient developmental lag in the first year of life.' *Child Psychiatry and Human Development*, **21**, 25–36.

St James-Roberts, I. (2000) 'Infant crying levels, and maternal patterns of care, in normal community and clinically referred samples.' *In:* Lester, B. (Ed.) *Biological and Social Aspects of Infant Crying.* New York: Plenum Press. *(In press.)*

—— Halil, T. (1991) 'Infant crying patterns in the first year: Normal community and clinical findings.' *Journal of Child Psychology and Psychiatry and Allied Disciplines,* **32,** 951–968.

—— Hurry, J., Bowyer, J. (1993) 'Objective confirmation of crying durations in infants referred for excessive crying.' *Archives of Disease in Childhood,* **68,** 82–84.

—— Conroy, S., Wilsher, K. (1995) 'Clinical, developmental and social aspects of infant crying and colic.' *Early Development and Parenting,* **4,** 177–189.

—— —— —— (1996) 'Bases for maternal perceptions of infant crying and colic behaviour.' *Archives of Disease in Childhood,* **75,** 375–384.

—— —— —— (1998) 'Links between maternal care and persistent infant crying in the early months.' *Child: Care, Health and Development,* **24,** 353–376.

Stahlberg, M-R., Savilahti, E. (1986) 'Infantile colic and feeding.' *Archives of Disease in Childhood,* **61,** 1232–1233.

Stifter, C.A., Bono, M.A. (1998) 'The effect of infant colic on maternal self-perceptions and mother–infant attachment.' *Child: Care, Health and Development,* **24,** 339–351.

—— Braungart, J. (1992) 'Infant colic: A transient condition with no apparent effects.' *Journal of Applied Developmental Psychology,* **13,** 447–462.

Talbot, E.M., Pitts, J.F., Dudgeon, J., Lee, W.R. (1992) 'A case of developmental glaucoma presenting with abdominal colic and subnormal intraocular pressure.' *Journal of Pediatric Ophthalmology and Strabismus,* **29,** 116–119.

Taubman, B. (1988) 'Parental counselling compared with elimination of cow's milk or soy milk protein for the treatment of infant colic syndrome: A randomized trial.' *Pediatrics,* **81,** 756–761.

Thomas, D.W., McGilligan, K., Eisenberg, L.D., Lieberman, H.M., Rissman, E.M. (1987) 'Infantile colic and type of milk feeding.' *American Journal of Diseases of Children,* **141,** 451–453.

Treem, W.R. (1994) 'Infant colic: A pediatric gastroenterologist's perspective.' *Pediatric Clinics of North America,* **41,** 1121–1138.

Trocinski, D.R., Pearigen, P.D. (1998) 'The crying infant.' *Emergency Medical Clinics of North America,* **16,** 895–910.

van den Boom, D.C. (1994) 'The influence of temperament and mothering on attachment and exploration: An experimental manipulation of sensitive responsiveness among lower-class mothers with irritable infants.' *Child Development,* **65,** 1457–1477.

van den Boom, D.C. (1995) 'Do first year intervention effects endure?' *Child Development,* **66,** 1798–1816.

—— Hacksma, J.B. (1994) 'The effect of infant irritability on mother–infant interaction: A growth-curve analysis.' *Developmental Psychology,* **30,** 581–590.

Wales, J.K.H., Primhak, R.A., Rattenbury, J., Taylor, C.J. (1989) 'Isolated fructose malabsorption.' *Archives of Disease in Childhood,* **65,** 227–229.

Wessel, M.A., Cobb, J.C., Jackson, E.B., Harris, G.S., Detwiler, A.C. (1954) 'Paroxysmal fussing in infancy, sometimes called "colic".' *Pediatrics,* **14,** 421–434.

Weston, J. (1968) 'The pathology of child abuse.' *In:* Helfer, R., Kempe, C. (Eds.) *The Battered Child.* Chicago: University of Chicago Press, pp. 77–100.

Wolke, D. (1993) 'The treatment of problem crying behavior.' *In:* St James-Roberts, I., Harris, G., Messer, D. (Eds.) *Infant Crying, Feeding and Sleeping: Development, Problems and Treatments.* Hemel Hempstead, Herts: Harvester-Wheatsheef, pp. 47–79.

—— Meyer, R. (1995) 'The colic debate.' *Pediatrics,* **96,** 165–166.

—— —— Ohrt, B., Riegel, K. (1995) 'Co-morbidity of crying and feeding problems with sleeping problems in infancy.' *Early Development and Parenting,* **4,** 191–207.

Zeskind, P.S., Barr, R.G. (1997) 'Acoustic characteristics of naturally occurring cries of infants with "colic".' *Child Development,* **68,** 394–403.

6
CRYING COMPLAINTS IN THE EMERGENCY DEPARTMENT

Steven Poole and David Magilner

The infant who is taken to an emergency department by parents concerned about excessive or prolonged crying often presents a difficult diagnostic dilemma. The infant may have a relatively benign condition such as infantile colic or a life-threatening condition such as occult head trauma from child abuse. Distinguishing serious from benign conditions in these infants can be very difficult and time-consuming, and a thorough diagnostic evaluation with careful follow-up is needed to make an accurate diagnosis. The professional who evaluates infants should be concerned if crying presents as: (1) an acute episode that is persisting longer than the usual crying periods for that infant without an apparent explanation; (2) recurrent episodes in an infant who does not appear to be healthy, well nourished or developing normally between episodes; (3) crying that does not fit the common pattern found in infantile colic; (4) excessive crying in the first week of life; (5) excessive crying beyond 4 months of age; and (6) crying in infants with fever. Each of these categories of presentation may indicate a serious, medical cause and should be evaluated by a physician experienced in assessing infants.

Colic

Colic is such a well-recognized cause of recurrent episodes of excessive crying that it is often over-diagnosed or misdiagnosed. The physician who evaluates a young infant for the first episode of excessive crying must be careful not to diagnose colic too quickly, since many medical conditions may resemble colic in the early stages. These conditions include: infections (such as ear infections, urinary tract infections, viral illnesses and mouth sores); hidden trauma (such as scratches to the eye or a foreign object in the eye or throat, insect bites, or broken bones or head injury from child abuse); gastrointestinal diseases (such as esophageal reflux disease or constipation); abnormalities of heart rate or function; neurological disorders (like hydrocephalus); and rare but serious metabolic disorders. Colic should not be diagnosed unless and until the following specific criteria are met (Poole and Doerck 1993):
- Recurrent crying spells that last more than 3 hours per day for at least 3 days a week
- Crying begins in the first three weeks of life
- The infant is developmentally normal and appears healthy and well nourished when not crying
- Crying periods occur at predictable times of day
- Crying is difficult to console by usual parental means.

From a medical standpoint, it often takes several days or nights of crying before the pattern of colic is recognized and the diagnosis can be made. Parents often require the reassurance associated with a physician's assessment, including a thorough physical examination, in order to feel comfortable with the diagnosis.

Management is difficult since there is no immediate cure, but only palliative treatment; and parents often require more special handling than the infants. Several techniques can be attempted to reduce crying in the infant. These include reducing overstimulation during those times when crying is anticipated, by putting the infant in a quiet, darkened room, perhaps with monotonous sounds and minimal handling. Rocking, walking, car rides, cuddling, swaddling and pacifiers may all reduce crying, as may keeping a predictable schedule with night-time sleeping (Poole and Doerk 1993). Although several medical interventions, including sedatives, antacids, anti-gas medications and antispasmodics, and changes in formula or maternal diet have been tried in the past, none has been shown to be effective, and some (like sedatives) are felt to be dangerous. These are therefore not recommended unless being used for a specific diagnosis. For the parents, effective counseling should: (1) emphasize the overall good health of the infant; (2) acknowledge the difficulty and stress involved in caring for such an infant; (3) reassure the parents that the colic will be self-limited; (4) identify and offer help for parental stresses that may lead to anxiety and exacerbation of colic; (5) encourage time away from the infant for the parent; and (6) reassure the parent that crying is not harmful to the infant.

Idiopathic crying
Another interesting phenomenon is referred to as idiopathic crying of infancy. It is a single, self-limited episode of excessive, prolonged crying for which the cause is not recognized. Typically the infant cries for one to three hours then suddenly, inexplicably stops crying and appears completely well. Much to the embarrassment of the parents, the improved status often develops after the parents and the infant have arrived at the emergency department. A brief period of observation in the emergency department is usually required to be certain that the crying was not due to a serious, intermittent medical condition. For example, intussusception is a condition in infants in which there is intermittent obstruction of the intestines early in the course of the illness. This can produce intermittent periods of crying with intervals in which the infant looks normal. Eventually the obstruction and crying become persistent and the illness life-threatening.

Infants with a self-limited episode of idiopathic crying probably have a self-limited, innocent source of pain that is not recognizable by the caretakers. However, very little is known about the etiologies and further research is needed.

The medical evaluation of the infant with excessive crying
Medical conditions that may manifest as excessive crying in infants are extremely varied, since crying is the primary pathway by which infants can express all pain or discomfort. The evaluation of a crying infant is challenging, since the infant usually does not manifest clues to help localize pain or the source of distress. It is only recently that the full breadth of potential diagnoses in infants with excessive prolonged crying has been established. In

TABLE 6.1

Diagnoses in 56 infants presenting to the Denver Children's Hospital emergency department with an episode of unexplained, excessive crying*

Diagnosis	No. with diagnosis
Idiopathic	10
Infectious	
Otitis media**	10
Viral illness with anorexia (poor oral intake), dehydration**	2
Urinary tract infection**	1
Mild prodrome of gastroenteritis	1
Herpangina (mouth sores)**	1
Herpes stomatitis (mouth sores)**	1
Trauma	
Corneal abrasion (scratch on the surface of the eye)**	3
Foreign body in eye**	1
Foreign body in oropharynx (back of throat)**	1
Tibial fracture (from child abuse)**	1
Clavicular fracture (accidental)**	1
Brown recluse spider bite**	1
Hair tourniquet syndrome (hair wrapped tightly around toe)	1
Gastrointestinal	
Constipation	3
Intussusception (a ballooning of one part of the intestine into another)**	1
Gastroesophogeal reflux (acid entering the esophogus from the stomach)**	1
Central nervous system	
Subdural hematoma (bleeding around the brain from child abuse)**	1
Encephalitis (viral infection of the brain)**	1
Pseudotumor cerebri (unexplained elevation of pressure in the fluid surrounding the brain)**	1
Drug reaction/overdose	
DTP reaction (from diptheria/tetanus/pertussis vaccine)	1
Inadvertant pseudoephedrine (cold medication) overdose	1
Behavioral	
Night terrors	1
Overstimulation	1
Cardiovascular	
Supraventricular tachycardia (very rapid heart rate)**	2
Metabolic	
Glutaric aciduria type 1 (a chemical derangement that may lead to brain damage)**	1
Total	56

*Adapted by permission from Poole (1991).
**Indicates conditions considered serious.

the only systematic study to date of these infants (Poole 1991), the final diagnoses involved an interesting array of conditions involving almost every organ system and ranging in severity from life-threatening to innocent conditions (Table 6.1). Figure 6.1 shows a suggested medical algorithm for the evaluation of the infant with excessive crying (Poole 1996).

INFANT WITH ACUTE EXCESSIVE CRYING

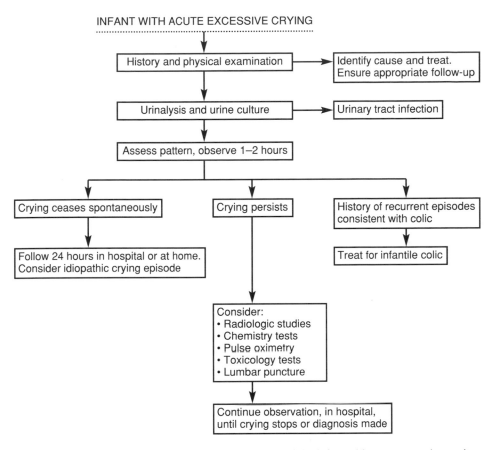

Fig. 6.1. Suggested algorithm for the medical evaluation of the infant with acute excessive crying. (Adapted by permission from Poole 1996).

It is important to remember that the infants in the above-cited study were evaluated in the emergency department of a large children's hospital. Many had been referred because crying was especially excessive. The parents or primary care providers may have felt that the pattern, duration or intensity of the crying made the diagnosis of idiopathic crying or colic less likely and that there was an increased probability of underlying pathology. For this reason, the proportion of infants with serious illness or injury (32 of 56 in the study by Poole 1991) is likely to be greater in this study than in the general population. The incidence of serious problems presenting to an emergency department will also be higher than in a primary provider's office. Nevertheless, the approach to history taking, physical examination and further diagnostic evaluation remains the same in all settings.

The history should seek to establish the duration and pattern of crying as well as any factors that may be contributing to it. An acute episode that lasts for several hours suggests a persistently painful acute medical condition or trauma. A gradual onset may indicate a metabolic, neurologic or endocrine cause, or perhaps a chronic illness. Infants with metabolic or neurologic disease may present with either persistent or intermittent excessive crying, but there are often associated clues to these diagnoses, such as developmental delay, poor growth, vomiting or changes in level of consciousness. Many children with these disorders will also have a positive family history for neurologic or metabolic disease (Fishman 1994). Infants with these disorders often have an abnormal, high-pitched cry that can provide an important clue. Despite these apparent associations of 'type' of crying with categories of etiology, the characteristics of the cry are not often reliably predictive of a specific type of etiology in any individual case.

The presence of fever is an especially important historical factor, even if it is absent at the time of clinical evaluation. A history of fever at home, even if the parent only felt the baby to be warm, accurately predicts an infectious cause approximately 80 per cent of the time (Hooker 1996). If fever is documented by a health care professional, the infant's fussiness is likely to be due to infection and the source of fever must be sought (see below for details of the evaluation). Other diagnostic clues in the history might include upper respiratory symptoms, constipation, diarrhea, blood in the stool, medications, red or tearing eyes, and trauma. At least one-quarter of the time, however, the symptoms are true but unrelated to the cause of the crying. For example, when an infant with a runny nose and cough develops sudden, excessive crying, it might be expected that the crying resulted from an ear infection that developed in association with the congestion. However, in a recent case seen by us with this set of associated symptoms, the infant had a speck of dirt under an eyelid causing a painful corneal abrasion. Consequently, associated symptoms may commonly mislead the evaluator.

Social factors that might be appreciated during the interview can also be important to the diagnosis. Overstimulation of the infant can lead to excessive crying. This might occur on the first day in a new daycare setting or at a large family gathering. Disturbance of sleep and/or feeding pattern can produce increased crying. This can occur if there are multiple caretakers who keep the infant on different schedules. This is more likely to be the case in instances of shared custody or if members of the extended family alternately care for the infant. Excessive parental anxiety, as is common with new or young parents or parents who have experienced the death of an infant in the family, may contribute to excessive crying in the infant. Some observations during the interview might raise concerns of child abuse. Concern about abuse might be raised if a parent is under a high degree of stress or is angry at the infant or at an older child. Similarly, it may be a concern with parents who appear disengaged and distant from the infant. Two of the 56 infants reported in our study (Poole 1991) were crying from injuries resulting from abuse that were not apparent on initial physical examination. Interestingly, all infants in our study (or identified since our study) whose excessive crying had resulted from child abuse had begun crying while in the care of their father, a sibling or a babysitter—never with the mother.

Vital signs can give important diagnostic clues. Temperature might be the first clue to serious infection. Abnormal heart rate might indicate heart rhythm abnormalities. An excessive respiratory rate might be the only sign of respiratory infection in a young infant. Growth parameters (height, weight, head circumference) should be noted because abnormalities may indicate a chronic condition such as neurologic or metabolic disease, chronic infection or nutritional deficiency.

A traditional physical examination will miss some important causes of excessive crying. Therefore, an extended examination is required that incorporates several assessments not routinely performed. The infant should be completely undressed so that thorough examination of the entire skin surface can be performed. Several of the diagnoses in Table 6.1 involved diagnostic findings that were readily apparent on close inspection of the infant, but were missed initially by parents or health care providers. A common phenomenon is the hair tourniquet syndrome in which a strand of hair (usually a caretaker's) becomes inadvertently and inexplicably wound around a young infant's toe, finger or penis, causing restriction of blood flow, swelling and pain (Vazquez Rueda *et al.* 1996). It is frequently missed when the infant is not completely undressed, including removal of the socks. Other evidence of trauma (scratches, bites, punctures, etc.) should also be sought.

Complete palpation (touching to identify tenderness or feeling for minor deformities caused by hidden fractures) can reveal serious problems that could easily be overlooked. Specifically, all bones, the fontanelle (soft spot) and the skull should be palpated. A 4-month-old girl recently evaluated in our institution for excessive crying had been evaluated at another hospital for more common causes such as urinary tract infection and corneal abrasion (a scratch on the eye). When no apparent cause was found, she was discharged home with a diagnosis of colic. When crying persisted, the mother brought her to our hospital where palpation of the thigh revealed a subtle deformity and tenderness of the thigh. An X-ray revealed a fracture of the femur, a condition that is usually the result of child abuse in a patient this young. It was ultimately determined that the 10-year-old sister, acting as a babysitter, had accidentally dropped her two days earlier and had been afraid to tell anyone.

The eyes should be evaluated with inspection, fundoscopic examination (looking through the pupil at the retina with an ophthalmoscope), eversion of the eyelids, and fluorescein staining (application of a dye to the cornea looking for evidence of occult injury). One of the more commonly missed causes of excessive crying in the young infant is corneal abrasion (Harkness 1989). This is usually the result of the infant scratching the eye. Some other clues to this diagnosis include red, tearing eyes, eyelids that have spasm, and scratches elsewhere on the face which indicate that the infant has indeed been scratching near the eye. These additional clues, usually associated with corneal abrasion in older children, are usually not present in infants. Fundoscopic examination might reveal bleeding from the small vessels in the back of the eye. This may be the only clue to significant head injury from child abuse. When this finding is discovered, it is usually the result of the 'shaken baby' syndrome in which a caretaker shakes the infant violently. When present, these broken blood vessels are nearly always indicative of child abuse.

Examination of the ear drums for infection should be performed. Many infants with ear infections will not have fever (Niemela 1994). Irritability alone is often the only symptom in an illness with ear infection.

Auscultation of the heart and lungs must be performed. A heart murmur or a too rapid heart beat may indicate an abnormality that results in decreased oxygen levels in the blood, one of the most serious and sometimes subtle causes of fussiness. Wheezing or other abnormal auscultatory sounds in the lungs would suggest decreased oxygen levels as a cause of excessive crying for the same reason.

The abdominal examination is required to identify signs that might be present in constipation, intestinal obstruction or hernia. Anal inspection may reveal fissures that are painful small tears, which are often caused by constipation. Digital rectal examination for hard or impacted stool might also reveal constipation. The stool should be tested for blood that could indicate obstruction or infection.

A complete neurological examination with emphasis on development should be performed. If there is any question about the infant's development, a full developmental screening test should be done. Subtle signs of developmental delay may be associated with specific congenital syndromes, metabolic diseases, other abnormalities of brain development or muscle disease. If there is any question of such abnormalities, the infant should be referred to a specialist in pediatric neurology for further testing.

Even after a thorough initial history and physical examination, as many as one in three infants will still have no apparent cause for their excessive crying (Poole 1991). Each of these infants should have a urinalysis and urine culture. This includes infants with apparent true infantile colic by history, since urinary tract infection can present with periodic fussiness and no fever. It is unknown what proportion of these infants actually have a urinary tract infection, but one series reported four infants who presented with typical infantile colic and had urinary tract infection (Du 1976). Another study showed that, of infants under 8 months of age admitted to hospital with a diagnosis of urinary tract infection, only 63 per cent presented with fever. 'Irritability' was present in 55 per cent of the infants. Unfortunately, this study did not document the percentage of infants who presented with irritability alone (Ginsburg and McCracken 1982). At least one authority currently recommends urinalysis and urine culture in all infants in whom the diagnosis of colic is being entertained, even in 'classic' cases (Henretig 1993). Other than urinalysis and urine culture, common screening laboratory tests for all infants with excessive crying, such as a complete blood count and electrolytes, have not proven to be useful.

If the diagnosis is still not apparent, and if the crying continues in the office or emergency department, a short period of observation lasting at least one to two hours is recommended. Many infants will cease crying during this time and may be discharged home if adequate observation and follow-up are ensured. These infants may be given a preliminary diagnosis of idiopathic acute crying. However, continued contact with these infants is important because many serious causes may have intermittent symptoms. This is likely to be the case with urinary tract infections, intestinal obstruction from any cause, and intermittent fast heart rhythms.

During the observation period, subtle or intermittent clues may become manifest that lead to a diagnosis. An example of this is provided by a 4-month-old boy seen in our institution. He continued to cry excessively during the initial history and physical examination, which were unrevealing. He had no fever. Urinalysis was negative. During the second hour of observation, the infant began to have diarrhea, and a diagnosis of gastroenteritis (intestinal infection) was made. He presumably had had abdominal pain from the infection that had been present before any other signs or symptoms. Another infant with continuing excessive crying did not begin to exhibit other signs of intestinal obstruction until the second hour of observation.

Infants who continue to cry through the observation period are likely to have a serious cause. In our study, approximately 60 per cent of infants who cried excessively after a two-hour observation period had a serious condition. The tests that are likely to be most useful at this stage tend to be invasive, difficult and expensive, so they should be chosen with considerable care and based upon the clues derived from the observation. Computed tomography of the head or skeletal X-rays may diagnose trauma that was not apparent by history or physical examination. Imaging studies to detect a foreign body in the airway or esophagus can be considered. Because serious infection without fever may occur, especially in younger infants, a lumbar puncture looking for meningitis should be considered. Other selected blood tests might be used to evaluate the likelihood of occult infection, anemia, electrolyte imbalance, metabolic conditions or poisoning. Pulse oximetry might reveal a decreased oxygen level in the blood, often from cardiac causes that may not be apparent on physical examination. Other tests of the heart, such as electro- and echocardiography, may also be revealing.

The febrile infant

In the infant with excessive crying and fever, the symptom of fever takes precedence over the symptom of excessive crying. The clinician must give primary consideration to determining the cause of the fever, since infection is by far the most common cause of both fever and crying in these infants, and because the infection is often potentially life-threatening. The evaluation of the febrile, crying infant is different from that of the infant with excessive crying alone.

In the infant under 2 months of age with fever, most experts recommend obtaining: (1) blood for complete blood count and culture; (2) urine for urinalysis and culture; and (3) cerebrospinal fluid (by lumbar puncture) for cell counts, protein and glucose concentrations, gram stain and culture. If the infant has any symptoms of respiratory disease, such as cough, runny nose or fast breathing, a chest radiograph should be done as well. There is some controversy in the literature about the exact age cut-off (6 weeks vs 8 weeks) below which this complete evaluation is required. However, the evaluation should be done regardless of clinical appearance of the infant, because even the expert clinician cannot accurately distinguish infants with severe infection from those with minor infection in this youngest age group.

In febrile infants over 2 months of age, clinical judgment is more reliable and should guide the laboratory evaluation. The first decision for the clinician is to determine if the infant appears relatively 'well' or significantly ill ('toxic'). This judgment is made by experienced clinicians while observing the infant, and is based on characteristics of the infant such as color, muscle tone, alertness, whether the infant makes eye contact with the parent, and degree of irritability. Excessive crying would be one clue to a 'toxic' infant, and should alert the clinician to the possibility of more serious infection. If an infant appears 'toxic', then a complete evaluation as described above for the infant under 2 months of age is warranted. If an infant appears relatively well, and a clear source of fever (such as viral upper respiratory infection or ear infection) is found by history and physical examination, no further laboratory evaluation is necessary. Debate in the literature exists, however, when an infant between the ages of 2 months and 2 years appears well, but no source of fever can be found on physical examination. Most experts agree that a urinalysis and urine culture (on a specimen obtained by catheterization) should be done on all infants who have fever with no source apparent on examination. Some also recommend a complete blood count and blood culture on these infants because of the risk of 'occult bacteremia', defined as bacteria infecting the bloodstream that causes fever without other symptoms. The decision regarding whether to do blood work in these infants is made by the clinician based on degree of illness ('toxicity').

On rare occasions, the excessive crying is the result of a condition that is separate and distinct from the cause of the fever. For example, a child with fever from pneumonia may be more irritable and difficult to care for, and therefore more likely to be mistreated by a caretaker. We have seen several cases in which the fever was the result of an infection and the excessive crying the result of nonaccidental trauma (child abuse).

Treatment
The treatment of colic and of idiopathic crying episodes has been described above. The treatment of the wide variety of medical conditions capable of causing excessive crying should be tailored to the diagnosis; its description is beyond the objectives of this chapter. There are several instances (perhaps 10 per cent of cases) in which there are multiple causes for the crying. When a single diagnosis is presumed rather than confirmed, care must be taken to observe the infant closely to confirm that treatment is definitely associated with reduced crying and irritability. In addition to responding to the specific cause of the crying, providers must remember to comfort the infant and parents. If a diagnosis is made that implicates pain in the infant, medication for pain should be considered for the infant.

Future research
Additional research is needed to better understand the predictors of serious causes of excessive crying episodes. For example, how useful are consolability or the nature of the crying (intermittent *vs* constant) in identifying specific causes or categories of causes? The relationship between characteristics of an infant's cry (intensity, pitch, volume, duration) and medical causes has not to our knowledge been thoroughly studied. A better understanding of the relationship between characteristics of the crying and severity of the etiology of the crying could be used to guide the pace and extent of the medical evaluation. Idiopathic excessive crying also needs further elucidation. We suspect that these infants include a very heterogeneous group with transient, innocent conditions that cause pain. Most clinical medical research in the next five years will focus on balancing cost-efficient evaluation and treatment with good clinical outcome. In the evaluation of the infant with excessive crying, attention will have to be paid to using historical, physical examination and visible clues during the observation period to identify only those infants who truly need invasive testing for serious disease. There is tremendous potential for collaborative research between medical

researchers and those who conduct developmental or psychological research in the area of excessive crying.

Conclusion

Excessive or prolonged infant crying is a common problem that often requires evaluation by the pediatrician, family practitioner or emergency physician. While infantile colic or transient, benign idiopathic, excessive crying may be the final diagnosis, the practitioner must be aware that many serious medical conditions may present with crying. Therefore, a thorough and systematic history and extensive physical examination, with emphasis on the signs and symptoms of potentially serious causes, must be pursued. For all infants in whom a diagnosis is not made by history and physical examination, urine should be obtained for analysis and culture. When the cause of the crying remains unclear, a period of close observation is needed. Perhaps as many as one-third of infants will require laboratory and/or radiologic evaluation. Because the list of potential diagnoses includes so many serious conditions, no persistently crying infant should be discharged home without a satisfactory diagnosis and appropriate treatment plan.

REFERENCES

Du, J.N.H. (1976) 'Colic as the sole symptom of urinary tract infection in infants.' *Canadian Medical Association Journal*, **115**, 334–339.
Fishman, M.A. (1994) 'Developmental defects.' *In:* Oski, F.A. (Ed.) *Principles and Practice of Pediatrics. 2nd Edn.* Philadelphia: J.B. Lippincott, pp. 2015–2019.
Ginsburg, C.M., McCracken, G.H. (1982) 'Urinary tract infection in young infants.' *Pediatrics*, **69**, 409–412.
Harkness M.J. (1989) 'Corneal abrasion in infancy as a cause of inconsolable crying.' *Pediatric Emergency Care*, **5**, 242–244.
Henretig, F.M. (1993) 'Crying and colic in early infancy.' *In:* Fleisher G.R., Ludwig, S. (Eds.) *Textbook of Pediatric Emergency Medicine. 3rd Edn.* Baltimore: Williams & Wilkins, pp. 144–146.
Hooker, E.A., Smith, S.W., Miles, T., King, L. (1996) 'Subjective assessment of fever by parents: Comparison with measurement by noncontact tympanic thermometer and calibrated rectal glass mercury thermometer.' *Annals of Emergency Medicine*, **28**, 313–317.
Niemela, M., Uhari, M., Jounio-Ervasti, K., Luotonen, J., Alho, O.P., Vierimaa, F. (1994) 'Lack of specific symptomatology in children with acute otitis media.' *Pediatric Infectious Disease Journal*, **13**, 765–768.
Poole, S. (1991) 'The infant with acute, unexplained, excessive crying.' *Pediatrics*, **88**, 450–455.
—— (1996) 'Acute or excessive crying in infants.' *In:* Berman, S. (Ed.) *Pediatric Decision Making.* St. Louis: Mosby–Year Book, pp. 202–205.
—— Doerck M. (1993) 'Infantile colic.' *In:* Eichenwald, H., Stroder, J. (Eds.) *Pediatric Therapy. 3rd Edn.* St. Louis: Mosby–Year Book, pp. 164–166.
Vazquez Rueda, R.F., Nuñez Nuñez, R., Gomez Meleno, P., Blesa Sanchez, E. (1996) '[The hair-thread tourniquet syndrome of the toes and penis.]' *Anales Españoles de Pediatria*, **44**, 17–20. *(Spanish.)*

SUGGESTED READING

Brazelton T.B. (1962) 'Crying in infancy.' *Pediatrics*, **29**, 579–588.
Heine, R.G., Jaquiery A. (1995) 'Role of gastroesophageal reflux in infant irritability.' *Archives of Disease in Childhood*, **3**, 121–125.
Schmitt, B.D. (1985) 'Diagnostic criteria of colic.' *Clinics in Perinatology*, **12**, 441–451.
St James-Roberts, I. (1991) 'Persistent infant crying.' *Archives of Disease in Childhood*, **66**, 653–655.

7

CRYING IN THE CHILD WITH A DISABILITY: THE SPECIAL CHALLENGE OF CRYING AS A SIGNAL

James A. Blackman

Crying is the earliest and most powerful form of communication. An infant's cry provides information about its biological status. Under usual circumstances, crying evolves into a social signaling system that guides parenting behavior. The function of a cry is to elicit responses from the environment that will meet the infant's physiological needs (Lester 1984). However, this function may go awry in an infant with a disability. The cry may be deviant or misinterpreted, leading to faulty communication and difficulties in parenting such a child.

Over the past 40 years, much has been learned about the characteristics of crying and its meaning for caregivers. Findings have included the following: crying is not a simple signal, but is graded (Wasz-Höckert *et al.* 1968, Wolff 1969); crying is consistently evaluated as undesirable (Harris 1979); experience plays a role in the responses that crying elicits from caregivers (Wasz-Höckert *et al.* 1964); the context of crying is involved in mothers' interpretation of it (Muller *et al.* 1974, Carey 1984); and soothing techniques, such as rocking, are effective in reducing crying (Elliott *et al.* 1988). All these factors are germane to interpreting crying correctly, especially in infants with developmental disabilities or chronic health problems, and to responding effectively. The objective of this chapter is to review our understanding regarding crying in very young children with disabilities due to neurological injury or chronic health impairments, and to discuss what practical implications these observations and related clinical research might have for clinicians.

Defining developmental disabilities

A developmental disability is, according to the World Health Organization (WHO 1980), any restriction or lack of ability to perform an activity within the range considered normal. Disability results from a physical, mental or emotional impairment that interferes with communication, mobility or social interaction or impedes the attainment of age-appropriate developmental milestones. The causes of developmental disabilities are numerous and may be preconceptual (gene defects), periconceptual (chromosome defects), embryonic (organ malformation), fetal (organ system injury or malfunction), perinatal (birth trauma), or post-natal (illness or accident). A significant impairment during gestation through the first two years of life is considered especially significant in that opportunity for development not realized during this time may result in permanent disability.

Most developmental disabilities result from a malformation of or injury to the brain. The problem may be global, as it usually is with birth asphyxia in which reduced delivery of oxygen or critical nutrients to the entire brain often leads to motor, sensory and cognitive dysfunction. Thus, sequelae might include cerebral palsy, visual or auditory compromise, or mental retardation. Alternatively, the problem may be selective with dysfunction limited to the motor or speech areas. The degree of involvement (which may range from mild to severe) and the anatomic location of the abnormality will greatly influence the infant's success in communicating through crying.

In addition to the primary disability, secondary disability or related health problems are common. An infant with cerebral palsy, for example, may develop soft tissue contractures from persistently high muscle tone. The contractures may lead to reduced mobility, hip dislocations, and pain. Recurrent otitis media, esophageal reflux, feeding problems with poor nutrition, and constipation are some of the other problems associated with cerebral palsy that result in chronic discomfort or pain. Poor nutrition may make an infant listless and unresponsive. Any of these factors in various combinations might affect the quantity or quality of crying.

A difficult case

The following case history illustrates the biological and social implications of crying in infants with, or at risk for, disabilities, and the challenges crying poses for parents, professionals and researchers.

CASE REPORT

Before his birth, A's parents were both in work, but his mother, who was 34, had planned to take three months off to stay home with him. This was their first child and they had spent a happy nine months preparing for him. Expectations were high, although the mother had had a feeling that something would go wrong. She was right.

A's fetal experience was unremarkable until the time of delivery. Then, several severe and prolonged bouts of fetal distress forewarned a difficult transition to extrauterine life. He was covered with thick meconium at birth and required mechanical ventilation with supplemental oxygen for five days. Grand mal seizures occurred within the first six hours of life and were difficult to control for several days. Since his suck was poor following extubation, he required nasogastric tube feeding for his first month of life. He was finally discharged from the hospital after six weeks.

A's mother had decided to go back to work while he was in the hospital in order to save her maternity leave for when he came home. She and her husband tried to visit as often as possible but the visits were quite unrewarding. A would either sleep or fuss most of the time. When they held him, he stiffened and screamed a high pitched cry. In response they would successively rock him, put a pacifier in his mouth, or change his diaper. Sometimes these measures calmed him; oftentimes they did not. Usually the parents would hand Andrew back to the nurses with a profound sense of failure or lay him back in his crib.

The nurses implied by their looks (or so the parents felt) that A's signals were not that difficult to read if only the parents were better attuned. He had a hunger cry, a pain cry and a dirty diaper cry just like the other infants in the nursery. To the parents, however, all the cries sounded alike (shrill), making them feel exasperated. How would they manage when the professionals were not around to guide them? They were extremely anxious and frightened.

The tension, anxiety and guilt experienced by those parents, and others like them, make the need for a better understanding of cry characteristics of developmentally disabled infants and the responses of their caretakers poignantly clear.

Review of research on cry sounds in healthy and sick infants

The first objective study of infant vocalization using sound recordings appeared over 90 years ago (Flatau and Gutzman 1906). After locating the basic pitch of normal neonates' crying at middle A (440 Hz), the investigators observed that the cry-pitch of one abnormal infant was one octave higher. There was a resurgence of interest in acoustic analysis of crying, especially among infants with neurological problems, in the 1950s and '60s. During this period, most studies of infant crying utilized the sound spectrogram. This technique was slow and required visual inspection of the output for interpretation (see Chapter 9).

The first extensive work on cry characteristics in children with disabilities, especially central nervous systems lesions, was conducted in Scandinavia (summarized by Wasz-Höckert et al. 1985) several decades ago as acoustic analysis techniques became more refined. Previous studies in the United States had shown that infants with diffuse brain damage require greater stimulation to produce a standard one minute crying response than do normal infants (Karelitz and Fisichelli 1962) and that the mean latency between pain stimulation and onset of crying is 1.6 s for normal and 2.6 s for abnormal infants (Fisichelli and Karelitz 1963). Fisichelli et al. (1966) also reported that infants with Down syndrome (Fig. 7.1) show significantly shorter, less active, and less differentiated cry outbursts than normal infants. The Scandinavian group reported that the cries of infants with cri-du-chat syndrome have a fundamental tone (pitch) significantly elevated above 500 Hz (Vuorenkoski et al. 1966). Michelson (1971) analyzed the pain-induced cries of asphyxiated and healthy term-born infants. She found that the pitch was higher and the cry longer in asphyxiated than in normal infants. The more severely asphyxiated the infant, the more marked the differences. Not surprisingly, it was found that the abnormal cries of babies with Down syndrome, cri-du-chat syndrome and birth asphyxia are perceived as more aversive than those of normal infants, possibly placing them at higher risk of tense infant–environmental interaction (Sagi 1982).

A study by Ostwald et al. (1968) was designed to determine whether two acoustic features—duration and pitch—of the expiratory cry sound would show any relationship to diagnostic ratings based on clinical evaluation of infants. It involved sonographic analyses of 356 expiratory cry utterances derived from 13 infants classified as normal, impaired or abnormal based on clinical data, behavioral development and neurological status. Duration measurements showed no consistent differences among the three groups. However, pitch measurements (as determined by the degree of closure of the vocal cords) showed a marked increase of the fundamental tone only among infants rated as impaired or abnormal. The authors postulated that this finding reflected a disorganization of innate adaptive mechanisms that ensure that infants can elicit appropriate social responses from their environment.

Acoustic analysis of cry sounds has undergone dramatic changes in the last 35 years, including the introduction of more than a hundred acoustic measures, largely focused on neonates with various medical problems or at risk for developmental delays. Golub and Corwin (1985) developed an automatic, computer-based signal-processing system based

108

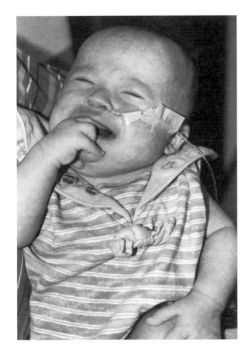

Fig. 7.1. Four-month-old girl with Down syndrome and persistent feeding problems. Sagi (1982) reported that the cries of infants with Down syndrome may be viewed as aversive. This infant was quite passive, crying infrequently and rather quietly.

on the physioacoustic model of cry. In this model, three peripheral sources determine the cry sound: the lower vocal tract (the subglottic system), the larynx, and the upper vocal tract (the supraglottal system). The original use of this system was to correlate medical abnormalities in the infant with the physical characteristics of the infant's cry.

The bulk of cry *perception* research has used as a stimulus the acoustic cry signal by itself. The result has been that work on crying has focused on the specific dimensions in the cry signal that yield information about the infant to the caregiver. Green *et al.* (1995) expanded the field by showing that visual–contextual as well as developmental factors affect adults' perceptions of infant sounds. When auditory and visual information conflicted (that is, when a videotaped non-cry face was paired with a cry sound or a cry face was paired with a non-cry sound), adults' judgments of whether the sound was a cry, a fuss or a laugh vocalization were often erroneous. This work raises an interesting research question about babies who cry but make no sounds, as occurs when infants are intubated or have tracheostomies (Fig. 7.2). Since they provide only visual cues of distress, how accurately are their 'soundless' cry signals interpreted? Green *et al.* (1995) also found that the ability to recognize cry sounds generally improves with the age of the infant, probably reflecting shaping by external responses to various cry types and learned behavior on the part of caretakers.

While fundamental frequency and other acoustic features (such as duration, sound quality and peak frequency) in cry perception are important (Gustafson and Green 1989), an alternative to the notion of cry types is the concept that cries are graded signals. Zeskind

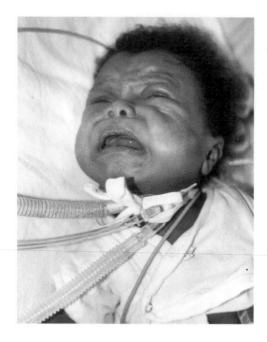

Fig. 7.2. This 8-month-old infant was hospitalized from birth with severe cardiac and pulmonary problems necessitating a tracheostomy and mechanical ventilatory support. He is obviously crying but there is no vocalization.

et al. (1985) investigated this concept by comparing adult ratings of initial, middle and final segments of pain and hunger cries. They found that different segments of cries resulting from the same stimulus provided different messages that communicated the level of infant arousal. That is, cry sounds reflect a general level of infant arousal rather than information about the specific stimulus that caused the crying. Perhaps there are fewer cry 'types' (hunger, startle, pain, anger, birth, pleasure) than generally thought. Furthermore, it is not clear that specific cries elicit specific caregiving responses. Gustafson and Harris (1990) found that the specific cause of crying (hunger or pain) was associated with few differences in caregiving behavior. Thus, it appears that cry sounds may communicate more accurate information about the general distress level of the infant than about specific causes. The caregiver attributes meaning to the crying by virtue of the context in which a particular level of arousal frequently occurs (*e.g.* uncomfortable stretching exercises for spastic muscles) rather than the acoustic characteristics of the sounds themselves.

Fuller *et al.* (1994) suggested that the cries of irritable infants are intrinsically distinct from those of non-fussy babies. They found that the cries of irritable infants were higher in jitter (difference in the durations of pitch cycles), shimmer (differences in the amplitudes of contiguous pitch cycles), proportion of noise, and tenseness than were the cries of control infants, indicating that infant irritability may be more than just excessive crying. Acoustic analysis of the cries of irritable infants was interpreted as revealing an increase in stress arousal that could support the concept of a state regulation disorder in these infants.

The association between excessive crying in infants and what has clinically come to be known as regulatory disorders has been examined by Maldonado-Duran and Sauceda-Garcia (1996). They argue that the essence of a regulatory disorder is that it is a distinct

110

maladaptive or dysfunctional behavioral pattern, together with clear difficulties in sensory reactivity, information processing, motor organization and attention control. Infants with this disorder may have difficulty remaining calm and, therefore, are fussy or irritable most of the time. They may be hypersensitive to certain types of sensory input, such as touch or sound. Preterm birth, *in utero* cocaine exposure and brain injury have been associated with regulatory disorder (Legido 1998).

The interactive nature of crying and caregiving

Most parents feel that they quickly learn to distinguish pain from hunger and fussing cries. Decades ago Wasz-Höckert *et al.* (1964) postulated that four basic cry types—birth, hunger, pain and pleasure—could be identified auditorily. Cries appeared best differentiated by adults who had had previous experience with infant cries, such as nurses on the pediatric wards and midwives. Training increased the ability to recognize different kinds of cries

Even a normal infant may find it difficult to learn to communicate effectively through crying. Drummond *et al.* (1993) described new mothers' assessments of their normal infants' cry behavior over a 16 month period. First time mothers were described as beginning with a reactive approach to their infant's cry signal of unknown meaning. They then moved through a utilitarian soothing approach and then to an implicitly understood, but nonetheless individualized, soothing response to the crying. Experienced mothers constantly sought to anticipate their infants' needs through acquainting themselves with their infants' individual characteristics. As the infant developed, the relation between crying and soothing expanded appropriately to include social–psychological development. The maternal responses to infant crying exemplified in this study are consistent with attachment theory, whereby signaling behaviors (including crying) in the infant promote proximity to the caregiver (Bowlby 1969).

Holaday (1982) has postulated that there are three distinct stages in the development of maternal interaction patterns in response to the cries. These stages are based on concepts derived from the Johnson Behavioral Systems Model (Holaday 1996) and observations and interviews of six pairs of mothers with chronically ill infants over three months beginning the week the infant reached 4 months of age. The illnesses these infants suffered included a variety of cardiac, pulmonary and physical abnormalities. According to Holaday, ill infants do not always provide clear cry signals. Thus, mothers are not always dealing with a distinctly identifiable cry, which might or might not be a pain cry.

Immediately after birth when these babies are in intensive care, Holaday found that mothers in Stage I will not or cannot respond to their infant's cry. Mothers feel highly frightened and intimidated, making contact limited. When the infant cries, the mother gives her/him back to the nurses. The parents described in the case study (p. 107) were at this first stage when their infant was discharged from the newborn intensive care unit.

In this first stage, mothers begin to develop simple, rigid, black-and-white rules for interpreting the type of cry. They see each cry as a sign of distress. There is no experience or conceptual basis available to them for generating other alternatives. The result is fast closure in the choice of intervention. Mothers seem almost intolerant of ambiguous situations and form quick judgments in such situations.

111

In Holaday's Stage II, mothers become less fixed in their interpretations of cries (usually pain) and are able to tolerate more ambiguity. Thus, they are able to generate alternative interpretations for the infant's cry. However, there is still inconsistency in the responses. Mothers with seriously ill infants first respond to crying by picking the infant up. If the infant does not quiet, the mother often responds with a barrage of interventions (talk to, change position, pat, bounce, rock, distract, offer bottle or pacifier) that show no consistent pattern.

Most mothers reach Stage III from two to six months after the infant's birth. During this stage more complex rules for comparing and relating alternative perspectives of the cry stimulus emerge. Mothers become more adept at discriminating among cry stimuli and can identify complex relationships between the infant's behavior and the cry. They also become more comfortable seeking more information before deciding on an intervention. They more easily strive to determine the reason for the infant's cry and attempt to understand the internal processes of the infant.

Different patterns of caretaking will have a marked impact on the child's ability to regain calm from a crying state. The importance of cry characteristics in eliciting caregiving responses is evident in Holaday's (1981) study in which she analyzed 388 cry bouts and maternal response episodes. She found that maternal response patterns to the crying of ill infants seemed to be determined by characteristics of the infant's cry rather than by specific infant characteristics (e.g. sex, ordinal position, degree of illness). She postulated that the different cry "may be part of biological systems designed to signal the mother that her infant needs special attention."

Since communication is an interactive process, the ability of the infant to send, and of the caretaker to receive and interpret, acoustic signals successfully will affect the early parent/child relationship. Some infants are better communicators than others, i.e. the acoustic qualities of their cries (and other sounds) are better defined. For other infants, these features are less clear. Parents, for their part, face the challenge of interpreting the meaning of their infant's crying and then responding appropriately. They vary in their ability to accomplish these tasks.

Lester et al. (1995) used acoustic analysis of the cries of 1-month-olds (both term and preterm) and mothers' perceptions of these cries to divide subjects into groups of 'matches' and 'mismatches' between infant cry characteristics and their mothers' perceptions of those cries. Approximately half of the mothers were 'matched' with their infants; that is, they had negative perceptions of infants with high-pitched cries or less negative perceptions of infants with lower-pitched cries. It is widely believed that both infant characteristics and parental caretaking behavior determine the developmental outcome of children. This seemed to be illustrated by the results in this study. Infants from the 'matched' groups, in which cries were correctly perceived as being high- or low-pitched, later scored higher on measures of language and cognitive performance than infants in the non-matched groups. Thus, a particular advantage was noted for infants in the matched group in which mothers accurately perceived higher-pitched cries. Thus, importantly for the issues discussed in this chapter, perhaps this means that these mothers were especially attuned to their infants, leading to more frequent and positive interactions.

However, the fact that half of the mothers in that study did not correctly perceive the sound qualities of their infants (including, for example, mothers who rated low-pitched [normal] cries negatively) may mean that it is not always easy for adults to interpret cries. It could also mean that interpretation of cries depends as much on the emotional state, self-esteem and social conditions of the perceiver as on the characteristics of the cry itself. This was dramatically illustrated in the case of one impaired infant described in the Ostwald *et al.* (1968) study cited above. This infant had such a remarkable cry that the resident physician was afraid the child was dying. In fact, however, the infant lived for another 4 months. At the time of death it was clear that the infant had been neglected. On one occasion when the child's screaming was being recorded his mother asked, "Isn't that the sound of a contented baby?" In this extreme example, it was determined that the mother had a history of severe mental illness.

Sending, receiving, interpreting and acting on cry signals is just one aspect of infant–parent interaction that can be understood in terms of the concept of 'goodness of fit'. According to Thomas and Chess (1977) working in the field of infant temperament, a good fit occurs when there is a match between characteristics of the child and characteristics of the parent, with positive developmental outcome the expected result. Mismatches lead to negative outcomes. Mothers who report that their infants cry more express irritation at the cry and a sense of failure (Michelsson *et al.* 1990). Also, mothers who report excessive crying also perceive a lack of positive reinforcement from their babies (Beebe *et al.* 1993). This potential disturbance in the child–parent relationship may have long-term consequences for the child's emotional development if not recognized and averted.

Parental emotional or experiential characteristics influence interaction with the infant (Fig. 7.3). Mothers and fathers who are depressed (due to lingering grief reactions), or stressed (due to recurring medical or developmental complications for their young child), or who were themselves the recipients of poor parenting may find it difficult to tolerate crying or to respond in a comforting manner. To the degree that mothers believe they are ineffective in managing infant crying, nonoptimal caregiving can arise that may result in negative consequences for the infant (Donovan and Leavitt 1992). First-time mothers are more aroused by the crying of difficult infants, and fathers express higher irritation with crying than mothers (Boukydis and Burgess 1982). Infant crying makes many fathers feel anxious and impotent (Wilkie and Ames 1986). The crying of an infant seems to be greatly affected by the anxiety and the tense atmosphere in the family (Makoi 1990). Interestingly, adolescent mothers rate the high-pitched cries of intrauterine growth retarded infants as more positive than adult mothers (Lester *et al.* 1989).

Finally, Frodi and Senchak (1990) examined responses to cries of atypical infants. Students and mothers were exposed to one of six types of infant cries coming from an adjacent room while their behavior and affective responses were observed. The cries were the pain cries of two normal newborns, one infant with cri-du-chat syndrome, one with Down syndrome, one asphyxiated infant with brain damage and one asphyxiated infant without brain damage. The results indicated that the six cries differentially affected the subjects' affective, self-reported and behavioral responses, as well as their tendency to report not hearing the cry. The highest-pitched cries (those of the asphyxiated infants) elicited more negative

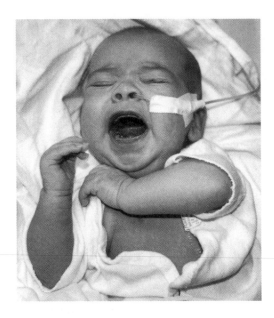

Fig. 7.3. At 2 months of age, this infant with cystic fibrosis and a colostomy required nasogastric tube feeding for poor weight gain. Her mother was 14, diagnosed with depression.

responses from listeners than the lowest-pitched cries (those of infants with Down syndrome or who were normal).

Behavior and disabilities

Behavior characteristics among children with disabilities are too varied to make generalizations that necessarily apply to an individual child. To understand how this contributes to the challenge that this presents to the parents, it is important to appreciate how a particular behavior may be altered or how a behavioral manifestation of a certain emotion may be altered due to a physical, sensory or cognitive impairment.

It has been reported that, although stereotypic personality traits do not inevitably accompany disabilities, certain characteristics such as irritability or low frustration tolerance may be unpleasantly exaggerated in children with disabilities (McDermott and Akina 1972). In a study of 29 boys who suffered birth asphyxia, Ucko (1965) found them to be more frequently constipated, more disturbed in their sleep, and more sensitive to noise than were control subjects. Furthermore, the same boys had more difficulties in adjusting to changes in routine and were rated by caretakers as 'very difficult' more often than were controls. Prechtl (1963) described two types of babies with minimal brain damage: hypoactive, apathetic babies who cry little, and excitable babies who overreact to mild stimulation and cry readily. In a study of 2-year-old physically disabled children, Wasserman *et al.* (1985) found them less likely to initiate social interaction, more distractible and passive, and less compliant than either term or preterm non-disabled toddlers.

All children manifest behavior problems, but children with disabilities may manifest them in a quantitatively or qualitatively different manner. Children with specific syndromes commonly have distinct personality types or behaviors. Infants with Down syndrome, for example, tend be passive, while children with Williams syndrome are excessively outgoing. Blackman (1989) asked the parents of 72 developmentally delayed (with a variety of diagnoses) and 70 normal children under 3 years of age to complete a questionnaire regarding the occurrence of common behavior problems (including 'crying often and easily'), their degree of concern about these and their understanding of their children's developmental status. Although the average number of reported problems was similar for both groups, the parents of the developmentally delayed group reported significantly more problems during the first year of life and that they lasted longer. In addition, those who specifically recognized intellectual or language delays in their children reported a comparatively greater number of problems. All of these parents of developmentally delayed children tended to have greater concern about these problems than did parents of normal children.

While Blackman's study included a broad array of common behavior problems in addition to 'crying often and easily', the other problems (*e.g.* constipation, irritability, stiffness and temper tantrums) are often associated with, or may even cause, crying. The findings illustrate how complex is the interaction between biological factors in infants with developmental problems (*e.g.* constipation and stiffness) and cognitive/emotional factors in the parent (*e.g.* greater concern about common behavior problems). Crying is likely to be an important link between these factors. These problems may heighten anxiety during a period when parents are coming to recognize developmental differences between their child and others.

Confusing signals from infants with disabilities

As summarized in Figure 7.4, a number of factors make it more challenging to read and interpret behaviors of young children with disabilities. Through personal experience, reading or advice from friends and family, parents expect certain behaviors at prescribed ages. Zero to 3-month-olds have colic, 9- to 12-month-olds first manifest stranger anxiety, and 1- to 2-year-olds display temper tantrums. Developmental delay or physical disability can confuse parents. An infant with spina bifida may scream with colic, but parents wonder whether there is malfunction in the ventriculo-peritoneal shunt used to treat the infant's abnormal physiological system. Similarly, a developmentally delayed 2-year-old may display the crying behavior more typical of a 1-year-old.

A child with a cognitive or motor disability may give unclear or atypical signals. Workers at the University of Virginia have adapted the Ainsworth and Wittig (1969) 'strange situation' to evaluate attachment in young children with motor impairments (R.S. Marvin *et al.* 1995, unpublished). In this testing procedure, an appropriately attached, motorically able toddler will physically reunite with a parent after a brief separation by moving to the parent and seeking comfort. Since a young child with cerebral palsy cannot independently walk or crawl to the parent, the security of attachment was assessed in other ways, such as cessation of crying, eye fixation or reaching hand gestures. The caregiver must learn to read these altered distress signals and go to the child for comfort-giving since the child cannot come to her/him.

Behavioral signals may be completely misread or misinterpreted. One example of such confusion involves car seats. Parents of a 3-year-old with spasticity may be confronted with

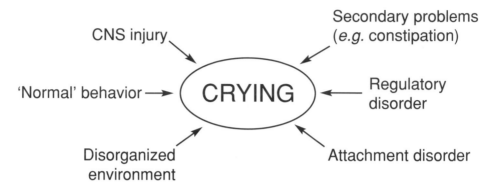

Fig. 7.4. Factors affecting crying and its interpretation in infants with disabilities.

crying and stiffening when the child is placed in an auto-restraint device. They interpret the behavior as stemming from reflexive hypertonia and discomfort from the disability. In reality, the child is exhibiting resistent behavior simply because s/he does not want to be restrained. The incorrect interpretation may result in the parent holding the child on the lap, which is unsafe, rather than insisting that the child not get her/his way.

Children with disabilities often have additional medical problems that can lead to true discomfort. Frequently recurring ear infections, reflux esophagitis, exaggerated startle responses, seizures and brittle bones with fractures will obviously lead to crying and irritability. When pain crying is frequent or persistent, parents may lose their ability to recognize the need for a doctor's evaluation.

Some infants with brain injury may be unusually quiet and placid. They are described as perfect babies, demanding little. They frequently have to be wakened for feedings. Other infants with brain injury or malformation are exceedingly irritable and inconsolable. They may have sensory regulatory disorders with reduced capacity to regulate behavioral state and autonomic function. Hypersensitivity to sensory stimulation can lead to frantic crying, color change and spitting up. The usual soothing and quieting response to rocking in normal infants often is not seen in these hypersensitive infants. An escalating cycle of crying, rocking and bouncing, more intense crying, and more vigorous rocking is commonplace.

Finally, cry quality may be affected by anatomic or motor variations. The cry of infants with congenital or acquired vocal tract abnormalities may be muted, hoarse or shrill. Trauma to the vocal cords from intubation often results in a weak, muffled cry. Children with chronic lung or neuromuscular disease may find it difficult to coordinate breathing, vocalizing and swallowing, resulting in an abnormal cry.

Early experiences can dramatically color parental interpretation and responses to crying. Sheeran *et al.* (1997) found that parents who are unable to resolve intellectually and emotionally the reality of their child's chronic medical diagnosis feel more stressed and less satisfied with their marital relationships. This has obvious implications for child–parent interactions. When parents are not functioning well, cry signals are likely to be ineffective, misinterpreted, ignored or even abhorred.

Children with developmental disabilities are at high risk for maltreatment (Goldson 1998). The altered quantity and quality of crying in some infants with disabilities may account for this observed phenomenon. Zeskind and Shingler (1991) concluded that crying is one part of an infant's behavioral repertoire that may contribute to the development of physically abusive parent–infant interactions.

Implications for clinical care

What researchers have taught us about crying in normal infants, as well as what we can learn from the less well studied problem of crying in infants with disabilities, should be helpful in guiding and supporting parents and other caregivers.

Crying in young children with disabilities is likely to be influenced by a variety of factors, some intrinsic to the child (brain injury, dependence on technology, chronic discomfort), others reflective of the caregivers or environment (parenting disorders, prolonged hospitalization, rotating attachment figures) (Fig. 7.4). Such children may cry more or less than usual, or have cries that are high-pitched and irritating. They may become aroused more quickly and calmed more slowly. Sensory impairments, anatomic anomalies of the vocal tract and muscle tone abnormalities interfere with cry production and its use as a signaling system. It is essential that the process of adjusting to these differences start early, before negative patterns of interaction develop and become established.

Both supportive professionals and researchers face significant challenges in sorting through these confounding variables, particularly with a view to identifying interventions that work. Nevertheless, careful assessment of the infant, caregiver, infant–caregiver interaction and environment may lead to clues that can be helpful. While there is still much to learn, the following examples of problems related to crying in infants with disabilities suggest possible solutions:

(1) Assume that behavior patterns, including crying, will be altered in quality and quantity in infants with central nervous system injuries (Bax 1985). These infants may be excessively irritable and difficult to console, with higher-pitched cries and prolonged episodes of crying. Their cries may be due to difficulties with internal state dysregulation, prolonged hospitalization in intensive care settings, or pain due to related medical problems such as esophageal reflux. Discuss this possibility ahead of time with parents so that they do not feel guilty or inept. Parents seem to adapt better if they recognize the abnormal cry characteristics of the infant.

(2) Assure parents that they can become more adept at reading cry signals even when the signals seem to be unclear, and that they can learn to assess the cause of crying and to use effective measures to calm their infant.

(3) A perfect fit may be unrealistic between an irritable infant and parents who may have difficulty resolving their emotional conflicts. Nevertheless, the interaction can become positive if parents are appropriately counseled and supported. Formal consultation with a psychotherapist may be indicated.

(4) Infants with neurological abnormalities are at higher risk for sensory regulatory disorders. DeGangi et al. (1991) have proposed three components of intervention for these disorders: (a) parent guidance that focuses on management of sleep, feeding and behaviors

in the home environment; (b) child-centered activity (*e.g.* reading a book, even to an infant) that fosters healthy parent–child interactions; and (c) sensory integrative therapy techniques that promote organized attention, adaptive behaviors and normalized responses to sensory experiences.

(5) Help parents understand their child's rate of developmental change. By focusing on developmental stage rather than chronological age, they are more likely to avoid a mismatch between their expectations and the child's actual performance.

(6) Provide a systematic step-by-step approach for evaluating irritability that includes the usual causes of crying, such as hunger, wetness or tiredness. Next, a variety of calming methods, typically employed with colicky infants, could be tried, recognizing that a reduction rather than an increase in tactile, vestibular, visual or auditory stimulation may be important for some infants who are especially sensitive. Finally, special instructions must be given for a child with certain medical conditions such as chronic constipation, esophageal reflux or shunted hydrocephalus.

(7) Help parents develop a sense of competency by successful progression through Holaday's (1982) stages of parental response to crying, briefly summarized earlier in this chapter. The goal is to broaden parental interpretation of their infant's crying and acceptable responses. For infants who require lengthy initial or recurrent hospitalization, this process should begin well before discharge.

Conclusions

The parents of infant A, described in the case study at the beginning of this chapter (p. 107), had neither the experience nor the typical signals from their infant to develop an understanding of his crying and its meaning. In Drummond's study (1993), as the mothers became more experienced, their understanding of the cry situation became more complete and their soothing was more effective.

A's parents could have been helped considerably by implementation of the clinical interventions suggested above. Long before A's discharge, a doctor should have explained the nature of the brain injury and what impact this might have on sensory and state regulation. A primary nurse who was with him for eight-hour shifts day after day should have shared the insights from her experience regarding what excited and what calmed him. Her silence reinforced their sense of incompetence. By sending the parents home unprepared, the medical staff initiated a probable cycle of unintelligible cry signals and ineffective responses, resulting in poor attachment, rejection, failure to thrive and suboptimal developmental progress.

Crying in the child with disabilities is as meaningful a signal as in the normal child. Professionals must understand the variations in crying of these children and how caregivers can most effectively interpret and react to this signal. Further research focused specifically on children with disabilities and their caregivers would aid these professionals immensely.

REFERENCES

Ainsworth, M.D.S., Wittig, B.A. (1969) 'Attachment and exploratory behaviour of one-year-olds in the strange situation.' *In:* Foss, B.M. (Ed.) *Determinants of Infant Behaviour, Vol. 4.* London: Methuen, pp. 111–136.

Bax, M. (1985) 'Crying: A clinical overview.' *In:* Lester, B.M., Boukydis, Z. (Eds.) *Infant Crying: Theoretical and Research Perspectives.* New York: Plenum Press, pp. 347–348.

Beebe, S.A., Casey, R., Pinto-Martin, J. (1993) 'Association of reported infant crying and maternal parenting stress.' *Clinical Pediatrics*, **32**, 15–19.

Blackman, J.A., Cobb, L.S. (1989) 'A comparison of parents' perceptions of common behavior problems in developmentally at-risk and normal children.' *Children's Health Care*, **18**,108–113.

Boukydis, C.F., Burgess, R.L. (1982) 'Adult physiologic response to infant cries: Effects of temperament of infant, parental status, and gender.' *Child Development*, **53**, 1291–1298.

Bowlby, J. (1969) *Attachment and Loss. Vol 1. Attachment.* New York: Basic Books.

Carey, W.B. (1984) '"Colic" – Primary excessive crying as an infant–environment interaction.' *Pediatric Clinics of North America*, **31**, 993–1005.

DeGangi, G.A., Craft, P., Castellan, J. (1991) 'Treatment of sensory, emotional, and attentional problems in regulatory disordered infants. Part 2.' *Infants and Young Children*, **3**, 9–19.

Donovan, W.L., Leavitt, L.A. (1992) 'Maternal self-efficacy and response to stress: Laboratory studies of coping with a crying infant.' *In:* Field, T.M., McCabe, P.M, Schneiderman, N. (Eds.) *Stress and Coping in Infancy and Childhood.* Hillsdale, NJ: Lawrence Erlbaum, pp. 47–68.

Drummond, J.E., McBride, M.L., Wiebe, C.F. (1993). 'The development of mothers' understanding of infant crying.' *Clinical Nursing Research*, **2**, 396–413.

Elliott, M.R., Fisher, K., Ames, E.W. (1988) 'The effects of rocking on the state and respiration of normal and excessive criers.' *Canadian Journal of Psychology*, **42**, 163–172.

Fisichelli, V.R., Karelitz, S. (1963) 'The cry latencies of normal infants and those with brain damage.' *Journal of Pediatrics*, **62**, 724–734.

—— Haber, A., Davis, J., Larelitz, S. (1966) 'Audible characteristics of the cries of normal infants and those with Down's Syndrome.' *Perceptual and Motor Skills*, **23**, 744–746.

Flatau, T.S., Gutzman, H. (1906) 'Die Stimme des Säuglings.' *Archiv für Laryngologie und Rhinologie*, **18**, 139–151.

Frodi, A., Senchak, M. (1990) 'Verbal and behavioral responsiveness to the cries of atypical infants.' *Child Development*, **61**, 76–84.

Fuller, B.F., Keefe, M.R., Curtin, M. (1994) 'Acoustic analysis of cries from normal and irritable infants.' *Western Journal of Nursing Research*, **16**, 243–253.

Goldson, E.J. (1998) 'Children with disabilities and child maltreatment.' *Child Abuse and Neglect*, **22**, 663–667.

Golub, H.L., Corwin, M.J. (1985) 'A physioacoustic model of infant cry.' *In:* Lester, B.M., Boukydis, C.F.Z. (Eds.) *Infant Crying: Theoretical and Research Perspectives.* New York: Plenum Press, pp. 59–82.

Green, J.A., Gustafson, G.E., Irwin, J.R., Kalinowski, L.L., Wood, R.M. (1995) 'Infant crying: Acoustics, perception and communication.' *Early Development and Parenting*, **4**, 161–175.

Gustafson, G.E., Green, J.A. (1989) 'On the importance of fundamental frequency and other acoustic features in cry perception and infant development.' *Child Development*, **60**, 772–780.

—— Harris, K.L. (1990) 'Women's responses to young infants' cries.' *Developmental Psychology*, **26**, 144–152.

Harris, J. (1979) 'When babies cry.' *Canadian Nurse*, **75**, 32–34.

Holaday, B. (1981) 'Maternal response to their chronically ill infants' attachment behavior of crying.' *Nursing Research*, **30**, 343–348.

—— (1982) 'Maternal conceptual set development: Identifying patterns of maternal response to chronically ill infant crying.' *Maternal–Child Nursing Journal*, **11**, 47–59.

—— Turner-Henson, A., Swan, J. (1996) 'Johnson Behavioral System Model: Explaining activities of chronically ill children.' *In:* Walker, P.H., Neuman, B. (Eds.) *Blueprint for Use of Nursing Models: Education, Research, Practice, and Administration.* New York: National League for Nursing Publications, pp. 33–63.

Karelitz, S., Fisichelli, V.R. (1962) 'The cry thresholds of normal infants and those with brain damage.' *Journal of Pediatrics*, **61**, 679–685.

Legido, A. (1998) 'Neurologic manifestations of children exposed to drugs in utero.' *International Pediatrics*, **13**, 70–83.

Lester, B.M. (1984) 'A biosocial model of infant crying.' *In:* Lipsett, L., Rovee-Collier, C. (Eds.) *Advances in Infant Research. Vol III.* Norwood, NY: Ablex, pp. 167–212.

—— Boukydis, Z, Garcia-Coll, C.T., Peucker, M., McGrath, M.M., Vohr, B.R., Brem, F., Oh, W. (1995) 'Developmental outcome as a function of the goodness of fit between the infant's cry characteristics and the mother's perception of her infant's cry.' *Pediatrics*, **95**, 51–57.

119

Maldonado-Duran, M., Sauceda-Garcia, J. (1996) 'Excessive crying in infants with regulatory disorders.' *Bulletin of the Meninger Clinic*, **60**, 62–78.

Marler, P. (1967) 'Animal communication signals.' *Science*, **157**, 769–774.

Makoi, Z. (1990) 'The crying infant and the family.' *Early Childhood Development and Care*, **65**, 91–94.

Marvin, R.S., Pianta, R.C. (1992) 'A relationship-based approach to self-reliance in young children with motor impairments.' *Infants and Young Children*, **4**, 33–45.

McDermott, J.F., Akina, E. (1972). 'Understanding and improving the personality development of children with physical handicaps.' *Clinical Pediatrics*, **11**, 130–134.

Michelsson, K. (1971) 'Cry analyses of symptomless low birth weight neonates and of asphyxiated newborn infants.' *Acta Paediatrica Scandinavica*, Suppl. 216, 1–45.

Michelsson, K., Paajanen, S., Rinne, A., Tervo, H., Kunnamo, I., Kiminkinen, T. (1990) 'Mothers' perceptions of and feelings towards their babies' crying.' *Early Child Development and Care*, **65**, 109–116.

Muller, E., Hollien, E.M., Murray, T. (1974) 'Perceptual responses to infant crying: Identification of cry types.' *Journal of Child Language*, **1**, 89–95.

Ostwald, P.F., Phibbs, R., Fox, S. (1968) 'Diagnostic use of infant cry.' *Biologia Neonatorum*, **13**, 68–82.

Prechtl, H.F.R. (1963) 'The mother–child interaction in babies with minimal brain damage.' *In:* Foss, B.M. (Ed.) *Determinants of Infant Behavior. Vol. 2.* New York: Wiley, pp. 53–66

Sagi, A. (1982) 'Adults' responses to the cries of normal and pathological infants.' *Journal of Preventive Psychiatry*, **1**, 359–364.

Sheeran, T., Marvin, R.S., Pianta, R.C. (1997) 'Mothers' resolution of their child's diagnosis and self-reported measures of parenting stress, marital relations, and social support.' *Journal of Pediatric Psychology*, **22**, 197–212.

Thomas, A., Chess, S. (1977) *Temperament and Development.* New York: Bruner/Mazel.

Ucko, L.E. (1965) 'A comparative study of asphyxiated and non-asphyxiated boys from birth to five years.' *Developmental Medicine and Child Neurology*, **6**, 27–31.

Vuorenkoski, V., Lind, J., Partanen, T.J., Lejeune, J., Lafourcade, J., Wasz-Höckert, O. (1966) 'Spectrographic analysis of cries from children with maladie du cri du chat.' *Annales Paediatriae Fenniae*, **12**, 174–180.

Wasserman, G.A., Allen, R., Solomon, D. R. (1985) 'The behavioral development of physically handicapped children in the second year.' *Journal of Developmental and Behavioral Pediatrics*, **6**, 27–31.

Wasz-Höckert, O., Partanen, T., Vuorenkoski, V., Valanne, E., Mickelsson, K. (1964) 'The identification of some specific meanings in infant vocalization.' *Experientia*, **20**, 154–156.

—— Lind, J., Vuorenkoski, V., Partanen, T., Valanne, E. (1968) *The Infant Cry: a Spectrographic and Auditory Analysis. Clinics in Developmental Medicine No 29.* London: Spastics International Medical Publications.

—— Michelsson, K, Lind, J. (1985) 'Twenty-five years of Scandinavian cry research.' *In:* Lester, B.M., Boukydis, C.F.Z. (Eds.) *Infant Crying: Theoretical and Research Perspectives.* New York: Plenum Press, pp. 83–101.

WHO (1980) *International Classification of Impairments, Disabilities and Handicaps.* Geneva: World Health Organization.

Wilkie, C.F., Ames, E.W. (1986) 'The relationship of infant crying to parental stress in the transition to parenthood.' *Journal of Marriage and the Family*, **48**, 545–550.

Wolff, P. (1969) 'The natural history of crying and other vocalizations in early infancy.' *In:* Foss, B.M. (Ed.) *Determinants of Infant Behavior. Vol. 4.* London: Methuen, pp. 81–109.

Zeskind, P.S., Shingler, E.A. (1991) 'Child abusers' perceptual responses to newborn infant cries varying in pitch.' *Infant Behavior and Development*, **14**, 335–347.

—— Sale, J., Maio, M.L., Huntington, L., Weiseman, J.R. (1985) 'Adult perceptions of pain and hunger cries: A synchrony of arousal.' *Child Development*, **56**, 549–554.

8

TODDLER TANTRUMS: FLUSHING AND OTHER VISIBLE AUTONOMIC ACTIVITY IN AN ANGER–CRYING COMPLEX

Michael Potegal

"A bold, fierce, and threatening Countenance, as pale as Ashes and in the same Moment as red as Blood."
> [From Seneca's description of anger in *De Irae* (trans. L'Estrange 1910).]

Temper tantrums are a common, if not ubiquitous, phenomenon of early childhood. Because young children tend to be more open about showing emotion, not yet having learned all the display rules in operation in their culture and having greater difficulty in masking emotional expression, tantrums provide a readily available opportunity to study the organization and expression of emotions so intense that they are not routinely observable or ethically elicitable in adults. As the quotation from Seneca implies, activation of the autonomic nervous system is regarded as one of the main, and in some views defining, elements of emotion. In some brief, interesting, but seldom cited observations on agonistic encounters among 3- to 5-year-old children in nursery school, Blurton Jones (1969) noted that a child who was hit or robbed of a toy often sat down and wept with reddened face and puckered brows. Blurton Jones likened these responses to tantrum behaviors. Crying is, in fact, one of the two most common tantrum behaviors (Einon and Potegal 1994). Blurton Jones's observations imply that flushing and the lacrimation associated with crying, each autonomic reactions readily observable on the face, may be important as emotion markers in children's tantrums.

Although tantrums have not been the subject of systematic study since Goodenough's (1931) classic work *Anger in Young Children*, a research interest in the autonomic concomitants of children's emotions dates back at least as far as Malapert (1902). He found that 47 per cent of French schoolchildren showed facial flushing (reddening of the skin) when angry. More recently, Stenberg and Campos (1990) reported that more than 90 per cent of 4- and 7-month-olds flushed during anger-inducing restraint. In a study of 4- and 7-month-olds briefly angered by withdrawal of a biscuit, Stenberg *et al.* (1983) noted that the occurrence of flushing predicted the persistence of a negative mood half an hour later. This finding is one indicator of the potential significance of autonomic activation as a predictor of and/or contributor to the intensity, duration and other characteristics of emotional expression. Such significance is implicit in William James' (1890) classic proposal that felt emotion is the consequence of bodily reactions to perceived situations. This notion gained popularity if not credibility with the demonstration by Schacter (1964) that anger (or mirth) could be augmented by 'nonspecific' autonomic activation, in this case, by an injection of epinephrine. Using more physiologically relevant manipulations, a number of investigators, notably Zillmann (*e.g.* 1994), have developed systematic evidence that increases of sympathetic activation can exacerbate both felt anger and expressed aggression (for review, see Potegal 1994). Autonomic activation theory suggests that there may be significant behavioral differences both between individuals who show autonomic reactions and those who do not (cf. personality differences between blushers and non-blushers—Leary *et al.* 1992) and within individuals on occasions when they show such reactions compared to occasions when they do not.

One classic objection to the proposition that autonomic reactivity mediates emotional responses is that autonomic reactions are, in general, slower than the voluntary activity by which emotion is expressed. Tantrums involve a sequence of more or less energetic physical actions. Since flushing can follow vigorous exercise, one might expect that flushing would appear later rather than earlier in the tantrum. If, as these lines of argument suggest, flushing appears only toward or at the end of a tantrum, its influence on tantrum behavior or duration is likely to be minimal. If it were to appear earlier in the tantrum, it would raise the possibility that autonomic feedback could exacerbate or otherwise dynamically alter the ways in which the tantrum is played out.

Our analysis of flushing and the other autonomic reactions in the tantrum data described below is informed by the work of Drummond and Lance (1987) on patients with Horner syndrome. These authors conclude that there are at least three anatomical pathways for facial flushing. Primary for both thermoregulatory flushing and embarrassment-induced blushing is a sympathetic vasodilator pathway usually running from the 2nd and 3rd thoracic roots to the scalp, forehead, chin and submandibular areas. There is also a sympathetic vaso-constrictor pathway. Reduction in the activity of this pathway is associated with reddening of ears and lips. A third, parasympathetic vasodilator pathway running via facial or glosso-pharyngeal nerves to the 'central mask' areas of the face is activated by gustatory stimuli. The most parsimonious hypothesis at the moment is that tantrum-associated flushing is a sympathetically mediated active vasodilation. Drummond and Lance also noted that flushing was routinely accompanied by sweating. Sweating is mediated by sympathetic activation of sudomotor glands. In contrast to flushing and sweating, the lacrimation associated with crying, one of the two most common tantrum behaviors (Einon and Potegal 1994), is para-sympathetically mediated. So are profuse salivation and rhinorrhea (secretions of the nasal mucosa—Cauna *et al.* 1972) that also occur during tantrums. The facial autonomic reactions visible during a tantrum are thus an exception to the rule that most autonomic end-organs are innervated by both the sympathetic and parasympathetic divisions of the autonomic nervous system. The sympathetic/parasympathetic division provides a natural grouping for the analysis of visible facial autonomic reactions.

To study the phenomenology of tantrum behavior, we have carried out a cross-sectional survey in which we asked parents of children preselected from birth-lists in the Madison, Wisconsin area to write a narrative of a tantrum had by their child, in as much detail as they could stand. This chapter briefly describes our general findings on tantrum composition and organization. Our instructions to parents included reporting on whatever autonomic activation was visible during the tantrum. In this chapter we extract some characteristics, correlates, and consequences of the reported autonomic activation and attempt to set them in a theoretical perspective.

The survey

Complete details of our initial survey methods and sample characteristics have been described elsewhere (Potegal *et al.* 1998a,b). In brief, names of parents of children in the noncontiguous age-groups of 18–24, 30–36, 42–48 and 54–60 months were obtained from newspaper announcements of births collated by the University of Wisconsin's Waisman Center for Human Development. Undergraduate interviewers conducted telephone interviews with over 1200 Madison, WI area parents, asking questions about tantrum incidence, frequency, duration and other characteristics. Tantrums were operationally defined as transient emotional events containing at least one of the following major behavior elements: crying, screaming, shouting, falling down, hitting and/or kicking, throwing something, or running away. Parents of 991 children reported that their child had had at least one tantrum in the previous month. Parents of these children were asked to estimate mean tantrum frequency in the last month along a scale of seven easily understood, roughly geometric steps: <1/month, 1–2/month, 1–2/week, 3–6/week, 1–2/day, 3–6/day, >6/day. Mean duration was similarly estimated along a seven step scale: <1 minute, 1–2 minutes, 2–4 minutes, 5–10 minutes, 10–20 minutes, 20–40 minutes, and >40 minutes.

At the end of the telephone interview, parents of tantrumers were asked if they would be willing to provide a written description of one of their child's tantrums. The narrative/ questionnaire packet included two 'representative' narratives that we wrote to indicate the level of detail we wished to have reported. The representative narratives, instructions and a list of terms drew parent's attention to signs of autonomic reactivity. (With regard to crying, we unfortunately did not ask parents to distinguish between vocalization patterns and lacrimation.) We also provided parents with a list of mood terms and their associated physical characteristics for describing pre- and post-tantrum mood. For the purposes of the present analysis, these are grouped into positive (pleasant, cheerful, playful, joking, laughing), neutral (normal, calm) and negative (angry, belligerent, defiant, sullen, dependent, nagging, upset, sad, scared) moods and an 'other' category (*e.g.* tired). Because of our interest in the issue of tantrum intensity, parents were asked to rate the intensity of the reported tantrum relative to their child's other tantrums in the past month using a five-point scale running from among the least intense (1), through average intensity (3), to among the most intense (5).

The narrative data and their analysis

We received 349 narratives of which 335 (178 boys and 157 girls) were usable. The parents providing the narratives were a largely white, college educated, middle-class sample of the population in and around Madison, WI. Tantrum durations in the sample varied from 0.5 to 39.5 minutes (median = 3.0 minutes, interquartile range = 1.5–5.0 minutes). The characteristics of the tantrums in the written sample closely resembled those of the larger telephone survey from which it was drawn. The tantrums were reconstructed in graphic

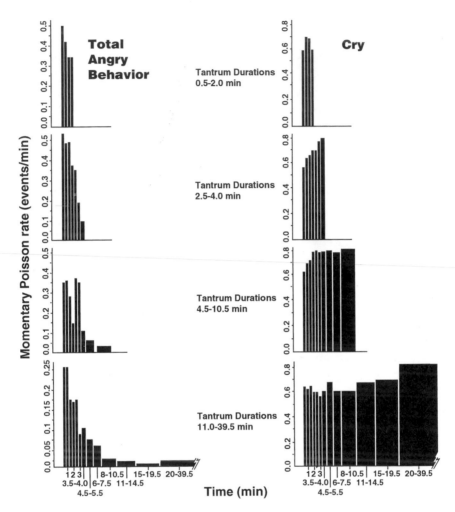

Fig. 8.1. Contrasting temporal profiles of physical expressions of anger (hitting, kicking, pulling/pushing, throwing and stamping combined) and of crying during tantrums. For the purposes of analysis, tantrums were partitioned into four duration groups, indicated by the vertical stacking of graphs. The probability of each behavior is indicated by the momentary Poisson rate for each time bin. Time bins for the first three minutes were set equal to the minimum 0.5 minute units originally used to score behavior. To offset the reduction in the number of tantrums still occurring at longer durations, time bins on the right side of the graphs for the last two duration groups were made progressively longer to include a larger sample of data from each remaining tantrum.

form as 'tantrugrams', time × behavior matrices in which time was partitioned into consecutive 0.5 minute units. Behavior in each of 14 different categories was scored as occurring or not occurring within each unit. A half minute was selected as the shortest possible time unit that could be plausibly discriminated from the narratives. We used momentary Poisson rates (MPRs)—the parameter of the best fitting Poisson distribution for each behavior within a time unit—to represent behavior probabilities in tantrums of varying duration (Potegal *et al.* 1996). The larger this parameter, the more probable was the behavior.

The physically *angry* behaviors—hitting, kicking, pulling/pushing, throwing, stamping—all had their maximum MPR at tantrum onset and declined thereafter. In contrast, *crying* MPRs increased over the course of the tantrum (Fig. 8.1). The time courses of these behaviors could be characterized by the skew of the MPR distributions; that is, the angry behaviors all had a positive skew, while crying had a negative skew. A multidimensional scaling analysis of the skews yielded a two-dimensional solution in which the angry behaviors clustered in one region of the mapping plane, while crying clustered with whining and consolation-seeking (*e.g.* clinging to mother) in a different region. Additionally, the distribution of the behaviors along the first (angry) dimension appeared to be related to their intuitive emotional intensity; that is, there was an ordering of hitting and kicking followed by throwing things followed by stamping.

A second, completely independent factor analysis was carried out on the log-transformed behavior durations. This analysis yielded a highly interpretable five-factor solution (with eigenvalues >1.0 and with loadings on major contributors to the factors >0.45) that collectively accounted for over 50 per cent of the variance in the observed behaviors. Furthermore, these factors were related in significant, orderly and comprehensible ways to tantrum variables that were, by design, not included in the factor analysis. The factor analysis confirmed the multidimensional scaling groupings (*e.g.* crying, whining and consolation-seeking formed a single factor) and extended it (*e.g.* the angry behaviors were subgrouped into three factors varying in emotional intensity). The two analyses converged on the following general tantrum model (Potegal *et al.* 1998a,b) suggesting an anger–crying complex represented graphically in Figure 8.1.

A model of tantrums

Distress and anger are the two main emotional/behavioral components of tantrums. The behaviors comprising the Distress factor—whining, consolation-seeking, crying—are distributed throughout the tantrum. Whining peaks in probability earlier followed by consolation-seeking; crying increases in probability over the course of the tantrum (see Fig. 8.1). The temporal sequence and relative emotional intensity of these three behaviors may reflect a progressive increase in distress as the tantrum continues. Tantrum duration increases strongly with increases in Distress duration.

The physical expression of anger is maximum at tantrum onset and drops relatively rapidly as shown in Figure 8.1. These angry behaviors are composed of three factors that are interpretable as levels of intensity. For High Anger (the first factor), screaming and kicking are the highest-loading (0.6-0.7) elements; hitting and stiffening of the body elements have slightly lower loadings (0.5). This factor presumably reflects the most intense level of anger. Crying also loads moderately (0.38) on High Anger. In the second factor, shouting and throwing characterize a presumptive level of Intermediate Anger. The third factor is defined by stamping, a presumptive Low Anger level. Among the reasons for this ordering of presumptive intensities is the consideration that hitting and kicking are aggressive behaviors requiring proximity to their targets and therefore entail the risk of immediate

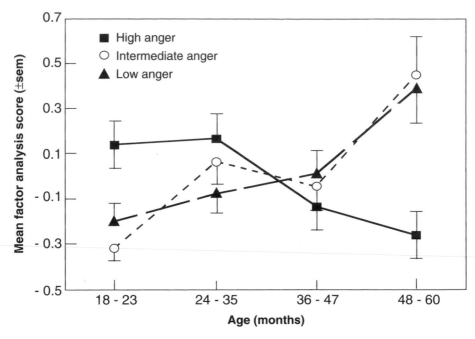

Fig. 8.2. The values of the high, intermediate and low anger factors for each tantrum were calculated. The plot of the mean values as a function of child's age is shown here. Error bars are standard error of the mean.

retaliation. Higher risk (and pain) tolerances are associated with higher levels of aggressiveness (Archer and Huntingford 1994, Bronstein 1994) and anger (Zachariae *et al.* 1991). Throwing, associated with Intermediate Anger, is usually done at a distance and involves a lesser risk. Stamping, the behavior defining Low Anger, is essentially a symbolic demonstration of anger for onlookers, involving no contact (proximal or distal) and the least risk.

High Anger is first expressed physically; screaming can than be added or switched to as a vocal expression of this intensity. High Anger is strongly correlated with tantrum duration, a correlation that is largely accounted for by the prolonged time course of screaming. Intermediate Anger is less strongly correlated with duration. Low Anger is uncorrelated with duration; indeed, if stamping occurs initially, it actually predicts shorter tantrums. High Anger was found to decrease with age (Fig. 8.2), apparently corresponding to the belief that children are better able to regulate their emotions as they mature. In contrast, Intermediate and Low Anger increased with age, suggesting a substitution of lower for higher anger levels rather than an overall reduction in the occurrence of anger.

Coping Style, the fifth factor in the factor analysis, was composed of high and oppositely signed loadings on running away and dropping to the floor. This factor, reflecting the child's often exclusive decision to either drop or run, is of ethological interest in that these behaviors are instances of submission and escape, the standard alternative coping strategies of losers in intraspecific agonistic encounters.

Observations on visible autonomic activity
VISIBLE AUTONOMIC REACTIONS

Flushing was by far the most frequent visible sign of autonomic activation, being reported in 26 per cent of tantrums. There was a slight trend for a reduction in the number of tantrums with flushing with age. There were no systematic differences between the sexes. Other autonomic reactions appeared in 2–6 per cent of tantrums. Listed in descending order of reported frequency, they were sweating, salivation (drooling and spitting), rhinorrhea (running nose), and other reactions (pupillary dilation, defecation). Respiratory distress in the form of gasping, panting or hiccuping was reported in 4.5 per cent of tantrums. Overall, one or more of these reactions was reported in 36 per cent of tantrums. Using instrumentation, Drummond and Lance (1987) found that flushing and sweating usually, but not invariably, co-ocurred. There was no trend for sweating to be associated with flushing in our reports. This lack of association may represent parental inattention, or it may just be that low levels of sweating are difficult to detect by visual inspection.

VISIBLE AUTONOMIC REACTIONS AND TANTRUM CHARACTERISTICS

The correlations of autonomic activation (as a dichotomous variable; that is, present or absent) with the High, Intermediate and Low Anger factors fell neatly in descending order (multiple regression β's of 0.31, 0.14 and 00.07, respectively), with only the first two being statistically significant. Distress was also significantly correlated with autonomic activation ($\beta = 0.17$); Coping Style was not.

In general, tantrums with one or more autonomic reactions were longer, contained more behavioral elements, and were judged to be more intense than those reported with no such reactions. An analysis (3-way MANOVA) that included duration, number of elements and intensity as dependent variables and with age, sex and the presence or absence of autonomic reactions as factors showed a significant difference between tantrums with or without autonomic reactions [Wilk's lambda = 0.86, $F(3,325) = 17.5$, $p<0.001$]. Follow-up univariate 3-way analyses of variance showed each of these effects to be individually significant. The presence of autonomic reactions was associated with greater judged intensity [$F(1, 317) = 27.1$, $p<0.0001$], greater numbers of behaviors [$F(1, 318) = 27.2$, $p<0.0001$], and longer durations (durations were log-transformed, with intensity and behavior number as covariates [$F(1,316) = 9.3$, $p<0.003$]). Although the interactions with age and sex were not significant, Table 8.1 suggests that the effect of autonomic activation on duration may be more pronounced for 2-year-olds, for whom visible activation was associated with a greater than two-fold increase in tantrum length.

ACUTE VERSUS CHRONIC FACTORS

How might we interpret this effect of autonomic activation on tantrum duration? At one extreme is the possibility that there are no consistent individual differences among children and that tantrum-prolonging autonomic activation occurs at random in about a third of all tantrums. At the other extreme is the possibility that children are strictly divided into consistent autonomic reactors with longer tantrums, and non-reactors with shorter tantrums. In a first test of these possibilities, we found that children whose tantrum narrative included

TABLE 8.1
Mean (±SD) tantrum duration (mins.) in the absence or presence of visible autonomic activation

		Age (years)			
		1	*2*	*3*	*4–5*
Visible autonomic activation:	Absent	3.7±5.6	3.0±3.5	4.7±6.7	4.0±4.2
	Present	5.9±7.7	7.4±8.3	5.9±5.9	5.8±5.3

one or more autonomic reactions also had estimated mean tantrum durations for the prior month that were significantly longer (mean ± SEM = 4.3 ± 0.4 mins.) than those with no such reactions (2.8 ± 0.2 mins. [$F(1, 315) = 13.9$, $p<0.0003$]). By comparison, there were no differences in estimated mean tantrum frequency.

We followed up the possibility that children may be consistent autonomic reactors or non-reactors by a small scale matched pair study in which 19 children who were reported to have flushed during the originally recorded tantrum were each paired with a child of the same age and sex who was not reported to have flushed. We re-interviewed by telephone the parents of these 38 children 7±4 months (mean±SD) after the described tantrum had occurred. At re-interview, when these children were between the ages of 22 and 48 months, we asked their parents to estimate the percentage of tantrums in the last month in which the child had flushed. We found no differences between original flushers and non-flushers in flushing or other autonomic activity either during the most recent month's tantrums or in response to other situations such as energetic play. This lack of consistency over an average period of seven months might be due to general decline in flushing with age. The correlation between age and the percentage of tantrums reported with flushing was –0.33 ($p<0.05$). This is a much stronger age effect than we originally observed, suggesting the unsurprising conclusion that the percentage of a *month's* tantrums with flushing is a more sensitive measure of individual differences than whether or not a child flushed during a single tantrum. This age-related decline in flushing parallels the age-related decline in High Anger noted above.

A possible caveat to the foregoing analysis is that the parents who noted autonomic reactions may have been more careful reporters than those who did not. The mean number of words (±SD) in the tantrum narratives of parents reporting autonomic reactions was 134 ± 63; narratives with no mention of reactions contained 107 ± 59 words. This difference was significant even when tantrum duration was used as a covariate [$F(1, 329) = 7.7$, $p<0.01$]. The average of 27 additional words could have been required to describe the autonomic reactions and additional behavioral elements. Alternatively, the association of autonomic activation with more elements and perhaps even with longer durations could be the consequence of more scrupulous reporting. However, such an artifact is unlikely to explain the association of autonomic activation with greater reported tantrum intensity that was a judgment relative to the child's own baseline. We presume that all three effects are veridical, but that more objective techniques of tantrum recording will be required to verify these findings.

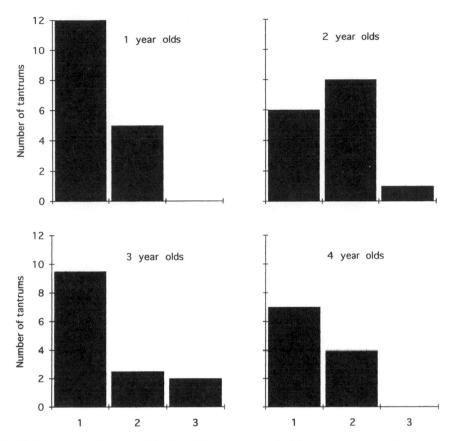

Fig. 8.3. Histograms indicating which third of the tantrum contained the onset of flushing. Each histogram is based on all tantrums ≥1.5 minutes in duration for which flushing onset could be determined. For tantrums in which it was unclear in which two of the three thirds flushing began, each of the possible thirds was credited with a score of 0.5.

THE TEMPORAL LOCUS OF FLUSHING

Another interpretation of the association between autonomic reactions and tantrum duration is that the more prolonged the tantrum, the more time these reactions have to occur or to reach thresholds of visibility. This raises the question of the temporal locus of flushing. Prior to carrying out this survey, we presumed that flushing was the *result* of vigorous and protracted tantrum activity and would therefore appear towards the end of the tantrum. The relative location of flushing in tantrums of varying length and content was determined by partitioning all tantrums of one and one-half minutes or longer into three consecutive segments of equal duration and noting the segment in which flushing was first reported. The results were contrary to our expectations. As shown in Figure 8.3, flushing clearly tends to be observed initially in the first third of the tantrum at every age. In our matched pairs follow-up, by contrast, parents reported that when flushing occurs in conjunction with vigorous exercise, it does so after about 10 minutes on average. This delay is longer than the duration of the majority of tantrums.

SYMPATHETIC AND PARASYMPATHETIC TONE

From the foregoing, it appears that the early, rapidly peaking anger component of tantrums has a predominantly sympathetic tone. This conclusion is consistent with the results of Stenberg and Campos (1990) who found flushing in over 90 per cent of 4- and 7-month-olds who were continuously restrained for up to three minutes. That this was an association of flushing with anger relatively unconfounded with distress was indicated by the observation that 28 of the 32 children in this study showed facial expressions of anger, but only three exhibited respiratory patterns of crying and only one expressed tears. In our survey, 10 per cent of the 287 narratives with crying also reported one or both of the other two parasympathetic reactions (nose running, drooling), whereas only one of 47 tantrums (2 per cent) without crying was reported with such reactions. While the existence of only a single case in one cell precludes a statistical analysis, it seems that the slowly developing Distress component may be associated with a more parasympathetic tone. These hypotheses are in keeping with the notion that intense emotions are associated with a sympathetic activation that can be followed by a burst of compensatory, arousal-reducing parasympathetic activity in the form of crying (for review, see Gross *et al.* 1994). In our data, however, as in the Gross *et al.* (1994) study of adults, there was also a significant association between one or more sympathetic reactions and crying [$\chi^2(1) = 5.7$, p<0.03], suggesting a simultaneous or partially overlapping sympathetic/parasympathetic coactivation.

Porges' (1995) related but more detailed and elaborate polyvagal theory emphasizes the role of fluctuations in vagal tone in emotion regulation. In this theory, acute rage (and panic) are associated with a massive withdrawal of the vagally mediated inhibitory influence of the nucleus ambiguus on the heart, as indicated by a complete loss of respiratory sinus arrythmia (George *et al.* 1989). The withdrawal of this 'vagal brake' produces a tachycardia that provides metabolic support for the classical fight-or-flight response. Because the nucleus ambiguus also influences the autonomic and somatic musculature that coordinates breathing with other laryngeal functions (*e.g.* swallowing, speech), the withdrawal of its vagal drive also leads to vocalizations of higher pitch (crying, screaming) and, it may be surmised, to respiratory distress. The subsequent return of vagal tone is associated with the relief of distress; that is, with quieting in crying infants (Porges 1995). Porges also suggests that during the period of nucleus ambiguus inactivation, output from the phylogenetically older and more primitive dorsal motor nucleus of the vagus may play a role in intensifying autonomic/somatic discoordination and distress.

Applying this model to the phenomenology of tantrums, physically expressed anger would be associated with sympathetic activation and the withdrawal of vagally mediated nucleus ambiguus output. A transition to high pitched screaming, deep sobbing, gasping and/or panting would be associated with assumption of control of vagal outflow by the dorsal motor nucleus of the vagus, while the eventual diminution in distress that signals the end of the tantrum would be associated with the return of vagal outflow control to the nucleus ambiguus. The foregoing conjecture refers to the roles of sympathetic and parasympathetic

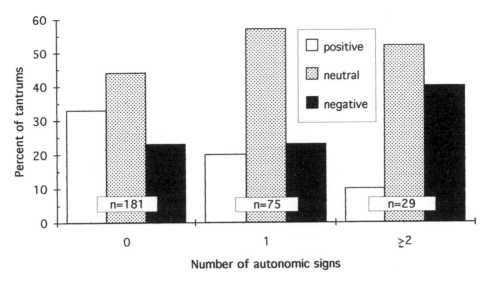

Fig. 8.4. Histogram showing a shift in post-tantrum mood as a function of the number of autonomic reactions reported in the tantrum. The numbers at the bottom of the bars indicate the total number of tantrums in the respective group.

activation in acute crises. Some data (*e.g.* Cole *et al.* 1996) suggest that increased vagal tone may account for the chronically reduced heart rate of children with 'externalizing' behavior problems (*e.g.* tantrums), but this complex issue is still under investigation (*e.g.* Mezzacappa *et al.* 1997).

AUTONOMIC REACTIONS AND POST-TANTRUM MOOD
As indicated in Figure 8.4, an increasing number of signs of autonomic activation during tantrums is associated with an increasing likelihood of a negative post-tantrum mood [$\chi^2(4) = 11.2$, p<0.025]. Thus, when no autonomic reactions were reported, the ratio of children with positive post-tantrum mood to those with negative mood was roughly 3:2. When two or more autonomic reactions were reported to be present during the tantrum, that ratio shifted to almost 1:4. This observation is entirely consistent with the Stenberg *et al.* (1983) report that flushing predicted the persistence of a negative mood in 4- and 7-month-olds one half hour after they had been angered. The fact that roughly half the children in each of the groups of Figure 8.4 showed no particular post-tantrum mood may indicate that, among 18- to 60-month-olds, there is a subgroup of especially mood-labile children who are susceptible to the persisting effects of autonomic activation.

Synopsis and some additional considerations
FLUSHING AND ANGER
Prior to carrying out our survey, we expected that if flushing appeared, it would either do so towards the end of the tantrum or else be randomly distributed within the tantrum.

Neither of these were reported. For most of the tantrums in which there was sufficient information to localize onset, flushing occurred early. This finding clearly rules out the interpretation that flushing is the *result* of vigorous, protracted tantrum activity. The early onset of flushing coincides with the peak of angry behavior. This observation fits with the traditional view, suggested by the quotation from Seneca at the head of this chapter, that autonomic activation is a major component of emotional experience including anger. Levenson (1992) cites seven recent studies of adults in which increases in heart rate and/or blood pressure were associated with the evocation of anger in a directed facial action or a relived emotions task. Some emotion theorists argue for the preeminence of bodily reactions, including autonomic ones, in defining emotion (for review, see Zajonc and Markus 1984). The present naturalistic observations contribute to the close association between flushing and anger. But is flushing obligatory in anger? Apparently, flushing intense enough to be visible to the parental eye is not. However, this does not preclude the occurrence of subthreshold flushing accompanying anger.

POSSIBLE AUTONOMIC FEEDBACK EFFECTS ON BEHAVIOR
Flushing appears to signal tantrums that are more prolonged, complex and intense. Experimental work showing that the sensorimotor feedback from facial expressions can intensify emotions (*e.g.* Izard 1990) and that sympathetic arousal can exacerbate anger and aggression (*e.g.* Zillmann 1994) suggests that flushing and/or other autonomic processes can actively contribute to these effects. It appears that autonomic activation is associated with an increased likelihood that children between 18 and 60 months of age will express a negative mood shift after the tantrum. This is entirely consistent with the observations of Stenberg and Campos (1990) in 4- and 7-month-olds. From the finding that older children and adolescents with externalizing disorder routinely have lower resting heart rate (Quay 1993), it may be inferred that when these individuals become angry, their increase in heart rate over baseline may be larger. The resulting greater cardiac (and perhaps other autonomic) feedback during anger may be more salient and/or effective in driving their aggressive behavior, which, as a consequence, is more extreme.

AGE TRENDS AND INDIVIDUAL DIFFERENCES
There may be consistent individual differences in flushing as there are in blushing (*e.g.* Leary *et al.* 1992). That is, there may be children who flush in every tantrum, no matter how mild, and others who fail to flush during any tantrum, no matter how intense. This raises the question of flush proneness, that is, whether children who were reported to flush during their tantrum were more likely to flush in other situations. In our small follow-up sample, we found no association between reported rates of flushing during tantrums and flushing from other causes, *e.g.* heat, cold, exercise or, for older children, embarrassment. The stability of the tendency to flush during tantrums may be limited by an age trend toward reduced flushing. The conjecture of an age trend is supported by the difference between our overall 26 per cent rate of flushing in children between 18 and 60 months and the greater than 90 per cent rate reported in 4- and 7-month-olds (Stenberg and Campos 1990). The parallel age-related declines in flushing and in High Anger imply that tantrums may become overlearned and

routinized with age and repetition, perhaps becoming less emotional and more deliberately manipulative. When we correlated the estimated frequency and duration of tantrums reported in the original telephone survey with the corresponding estimates reported weeks later in the returned questionnaire, we found that the correlations increased systematically with the age of the child. This is consistent with the notion that tantrums gradually become routinized.

WHAT FLUSHING MEANS

From a functionalist perspective, it has been suggested that blushing is a visible signal of embarrassment that serves to disarm those who may have been offended by the act or event that occasioned the blush (Leary *et al.* 1992, Miller and Leary 1992). Is it possible that flushing also has a display value in interpersonal interactions, *i.e.* that it might be an involuntary threat display of anger and therefore of incipient attack? An alternative possibility is raised by Blurton Jones' (1969) observations of conflict over toy possession in nursery school. A child robbed of a toy often shouted a low-pitched "No" immediately after it had been grabbed. Blurton Jones describes the behaviors during the resulting struggle in some detail, including some instances of apparently inhibited attack. "Occassionally a robbed child would scream long and loud, a lowish-pitched scream or roar, and, red in face, beat at, with closed fist, but not hit, and not approach its opponent" (Blurton Jones 1969, p. 447). More often, a child who is hit or is being robbed of a toy gives a high-pitched scream usually followed by a call for help, retaliation, or a letting go of the toy followed by immobility (typically sitting down), weeping, puckering of the brows and reddening of the face. While neither systematic nor supported by presentation of data, these accounts suggest that flushing is usually associated more with frustrated anger than with aggressive responding itself. A somewhat indirect argument in support of this hypothesis can be drawn from the generalization that when the child's initial response to a transgression was associated with some display of counteraggression, the accompanying vocalizations tended to be low-pitched. When no counteraggression was displayed, vocalizations were high-pitched. This is consistent with Frick's (1986) finding in adults that angry utterances of lower pitch are identifed as threat while those with higher perceived pitch are interpreted as signs of frustration. Blurton Jones (1969, p. 449) comments on the resemblances between these conflicts and temper tantrums: "I would speculate that a temper tantrum is the behaviour shown when attack is stimulated but the opponent is overwhelmingly powerful and/or a friend (*e.g.* a parent; in my observations it has been a child opponent, but a playmate and one who usually wins his fights)." From the current perspective, an important point about the behavior described by Blurton Jones is that the child's weeping reflects distress but flushing indicates anger. In the case of the child who sits down after being attacked, flushing is the only sign of anger.

Directions for future research

CONFIRMATION OF THE PRESENT FINDINGS

Traditional studies of autonomic involvement in emotional behavior have used measures such as blood pressure and heart rate. Thus, most of the data that supports the autonomic/ behavioral feedback hypothesis have been generated in laboratories under the restrictive conditions required by the traditional instrumentation for the measurement of autonomic physiology. Their generalizability to the real world is accordingly questionable. This report on visible autonomic effects during tantrums provides information on the role of autonomic activation in real world situations. In asking parents to describe their children's tantrums, we have returned to the venerable tradition of guided naturalistic observation. Along with the several advantages of this tradition comes the disadvantage of unknown and unknowable biases. Objective data in the form of video and audio recording and/or observers in the home will be needed to confirm and extend these findings.

TANTRUMS, TEMPERAMENT, AGGRESSION AND PSYCHOPATHOLOGY

Jenkins *et al.* (1984) reported that 2- and 3-year-old children having more than four tantrums a day were likely to be rated by their mothers as attention-demanding and difficult to manage. Factor analytic studies of the behavior of normal and clinical samples of children aged 4 to 16 years have found that tantrums load highly on a factor identifiable as aggression (Achenbach 1978, Elithorn 1974). In a survey carried out in England, Einon and Potegal (1994) found that children having more than five tantrums a day had a higher incidence of aggressive behaviors both within the tantrum (hitting objects and people, biting) and in peer relations (retaliating against and bullying others). In an experimental study of the temperamental correlates of tantrums, we compared 4-year-olds with chronic severe, frequent and/or prolonged tantrums to those whose tantrums were mild, brief and infrequent (Potegal *et al.* 1998a,b). Our laboratory assessment of response to mild provocations (*e.g.* brief restraint by a parent) found that the angry facial expressions of the tantrum-prone children were significantly more intense. This finding was confirmed by a parent questionnaire on which these children were reported to be generally more angry. They were also reported to be more active and less persistent (more distractible) than their non-tantrum-prone counterparts. In short, selection for extreme tantrum proneness brought with it a subclinical version of externalizing disorder. Tantrums are, in fact, a prominent early feature of externalizing behavior (*e.g.* Patterson *et al.* 1992), and it is therefore appropriate that they appear as an item in rating scales for this form of psychopathology (Achenbach 1991, Eyberg 1992). Hinshaw *et al.* (1993) have proposed that tantrums at age 5 years are a 'gateway' to the development of subsequent conduct disorder, while Caspi *et al.* (1987) have found that tantrums persisting to age 8 are, by themselves, a reliable predictor of poor life adjustment and of psychopathology such as conduct disorder and adult antisocial personality.

Prolonged, weepy tantrums, as opposed to frequent angry tantrums, may be a prognosticator of a different form of psychopathology. In contrast to the children with very frequent tantrums, the children in the Einon and Potegal (1994) survey whose reported tantrums lasted 20 minutes or more looked angry but were less likely than the average child to act aggressively within the tantrum or towards other children outside the tantrum. They were almost twice as likely to be picked on by other children. Because the probability of anger declines and crying increases over the course of the tantrum, such long tantrums are likely to be associated with the experience of greater distress. They may also be indicators of clinically significant internalizing disorder.

ACKNOWLEDGEMENTS

Early stages of this project were supported by a grant to M. Potegal from the Harry Frank Guggenheim Foundation. Later stages were supported by National Research Service Awards to M. Potegal from the National Institute for Neurological Disorders and Stroke (F33 NS09638) and the National Institute of Child Health and Human Development (F33 HD08208). Many University of Wisconsin undergraduate psychology students participated in data collection and analysis. Alyssa Axelrod helped in the collection of the matched pair follow-up sample. Special thanks are due Sara Woboril, Julie Arendt and Rebecca Strauss for their organization of the other students' work.

REFERENCES

Achenbach, T.M. (1978) 'The child behavior profile: I. Boys aged 6–11.' *Journal of Consulting and Clinical Psychology*, **46**, 478–488.

—— (1991) 'Parent child behavior check list.' *In:* Achenbach, T.M., Edelbrock, C. (Eds.) *Manual for Child Behavior Check List and Revised Child Behavior Profile.* Burlington, VT: University of Vermont, Dept of Psychiatry, p. 12.

Archer, J., Huntingford, F. (1994) 'Game theory models and escalation of animal fights.' *In:* Potegal, M., Knutson, J. (Eds.) *The Dynamics of Aggression: Biological and Social Processes in Dyads and Groups.* Hillsdale, NJ: Lawrence Erlbaum, pp. 3–31.

Blurton Jones, N.G. (1969) 'An ethological study of some aspects of social behaviour of children in nursery school.' *In:* Morris, D. (Ed.) *Primate Behavior.* Garden City, NY: Doubleday, pp. 437–463.

Bronstein, P. (1994) 'Aggression waxing (sometimes waning): Siamese fighting fish.' *In:* Potegal, M., Knutson, J. (Eds.) *The Dynamics of Aggression: Biological and Social Processes in Dyads and Groups.* Hillsdale, NJ: Lawrence Erlbaum, pp. 113–122.

Caspi, A., Elder, G.H., Bem, D.J. (1987) 'Moving against the world: Life course patterns of explosive children.' *Developmental Psychology*, **23**, 308–313.

Cauna, N., Cauna, D., Hinderer, K.H. (1972) 'Innervation of the human nasal glands.' *Journal of Neurocytology*, **1**, 49–60.

Cole, P.M., Zahn-Waxler, C., Fox, N.A., Usher, B.A., Welsh, J.D. (1996) 'Individual differences in emotion regulation and behavior problems in preschool children.' *Journal of Abnormal Psychology*, **105**, 518–529.

Drummond, P.D., Lance, J.W. (1987) 'Facial flushing and sweating mediated by the sympathetic nervous system.' *Brain*, **110**, 793–803.

Einon, D.F., Potegal, M. (1994) 'Temper tantrums in young children.' *In:* Potegal, M., Knutson, J. (Eds.) *The Dynamics of Aggression: Biological and Social Processes in Dyads and Groups.* Hillsdale, NJ: Lawrence Erlbaum, pp. 157–194.

Elithorn, A. (1974) 'Sources of aggressivity in epileptic children.' *In:* de Wit, J., Hartup, W.W. (Eds.) *Determinants and Origins of Aggressive Behavior.* The Hague: Mouton, pp. 325–336.

Eyberg, S. (1992) 'Parent and teacher behavior inventories for the assessment of conduct problem behaviors in children.' *In:* VandeCreek, L., Knapp, S., Jackson, T.L. (Eds.) *Innovations in Clinical Practice: A Source Book. Vol. 11.* Sarasota, FL: Professional Resource Press, pp. 377–382.

Frick, R. (1986) 'The prosodic expression of anger: Differentiating threat and frustration.' *Aggressive Behavior*, **12**, 121–128.

George, D.T., Nutt, D.J., Walker, W.V., Porges, S.W., Adinoff, B., Linnoila, M. (1989) 'Lactate and hyperventilation substantially attenuate vagal tone in normal volunteers: A possible mechanism of panic prevention.' *Archives of General Psychiatry*, **46**, 153–156.

Goodenough, F. (1931) *Anger in Young Children.* Minneapolis: University of Minnesota Press.

Gross, J.J., Fredrickson, B.L., Levenson, R.W. (1994) 'The psychophysiology of crying.' *Psychophysiology*, **31**, 460–468.

Hinshaw, S., Lahey, B., Hart, E. (1993) 'Issues of taxonomy and comorbidity in the development of conduct disorder.' *Developmental Psychopathology*, **5**, 31–49.

Izard, C. E. (1990) 'Facial expressions and the regulation of emotions.' *Journal of Personality and Social Psychology*, **58**, 487–498.

James, W. (1890) *Principles of Psychology. Vol. 2.* New York: Henry Holt.

Jenkins, S., Owen, C., Bax, M., Hart, H. (1984) 'Continuities of common behaviour problems in preschool children.' *Journal of Child Psychology and Psychiatry*, **25**, 75–89.

Leary, M.R., Britt, T.W., Cutlip, W.D., Templeton, J.L. (1992) 'Social blushing.' *Psychological Bulletin*, **112**, 446–460.

Levenson, R.W. (1992) 'Autonomic nervous system differences among emotions.' *Psychological Science*, **3**, 23–27.

Malapert, P. (1902) 'Enquête sur le sentiment de la colère chez les enfants.' *Année Psychologie*, **9**, 1–40.

Mezzacappa, E., Tremblay, R.E., Kindlon, D., Saul, J.P., Arsenault, L., Pihl, R.O., Earls, F. (1997) 'Trait anxiety, aggression and delinquency, heart rate and regulation of heart rate variability in adolescent males.' *Journal of Child Psychology and Psychiatry and Allied Disciplines*, **38**, 457–469.

Miller, R.S., Leary, M.R. (1992) 'Social sources and interactive function of emotion.' *In:* Clark, M.S. (Ed.) *Emotion and Social Behavior.* Newbury Park, CA: Sage, pp. 202–221.

Patterson, G.R., Reid, J.B., Dishion, T.J. (1992) *A Social Interactional Approach. Vol. 4. Antisocial Boys.* Eugene, OR: Castilia Publishing.

Porges, S.W. (1995) 'Orienting in a defensive world: Mammalian modifications of our evolutionary heritage. A polyvagal theory.' *Psychophysiology*, **32**, 301–317.

Potegal, M. (1994) 'Aggressive arousal: The amygdala connection.' *In:* Potegal, M., Knutsen, J. (Eds.) *The Dynamics of Aggression: Biological and Social Processes in Dyads and Groups.* Hillsdale, NJ: Lawrence Erlbaum, pp. 73–111.

—— Kosorok, M.R. (1995) 'Temper tantrums in young children.' *In: Proceedings of the 61st Meeting of the Society for Research in Child Development, Indianapolis, IN, March/April 1995*, p. 82

—— —— Davidson R.J. (1996) 'The time course of angry behavior in the temper tantrums of young children.' *Annals of the New York Academy of Sciences*, **794**, 31–45.

—— Davidson, R.J., Goldsmith, H.H., Chapman, R.S., Senulis, J.A. (1998a) 'Tantrums, temperament and temporal lobes.' *In: Proceedings of the XIIIth World Meeting of the Internatioonal Society for Research on Aggression, Mahwah, NJ, July 1998*, p. 36.

—— Kosorok, M.R., Davidson R.J. (1998b) 'Anger and distress in temper tantrums.' *In: Proceedings of the XIIIth World Meeting of the Internatioonal Society for Research on Aggression, Mahwah, NJ, July 1998*, p. 18.

Quay, H.C. (1993) 'The psychobiology of undersocialized aggressive conduct disorder: A theoretical perspective.' *Development and Psychopathology*, **5**, 165–180.

Schacter, S. (1964) 'The interaction of cognitive and physiological determinants of emotional state.' *In:* Berkowitz, L. (Ed.) *Advances in Experimental Social Psychology. Vol. 1.* New York: Academic Press, pp. 49–80.

Seneca (*ca.* 41AD) 'De Irae.' [Translated by L'Estrange, R. (1910) *In: The Latin Classics. Vol. 1. Drama, Ethics.* New York: Vincent Parke, pp. 378–428.]

Stenberg, C.R., Campos, J.L. (1990) 'The development of anger expressions in infancy.' *In:* Stein, N.L., Leventhal, B., Trabasso, T. (Eds.) *Psychological and Biological Approaches to Emotion.* Hillsdale, NJ: Lawrence Erlbaum, pp. 247–282.

—— —— Emde, R.N. (1983) 'The facial expression of anger in seven-month-old infants.' *Child Development*, **54**, 178–184.

Zajonc, R.B., Markus, H. (1984) 'Affect and cognition: The hard interface.' *In:* Izard, C.E., Kagan, J., Zajonc, R.B. (Eds.) *Emotions, Cognition, and Behavior.* Cambridge/New York: Cambridge University Press, pp. 73–107.

Zachariae, R., Bjerring, P., Arendt-Nielsen, L., Gotliebsen, K. (1991) 'The effect of hypnotically induced emotional stresses on brain potentials evoked by painful argon laser stimulation.' *Clinical Journal of Pain*, **7**, 130–138.

Zillmann, D. (1994) 'Cognition–excitation interdependencies in the escalation of aggression.' *In:* Potegal, M., Knutson, J. (Eds.) *The Dynamics of Aggression: Biological and Social Processes in Dyads and Groups.* Hillsdale, NJ: Lawrence Erlbaum, pp. 45–72.

9
ACOUSTIC CRY ANALYSIS, NEONATAL STATUS AND LONG-TERM DEVELOPMENTAL OUTCOMES

James A. Green, Julia R. Irwin and Gwen E. Gustafson

The challenge in this chapter in to synthesize three different literatures—on the acoustic analysis of cry sounds, on physiological models of crying, and on predictions of adverse outcomes from cry analysis. Rather than creating a crazy-quilt of separate pieces stitched together, we hope to depict in a more coherent framework how crying might relate to early health and development. This task at first appears rather straightforward, but we have discovered some formidable obstacles.

At least part of the difficulty in synthesizing these literatures arises from the simple fact that our understanding of crying is enhanced in only a limited way by reductionist analyses, that is, by breaking the cry into elemental parts and studying each in isolation. Although much can be gained from researching the acoustics, physiology, perception or social effects of crying, a synthesis requires more. Indeed, putting these elements back together may require concepts not inherent in any of the literatures themselves. Despite many years of research, the field still struggles to develop adequate constructs to describe the activity we call 'crying' and the effects that it has on the environment.

This view of crying as an emergent, irreducible phenomenon is relatively recent, however. Early studies of infant crying had an aura of certainty and hope that cry analysis would be useful in the diagnosis of certain neonatal disorders (*e.g.* Wasz-Höckert *et al.* 1968). Some of that early optimism carried through to 1986, when there was discussion at the 2nd International Workshop on Infant Cry Research about what elements would be necessary to build an automatic cry screening device for neonatal nurseries, and even into the early 1990s, when a multicenter study was funded in the United States to evaluate cry acoustics as a screening tool for sudden infant death syndrome (Corwin *et al.* 1995).

The story of what happened to these plans to use cries as an index of health and development lies, in part, in the findings and models we will review below. To tell that story, we first need to examine how cries are analyzed acoustically, and what models have been proposed to account for cry production. With this background, we will then examine some of the literature relating acoustic features to neonatal disease and to developmental outcome. We conclude by suggesting research directions we believe will be profitable in the future, especially toward the broad goal of understanding crying as a dynamic developmental phenomenon.

Acoustic analysis of infant cry sounds

OVERVIEW

Crying is a multimodal, dynamic behavior. It involves characteristic vocalizations, facial expressions and limb movements, all of which change and, probably, covary over time. Although research addressing crying as a communicative act has begun to take into account these complexities (*e.g.* Green *et al.* 1995), research on crying as an indicator of CNS functioning has focused almost exclusively on the cry sound. There are both historical and theoretical reasons for this focus. Historically, the methods for acoustic analysis became available shortly after World War II (Potter *et al.* 1947), long before there were systematic methods for coding facial expressions and movement. From a theoretical point of view, the muscles of the larynx are controlled partially by areas of the brainstem that are also involved in heart rate and respiration (Golub 1980, Porges *et al.* 1994). Therefore, the sound of the cry is likely to be more closely related to autonomic functioning than are the facial expressions and limb movements associated with crying.

Focusing on the sound of the cry helped to make manageable the task of relating crying to health and developmental status. However, even further constraints were necessary to narrow the research focus. First, the majority of studies have examined full-blown cry sounds, ignoring the fussing and grunting noises that are characteristic of longer bouts of crying. Second, in order to help standardize the analytic process, the cry sounds have often been elicited by (presumably) painful stimuli, such as injections, heel lances, rubber band snaps to the heel, and pinching. Third, because the goal has been to aid in the diagnosis of neonatal dysfunction, most studies have been done in the immediate postpartum period. Finally, serial investigations of changes in cry sounds have been virtually absent, with research concentrating on cry measurements made at a single point in time. We shall return to some of these issues when discussing directions for future research. For now, it is worth noting that the constraints that made much of the research on crying and neonatal health possible should now probably be viewed as limitations to be overcome in future research.

BASIC ACOUSTICS

Despite years of research, the acoustic analysis of cry sounds remains a complex, unstandardized endeavor. This state of affairs is due both to the complexity of the sound itself and to the complexity of the act of crying.

A pure tone or sine wave (Fig. 9.1) can be described fully by its single frequency (number of cycles per second) and amplitude (amount of excursion of the wave). In general, we perceive the frequency of such a wave as pitch and the amplitude as loudness. The greater the number of cycles per second, the higher the pitch of the tone. The larger the excursions, the louder the tone (for an extended introduction to speech acoustics, see Denes and Pinson 1973).

Unfortunately, there are no such pure tones produced by nature. Even the relatively simple, stereotyped calls of some songbirds are best represented by multiple acoustic features in multidimensional space (Nowicki and Nelson 1990). For a typical cry from a human neonate, a plot of time × amplitude of the cry (Fig. 9.2) shows much more complexity than the pure tone. A frequency × amplitude plot (Fig. 9.3) for a small segment of this cry

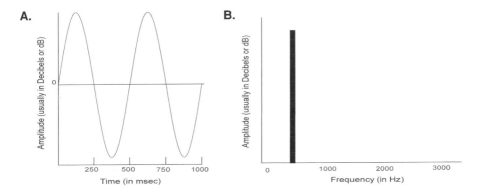

Fig. 9.1. A. Time × amplitude representation of a sine wave or pure tone. **B.** Frequency × amplitude representation of the same wave. A sine wave oscillates at only one frequency.

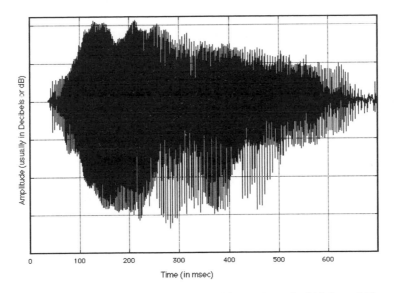

Fig. 9.2. A time × amplitude plot of a single cry sound from a 1-month-old infant; cf. Figure 9.1A.

shows energy in frequencies ranging from 100 to 5000 Hz. For even a single, 1 second cry sound, there are complex changes in the distribution of energy over time, such that it is possible to derive 100 or more measures for any cry sound.

HISTORICAL SKETCH

In the 1960s and '70s, the sound spectrogram was the major tool for analyzing cry sounds. Produced by an analog device, a spectrogram plots time on the *x* axis and frequency on the *y* axis, and encodes amplitude as the darkness of the frequency lines (Fig. 9.4). Elaborate

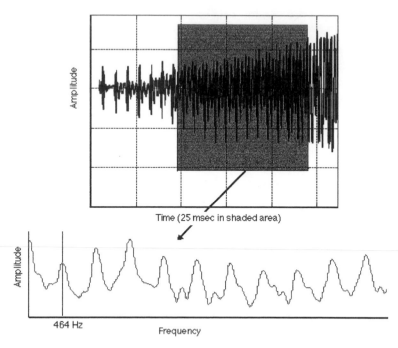

Time (25 msec in shaded area)

464 Hz

Frequency

Fig. 9.3. Top figure shows a time × amplitude plot of a small segment from the beginning of the cry shown in Figure 9.2. Bottom figure shows a frequency × amplitude representation obtained via a fast Fourier transform of the 25 ms portion of wave shown at top. Compare with Figure 9.1B.

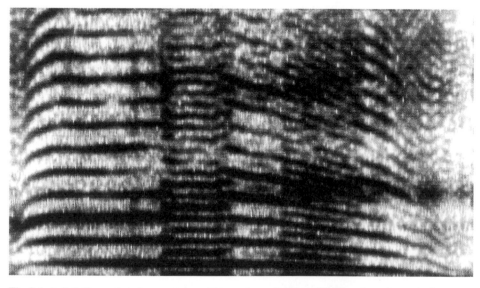

Fig. 9.4. A digitally-produced spectrogram of the cry shown in Figure 9.2. Time is on the *x* axis, frequency on the *y* axis, and amplitude is encoded in the darkness of the bars.

coding schemes were developed, particularly by the Scandinavian researchers (*e.g.* Michelsson *et al.* 1984), to capture the rich information displayed in the spectrogram. Details of those schemes will be presented shortly.

In the 1980s and '90s, cry researchers turned toward computers to quantify information about the cry sound. In computer analyses, taped cry sounds are digitized (*i.e.* their amplitude is measured repeatedly, usually about 25,000 times per second), and then one of several methods is used to extract frequency and temporal information from the sampled cries.

The fast Fourier transform (FFT) is the most common algorithm for creating a frequency × amplitude display. Typically, the FFT is performed on a small window or 'slice' of the cry (say 25 or 40 ms), so that many FFTs are required to analyze even a single cry sound. For example, forty 25 ms time segments comprise a 1 s cry sound. Thus, it is necessary to generate many displays to capture changes in frequencies over time. However, many sound analysis programs can create spectrographic images from the digitized cries (*e.g.* Fig. 9.4), and these spectrograms are still considered a useful device for visualizing the entire cry.

The use of digitization and computer analysis added quantification and precision to cry measurement. It also added variability, as there are many parameters to set in performing the many FFTs necessary to analyze a cry sound, including the frequency range, the type of weighting function to apply to the beginning and end of the samples, the number of FFTs to perform, what to do with sound waves that do not repeat themselves (*i.e.* are aperiodic), and so on. For these and other reasons, computer aided cry analysis appeared to proceed without much input from spectrographic analyses, focusing instead on analysis of fundamental frequency, formant frequencies (resonant frequencies of the vocal tract), dysphonation (aperiodic vibration of the vocal folds), and duration (*e.g.* Golub and Corwin 1985, Green and Gustafson 1989, Zeskind *et al.* 1996).

MEASURES FROM SOUND SPECTROGRAMS

The most elaborate system for using sound spectrography to analyze cries came from the Scandinavian research group (*e.g.* Michelsson *et al.* 1977). The system they used to generate these spectrograms was analog based, and the output was a piece of paper with the spectrogram literally burnt into it. To describe their measurement system, they developed a schematic spectrogram depicting the acoustic features they found useful in distinguishing normal and abnormal cries (Fig. 9.5).

One of the many interesting aspects of this analytic scheme is that so many of the features involve changes in the distribution of frequencies over time. Note that shift, vibrato, double harmonic break and gliding all are depicted as changes in the pattern of bands over time. It is precisely this kind of patterning that is difficult to quantify. Thus, at least some of the cry features that the Scandinavians found so useful are not the same ones that have occupied cry researchers using digital analysis techniques.

The cry features common to almost all analytic systems include cry duration and various parameters of the fundamental frequency of the cry. Especially important aspects of the fundamental frequency include its minimum and maximum value during the cry, the melody type (*e.g.* falling, rising, or rising–falling), and the occurrence of very low frequency voiced sounds (called glottal rolls in the spectrographic literature).

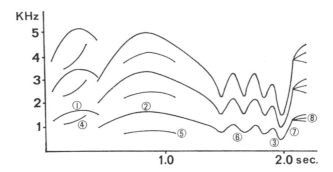

Fig. 9.5. A schematic spectrogram illustrating the features studied by the Scandinavian researchers (*e.g.* Michelsson *et al.* 1977) in preterm and term infants. 1 = shift; 2 = maximum pitch; 3 = minimum pitch; 4 = biphonation; 5 = double harmonic break; 6 = vibrato; 7 = glide; 8 = furcation.

The spectrogram is a very rich visual display, capturing three dimensions (time, frequency and amplitude) in a two-dimensional display. However, cry analysis via spectrography is basically a qualitative endeavor. The researcher must be trained to read the spectrograms; in fact, the analysis system described above was developed in collaboration with phoneticians and acousticians. Thus, learning to use the system effectively may be too burdensome for many researchers and/or clinicians. We could find no data on the amount of training necessary to reach adequate levels of expertise or interobserver agreement using this system.

MEASURES FROM DIGITAL FREQUENCY ANALYSES

Digital analysis of cry sounds relies on computers to manipulate huge quantities of information quickly and to distill it to a few summary measures. Most analysis systems rely on the fast Fourier transform (see above) as the basic analytic algorithm. It is in the reduction of the information obtained from the many FFTs performed on each cry sound that various laboratories differ.

Perhaps the most frequently used digital analysis system has been that of the Pediatric Diagnostic Service (PDS), a private company using Golub's (1980) model to analyze cries. The system used by the PDS is automated and, thus, confers the great advantage of speed in analyzing large numbers of cries. The system concentrates on a few acoustic parameters, especially duration of cry segments, fundamental frequency of the cry, percentage of time that the cry is phonated, dysphonated or hyperphonated, and estimated formant frequencies. These acoustic parameters are quite similar to those measured in other laboratories (*e.g.* Gustafson and Green 1989, Zeskind and Barr 1997).

The cry features measured from the spectrograph, and found to relate to neonatal health, are generally different from the cry features measured by computer. Furthermore, the cry features that are common to both analysis systems, such as fundamental frequency (F_0), are viewed in slightly different ways. In spectrographic analysis, melody type, shifts in fundamental frequency and vibrato of F_0 are measured in addition to maximum and minimum

F_0. In the digital analysis systems, it is more common to find *average* F_0 measured along with maximum and minimum F_0, while melody type, vibrato and shift are ignored.

In conclusion, the acoustic analysis of cry sounds remains largely unstandardized (for similar comments, see Raes *et al.* 1990). Not only are there very basic differences between spectrographic and digital analyses, but different laboratories may employ slightly different techniques for measuring the same parameter. Despite these differences, some consistent findings do emerge. These consistencies may be accounted for by the relation of certain cry features to CNS functioning, so it is appropriate to turn now to physiological models of cry production and their predictions about cry acoustics.

Models of cry production
The theory that underlies most acoustic analyses of cry sounds is the source–filter theory (Flanagan 1965, Fant 1973, Stevens 1998). This suggests that the waveform that impinges upon the listener's ear is a function of the characteristics of the source (in this case, the vibrating vocal cords) and its filters (in this case, the resonances of the supraglottal vocal tract and the radiation characteristics from the lips). Thus, the cry sound that one hears has acoustic characteristics that are attributable to the vocal cords, the nasopharyngeal pathway and radiation from the mouth across the air. (In most cry studies, the radiation effects are minimal, as cries are typically recorded at close distance to the infant; but see Gustafson *et al.* 1994).

Golub's (1980) physioacoustic model of crying was designed to select acoustic features that would identify infants at medical risk. The model assumes the source–filter theory, that is, that the acoustic waveform radiating from the infant's mouth is a function of its source, air from the lungs being pushed through the vocal folds of the larynx, and its filters, the rest of the vocal tract (Fig. 9.6).

The development of the physiological basis for cry *production* is the more interesting aspect of Golub's model. This physioacoustic model assumes three levels of central processing of the muscles contributing to the source and filters of crying. These three levels are identified as the upper, middle and lower processors. The upper processor is implicated in determining the state of the infant (*e.g.* fussiness). The middle processor is involved with the infant's vegetative states, such as swallowing, coughing, digestion and crying. The lower processor involves control of many muscle groups, including the subglottal, supraglottal, glottal and facial muscles. These muscle groups are coordinated in the act of crying.

A major assumption of the model is that the subglottal (respiratory), supraglottal (filter) and glottal (laryngeal) muscles are controlled independently. This assumption leads to the central hypothesis of the model, namely, that if these three muscle groups are controlled independently, then differences in the cry caused by any one of them can lead to the identification and diagnosis of abnormality specific to a pathology in that area. In fact, Golub proposed several cry 'tests' (Golub 1980, Golub and Corwin 1985) based on constellations of acoustic features. For example, there is a test for glottal instability, a test for constriction of the vocal tract, and a test for abnormal respiratory effort. These tests should reflect abnormalities in different locations in the CNS (Golub 1980), as the muscles associated with the glottis and the nasopharyngeal pathways are independently controlled. In particular,

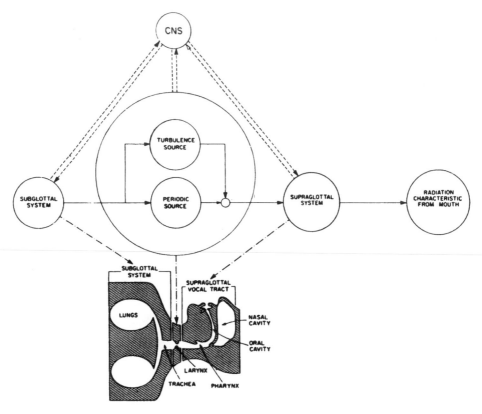

Fig. 9.6. A representation of Golub's physioacoustic model of infant crying.

Golub suggested that cranial nerve X (the vagus) is crucial in influencing glottal muscle processes and, hence, the modes of phonation of the cry and its fundamental frequency.

There have been elaborations of Golub's model, most importantly by Lester (1987), who adds cranial nerves IX, XI and XII to the vagus (X) as important to cry acoustics. These cranial nerves influence the muscles of the larynx, pharynx, chest and neck. Lester also suggests that the phrenic and thoracic nerves, and the source nuclei for these pathways, will affect cry acoustics. This elaboration of Golub's physioacoustic model continues to emphasize the fundamental frequency (both its average and variability) and the formant frequencies associated with the cry as critical measures reflecting CNS functioning.

A second physiological model that bears on cry production and acoustics is the physiological regulatory model of Porges *et al.* (1994). This model posits *vagal tone* as important to the expression and regulation of emotion. Research has shown that infant vagal tone is correlated with appropriate responses to novelty, with maternal ratings of difficultness, and with various developmental outcomes (Porges *et al.* 1995, Porges and Doussard-Roosevelt 1997).

The vagal system consists primarily of the vagus (the Xth cranial nerve), which has two branches. Each of the branches has two source nuclei, with fibers that originate in either the dorsal motor nucleus or the nucleus ambiguus. The nucleus ambiguus, the source nucleus of the right vagus, controls the larynx and sino-atrial node of the heart and is important, therefore, to both vocal intonation and vagal tone. Thus, vagal control of the right side of the larynx produces changes in vocal intonation as well as changes in heart rate, creating a cardiovascular state associated with specific emotions.

Porges' model proposes that emotions may originate either centrally or peripherally. That is, an emotion can be initiated by some internal event (*e.g.* illness) or by an external stimulus, and the course of emotional responding is then regulated (at least in part) by afferent feedback from visceral organs. However stimulated, the cerebral cortex activates the amygdala, after which the central nucleus of the amygdala stimulates the nucleus ambiguus. The nucleus ambiguus controls the vagus, which in turn regulates heart rate and vocal intonation by communicating with the sinoatrial node of the heart and the right side of the larynx.

This model suggests that the vagal system should be involved in the 'vocal intonation' associated with emotion. Although it is not stated explicitly in the model, one presumes that fundamental frequency is the main acoustic feature likely to be affected by vagal processes. Indeed, Porter *et al.* (1988) have shown a relation between baseline vagal tone and changes in fundamental frequency during neonatal circumcision. Developmental work involving the vagal system suggests that autonomic vagal control increases as the nervous system develops (Porges *et al.* 1996, Doussard-Roosevelt *et al.* 1997).

Yet another model of autonomic control of cry features is the two-part, 'biobehavioral' model of Lester and Zeskind (1982). Lester and Zeskind, building on the work of Truby and Lind (1965), distinguish between the *act* of crying and the *sound* of crying. The cry act and cry sound in this conceptualization tap different behavioral systems. Cry production is thought to be driven by the sympathetic nervous system, which is implicated in excitatory responses, and is thought to influence production characteristics such as the threshold to cry and the duration of sustained crying. Spectral components of the cry are driven by the parasympathetic nervous system, which is involved in inhibitory responses and influences acoustic characteristics of the sound (*e.g.* fundamental frequency, dysphonation) through regulation of the vagus.

According to this model, sympathetic and parasympathetic systems, acting in opposition when the infant is aroused, lead to acoustic outcomes such as frequent pitch shifts (*e.g.* from phonation to hyperphonation), thought to reflect poor organization/modulation of these systems in the infant. Thus, departures from the mean on either cry production (sympathetic system) or spectral characteristics (parasympathetic system) could reflect poor biobehavioral functioning.

In summary, all three models of cry production imply that the vagal system is the primary source of variations in cry acoustics. Deficits in either brainstem functioning or higher brain functioning may affect vagal control of the cry, producing abnormalities in cry acoustics, especially fundamental frequency. Golub suggests that respiratory influences are independent of laryngeal influences on cry acoustics. Although Porges' model is silent on this score, a logical extrapolation would be that respiratory and laryngeal functioning should *both* be affected by changes in activity of the right branch of the vagus. Finally, Zeskind's model adds arousability to crying as an additional feature of cry analysis, one that ought to reflect sympathetic influences of the CNS and be independent of parasympathetic influences on cry acoustics.

We turn now to look at how cry acoustics have been studied in relation to neonatal disease.

Relation of cry acoustics to health and development

It is noteworthy that these physiological models of cry production are relative latecomers on the cry research scene. Early cry researchers were interested in discriminating sick from healthy infants, but the rationale for these studies generally stemmed from anecdotal reports of sick infants having 'sick sounding' cries (Illingworth 1955; Karelitz and Fisichelli 1962; Lind 1965; Truby and Lind 1965; Wasz-Höckert *et al.* 1963, 1964a,b). An excellent review of early studies relating cry acoustics to disease has been published by Corwin *et al.* (1996). Rather than review these same studies again, we will summarize a few representative papers, concentrating on the value of cry analysis as a screening tool.

CRIES AND NEONATAL DISEASE

In 1971, Michelsson published a comprehensive study of cry analyses in 360 infants, aged 0–10 days. The infants were divided into three groups: 105 infants were 'low birthweight' (740–2500 g) without complications and with no signs of distress; 205 infants were 'asphyxiated', suffering respiratory failure or distress immediately after birth; and 50 were healthy, term neonates. Follow-up data revealed that three of the low birthweight infants *vs* 31 of the asphyxiated infants had died in the neonatal period. An additional 27 of the asphyxiated infants were neurologically abnormal at follow-up.

Spectrographic analysis was completed on pain cries elicited during the first 10 days of life. In the low birthweight group, there was more gliding (rapid change in F_0), more biphonation (evidence of two sound sources), and fewer glottal plosives (short phonations during the cry expiration) compared with the normal cries, as well as a higher maximum fundamental frequency (see Fig. 9.5). In the asphyxiated infants, there were longer durations of the cry sound, higher maximum F_0, more gliding, more bi-phonation and fewer glottal plosives. Furthermore, there appeared to be a relation between the degree of distress suffered by the asphyxiated infants and the amount of elevation in F_0 and increase in duration. This latter finding led to a scheme for scoring the number of abnormalities in a cry and relating that score to clinical outcome (more on this scheme is reported below).

Michelsson concluded this work with the suggestion that cry analysis might be useful in identifying infants who should be followed more closely after discharge from the hospital. Another suggestion was that cry analysis might be useful in judging the degree of distress, at least for infants with a peripheral locus of respiratory distress. Michelsson did not suggest that cry analysis would be helpful in the diagnosis *per se*, but rather, in helping the pediatrician make decisions about severity or risk.

Karelitz and Fisichelli (1962) studied 63 'unquestionably abnormal' infants and 201 healthy infants between the ages of 1 and 3 years. They elicited, or attempted to elicit, one minute of sustained crying from each infant, and then compared the groups on a set of measures relating to cry arousal. A hierarchical procedure was used to elicit the sustained cry. The first stimulus was the snap of a rubber band to the heel. For those infants who did not cry after five snaps, heel 'scratching' or 'flicking' was used in order to elicit a sustained cry.

The major summary variable in this study was whether the infant cried continuously for one minute. Only 53 of 201 normal infants failed to meet this criterion, but 48 of the 63 brain-damaged infants failed. Putting these numbers into a standard screening performance table, this cry 'test' yielded a sensitivity of 0.76 and a specificity of 0.74. (Predictive value is impossible to calculate without a prevalence estimate for their definition of 'abnormality'; however, estimating a prevalence of 5 per cent yields a predictive value of 0.13.)

The authors concluded that the amount of stimulation required to elicit sustained crying may be useful in diagnosing brain damage. They noted that predictive performance improves slightly when the youngest infants (0–4 days) are excluded and that the one-minute criterion may be too severe for infants older than 1 year.

Karelitz and Fisichelli's work served as part of the rationale for Zeskind's addition of sympathetic influences to his biobehavioral model of crying. In fact, Zeskind *et al.* (1996) used procedures very similar to those of Karelitz and Fisichelli in a recent study investigating the relation between amount of stimulation required to elicit crying and CNS regulation. Zeskind *et al.* divided a sample of 64 newborn infants into a normal threshold group and a high threshold group. The normal group required only one rubber band snap to elicit a 10 second sustained cry sample and the high group required three or more snaps (10 infants fell into the intermediate group and were excluded from the analysis). Infants in the high threshold group showed a different time series in their heart rates, measured over a two-hour period, as well as more behavioral startles and fewer state changes. The authors concluded that the heart rate and state data are indicative of homeostatic and regulatory irregularities and called for developmental investigations of both cry threshold and regulatory processes as they relate to temperament and other behavioral dimensions.

A final example of a study relating cry acoustics to concurrent measures of CNS function concerned lead exposure and cry acoustics. Rothenberg *et al.* (1995) correlated blood lead levels with several cry measures in a portion of the sample recruited for the Mexico City Prospective Lead Study. Blood lead levels were obtained during prenatal weeks 12, 20, 28 and 36, during delivery, and from the umbilical cord. Lead levels averaged about 9 mg/dL (SE about 0.5 mg/dL). Cry measures included median fundamental frequency, percentage of nasalization of the cry, and number of cries resulting from a heel flick at 2, 15 and 30 days after birth. Bivariate correlations and multiple regressions were employed to analyze the data. Sample sizes varied between 51 and 124 infants, depending on the date of the blood sample and age at the time of the cry recording. At least one of the cry measures was correlated with at least one of the lead measurements during at least one of the testing periods. Although it is difficult to know exactly how many correlations were computed, it appears that 11 of 54 possible correlations were statistically significant, with the median significant correlation being 0.165. A series of multiple regressions yielded adjusted R-square values in the range of 0.01–0.15, suggesting that no more than 15 per cent of the variance in cry acoustics could be accounted for by demographic variables and blood lead levels.

Given that other studies have shown the same kinds of relations between cry acoustics and prenatal cocaine, alcohol and marijuana exposure, the authors concluded that cry acoustics may provide an early marker of CNS damage by several toxic agents.

At the end of their review of studies relating cry acoustics to disease or developmental outcome, Corwin *et al.* (1996) conclude that studies of infants with known medical problems have "served to validate the concept that medical problems that affect the cry-production system do indeed result in changes in the acoustic characteristics of the cry" (p. 325). In other words, when infants are already *known* to have brain damage, their cries often have abnormal characteristics. These same characteristics, however, often appear in the cries of normal infants. Thus, the relations are not strong enough, either for measures of cry production or cry sound, to suggest that the cry, by itself, can be used as a screening tool.

CRIES AND SUDDEN INFANT DEATH SYNDROME (SIDS)

Given that a diagnosis of brain damage is never made on the basis of the cry alone, the more interesting problem concerns the value of the cry as a prognostic aid. One syndrome that has been of great interest to cry research is SIDS. Several case studies suggested that there were abnormal features in the cries of infants who died of SIDS (Stark and Nathanson 1975, Colton and Steinschneider 1980, Golub and Corwin 1982). These studies were the basis for a large prospective study conducted by Corwin *et al.* (1995).

Over a two-year period, cries from 21,880 infants were recorded in the newborn nurseries of 13 participating hospitals. Cries were elicited during routine blood studies or by heel flick and were analyzed by an automated computer program. Variables related to the timing of the cry sounds over a 30 second period, the modes of phonation of the cry (*e.g.* phonated, dysphonated, hyperphonated) and the cry frequencies were measured using the automated system at Pediatric Diagnostic Services. Twelve of the infants died of SIDS during their first year, or 0.6 per 1000. Only two acoustic variables were related to SIDS deaths; a high first formant and a high number of changes in mode of phonation. Combining these two features, 50 per cent of the SIDS deaths were correctly classified (sensitivity = 0.50) and there were 3729 false positives (specificity = 0.78). The best possible prediction system, using information obtained from the smaller set of infants who had two cry recordings, yielded a sensitivity of 0.556, a specificity of 0.963, and a predictive value of 0.01 (only five of 530 infants with abnormal cry features died of SIDS).

Given the low predictive value, the authors concluded that, at the present time, cry analysis is not a practical SIDS screening tool. They suggested, however, that cry analysis might improve prediction of SIDS when used in combination with other physiological measures, such as heart rate variability.

Summary of acoustics and neonatal disease

It is apparent from this large literature that infants with obvious brain damage often have cries that sound abnormal. Further, these cries show a variety of abnormal cry features, whether measured spectrographically or digitally. Specific cry features, however, have not been tightly linked to specific types of brain damage, and cry analysis does not appear to be a viable mechanism of screening for brain damage or other neonatal injuries and diseases.

Part of the 'fuzziness' in linking cry acoustics to neonatal outcomes lies in our level of understanding of the mechanisms of cry production. It is almost certain, for example, that a key assumption of Golub's physioacoustic model is incorrect: subglottal and glottal control processes are not independent. In fact, some recent work has suggested that the model of three independent components underlying cry production does not fit the acoustic data (Green *et al.* 1998). Further, the model of emotion regulation proposed by Porges is not specific enough to yield predictions about the vocal 'melodies' associated with abnormal vagal processes.

The broad distinction that Lester and Zeskind (1982) and Zeskind (1983) have made between parasympathetic control of cry acoustics and sympathetic control of cry arousal is intriguing and may provide another avenue for exploring the usefulness of cry analysis. An early study by Karelitz and Fisichelli (1962) showed that poor arousability is associated with brain damage. Zeskind *et al.* (1996) showed that infants who are difficult to arouse to a sustained cry have heart rate rhythms that are less complex, with fewer spectral peaks. These characteristics, Zeskind *et al.* argue, are like those of infants with regulatory disorders.

We suspect that analysis of cry acoustics, like so many other neonatal measures, will not stand on its own as a useful screening tool. The sound of the cry is the outcome of a complex interaction among specific CNS activity, general arousal level, the peripheral motor system and other unknown variables. Michelsson *et al.* (1977) suggested that cry analysis might be one more 'expedient' in the diagnosis of dysfunction. At this point, however, it remains unclear exactly what that role might entail. Used by an experienced clinician and cry researcher, the cry spectrogram may help to identify infants with more severe problems or who require more intense surveillance. Certainly, additional studies of cries, especially from a developmental point of view, will be useful in evaluating such a role.

Relation of cry acoustics to long-term outcome

Only two published studies were found that related neonatal cry features to long-term outcome. The first was that of Michelsson *et al.* (1977), who followed 45 newborns meeting criteria for asphyxiation until they were 2–8 years of age. One hundred and fifteen cries from these 45 infants were recorded in the neonatal period. Seventy-five control cries from 75 healthy infants were compared with the cries from the asphyxiated infants. Cries were elicited by a pinch to the upper arm or ear.

Data analysis indicated that the asphyxiated infants had significantly briefer cries, higher maximum and minimum fundamental frequencies, different melody patterns (primarily falling or rising–falling in controls, but frequent rising or falling–rising in asphyxiated infants) and more abnormal modes of phonation. These features are all consistent with brain damage.

Perhaps more interesting was their comparison of asphyxiated infants who were later healthy (32 infants yielding 70 cries) *vs* those with later neurological sequelae, including epileptic convulsions, mental retardation and even death (13 infants yielding 45 cries). There were differences between these two subgroups in the duration of cry sounds (shorter in damaged infants), minimum and maximum fundamental frequencies (higher in damaged infants), unstable fundamental frequencies (more frequent in damaged infants), and the likelihood of glottal rolls (less frequent in damaged infants). (Glottal roll is defined as a 'low frequency voiced sound'.)

Michelsson *et al.* concluded that cry analysis might be one additional way to assess the severity of brain damage resulting from severe asphyxia. They also suggested that the value of cry analysis can be enhanced by repeated recordings. Using two cases, they showed that an infant with abnormal cries at 2 days who had normal cry features at 8 days turned out to be healthy, whereas an infant with abnormal cry features at both 2 and 8 days developed cerebral palsy.

This critical follow-up study illustrates the difficulties inherent in relying on spectrographic methods for cry analysis. Although it is possible to see *differences* between asphyxiated infants who are later normal and those who are damaged, it is difficult to *quantify* the degree of abnormality of a given cry. It is possible, in principle, to have an expert (or an expert panel) categorize a cry spectrogram as abnormal, and thus trigger a surveillance or diagnostic regime for an infant. However, there are few qualified individuals available to make such judgments. Thus, the value of qualitative analysis in screening or diagnosis based on cry spectrograms is quite limited.

Michelsson *et al.* (1984) attempted to develop a cumulative cry score system using groups of preterm and term infants. Using the standard deviation of the acoustic characteristics of term infants' cries to create cut-offs, six different cry characteristics were scored as 0 (normal), 1 (1 SD away from the full-term cries), or 2 (2 SD away) for the preterm infants. These characteristics were duration, maximum and minimum fundamental frequencies, maximum pitch of shift, melody type, and phonation mode. Thus, a cry could be given a score ranging from 0 to 12.

The cry scores were then grouped into the categories of 0–1, 2–3, 4–5, and 6 or more. The subgroup of preterm infants with the most frequent cry abnormalities was the group with congenital hydrocephalus. Classifying the 84 cries from these 21 infants along with the 104 cries from 27 healthy term infants, it was possible to generate sensitivity and specificity scores for such an analysis system. Using a cry score of 2 or more as indicating abnormality, the sensitivity of this scoring system was 0.68, with a specificity of 0.64. While respectable, these values would not be clinically useful, with too many under-referrals (false negatives) and over-referrals (false positives). Furthermore, it should be noted that these clinical indices must be considered upper bounds, as the cut-off values for the cry features were generated using these very same data, and these infants showed the clearest abnormalities.

Spectrographic analysis of crying reached its zenith in the work of Michelsson *et al.* and the cry score scheme just outlined. Indeed, the results obtained for the prediction of adverse outcomes were quite impressive. As noted above, however, this technique is probably not widely applicable. The primary reason is time and effort. In order to apply this scheme, individuals with a great deal of training and experience are required to 'read' the spectrograms properly. Furthermore, a larger database of normal infants' cries would be required to establish its usefulness

A very different approach was taken by Lester (1987), in the second of the two studies that have used neonatal cry analysis to predict long-term outcome. Lester compared a sample of 13 normal, healthy newborns with a heteogeneous sample of 18 preterm infants. The preterm infants included a group with respiratory problems, a group with neurologic problems, and a group without problems. All of the preterm infants were born at less than 34 weeks gestational age (mean GA = 31.4 weeks, mean birthweight = 1614 g).

Although the age at cry recording was not specified, all preterm infants had to be in an open crib and free of intravenous catheters, and not past their expected due dates. Cries were recorded during the administration of the Brazelton Neonatal Behavioral Assessment Scale (Brazelton 1973). Additional neonatal measures included assessments of neurological and obstetric/postnatal complications. Developmental outcome was measured at 18 months corrected age using the Bayley Scales of Infant Development (Bayley 1969) and again at 5 years using the McCarthy Scales of Children's Abilities (McCarthy 1972). Cries were analyzed by an automated computer system (at Pediatric Diagnostic Service, Cambridge, MA). Acoustic features were grouped into three categories based on Golub's physioacoustic model, that is, into respiratory, glottal and nasopharyngeal measures.

For data analysis, the term and preterm infants were combined, and the combined group was divided at the median on the Bayley scales. The group was apparently also split at the median on the acoustic features. Using this procedure, 14 of 16 infants having high average fundamental frequencies scored low on the Bayley, compared with only one of 15 infants who had low average fundamental frequencies (sensitivity = 0.88, specificity = 0.93). Three other acoustic measures also significantly discriminated infants who scored high *vs* low on the Bayley, but not as impressively as the average fundamental frequency.

Similar procedures were used to relate acoustic measures to McCarthy scores for the 21 infants followed to 5 years of age. There was a statistically significant relationship between acoustic features and McCarthy scores for the General Cognitive Index (GCI) as well as the Verbal, Perceptual and Quantitative subscales. The strongest relationship appeared to be between average amplitude of the cry and the McCarthy GCI, with nine of 11 infants who had low-amplitude cries scoring low on the McCarthy (sensitivity = 0.82). In contrast, only one of 10 infants with high amplitude cries scored low on the McCarthy (specificity = 0.90).

There are several methodological issues that suggest these results should be viewed as preliminary. First, the sample sizes are very small. Second, the predictive value of the cry measures could not be assessed because of the sampling procedure. The prevalence rate is difficult to ascertain for a poor outcome defined in this manner, that is, as the bottom half of a sample distribution. Third, and related to this issue, is the definition of a poor outcome. No data are reported on the Bayley or McCarthy means for any of the groups, so it is unclear whether any of the infants met more traditional criteria of poor outcome, *e.g.* scoring 1 standard deviation below the mean. It is possible that all infants were functioning within the normal range. Finally, the groups were combined for the analysis, so it is possible that the relationship between cry and outcome is actually a relationship between preterm birth and outcome.

Lester reported that there were no significant correlations between acoustic features and the other neonatal measures (neurological risk, obstetrical complications) or with socioecomic status (SES), and it was not stated whether correlations between any of these measures and Bayley or McCarthy scores were calculated. It is unfortunate that no actual values were reported for these correlations. Given that the sample size was so small, a correlation of 0.40 between SES or birthweight and McCarthy GCI would be considered nonsignificant. Thus, it is possible that modest relationships between cry acoustics, other neonatal measures and developmental outcomes were present but not reported because the correlations did not reach conventional significance levels. It is also unfortunate that these possible moderating variables were not treated in the same manner as the acoustic variables (that is, with median splits and chi-square analysis), because it is impossible to compare the predictive value of cry acoustics versus SES, birthweight and other common predictors of poor developmental outcome.

Although tantalizing, the Lester (1987) study is very preliminary (as noted by the author). Lester used a very different cry analysis system than that employed by Michelsson *et al.* (1977). However, both studies reached similar conclusions, namely that cry analysis alone will not be a useful long-term predictor of developmental outcomes.

Future directions

We have reviewed the theory and practice of cry acoustic analysis, models of cry production, and representative empirical research relating cry acoustics to health and development. The questions now are what are the most profitable directions for future research, and what are the results likely to tell us? As noted at the beginning of the chapter, the study of newborn crying has largely been the study of the sound of single cry expirations following application of a painful (or perhaps startling) stimulus. Several directions for future research are outlined below.

(1) Systematic acoustic comparisons are needed between spontaneous cries and those elicited by painful stimuli. We simply do not have enough information to know whether crying initiated by external stimulation differs from that initiated by the infant. Although one can conceptualize all crying to be the result of some manner of stimulation, snaps of rubber bands, pinches and the like are relatively discrete, intense, exogenous stimuli and may initiate physiological and/or behavioral events that are different from continuous, endogenous stimuli such as hunger or an ear infection. Cries initiated by the pain of circumcision are *perceived* differently from those emitted before a feeding (G.E. Gustafson and J.A. Green, unpublished observations), but the acoustic features underlying that difference have not been clearly described.

(2) An additional window on CNS functioning might be provided by systematic comparisons of *changes* in the acoustics of cries over the course of a bout of crying. Most studies to date have examined either the first one or two expirations following a painful stimulus or have averaged over several expirations to arrive at summary measures of cry acoustics. Yet, the acoustics of cries elicited by painful stimuli change over the course of the first few expirations (Thodén and Koivisto 1980), and the time course of these changes may reflect self-regulatory abilities of the infant and even the balance of sympathetic and parasympathetic activity.

(3) The motor components of crying should be studied along with the acoustic components. Facial expressions and limb movements have been shown to affect how cries are perceived

(Irwin *et al.* 1997), but there has been no research on possible linkages between these components of crying and CNS activity.

(4) Developmental studies of crying are sorely needed. Although there have been developmental investigations of *amount* of crying (see Barr 1990), there are precious few developmental investigations of cry acoustics (for a review, see Chapter 11). It is noteworthy that Michelsson *et al.* (1977) and others have suggested that the value of cry analysis in infant diagnosis will be greatly enhanced through longitudinal investigations of crying that examine the relationships between changes in cry acoustics and changes in infant health.

(5) New technologies for the acoustic analysis of cries should be pursued. For example, 'jitter' and 'shimmer' are two measures of small, rapid changes in the fundamental frequency measurable from digitized cry samples (Grauel *et al.* 1990, Lüdge and Rothgänger 1990, Fuller *et al.* 1994). Jitter is a measure of peak-to-peak differences in the duration of each cycle of the fundamental frequency, whereas shimmer is a measure of peak-to-peak differences in the amplitude of each cycle of the fundamental frequency.

Grauel *et al.* (1990) presented data on 36 infants, 14 born at term and 22 preterm. Using independently derived cut-off values for normal, intermediate and abnormal jitter scores, Grauel *et al.* compared outcome at 2 years for the infants classified into the three jitter categories. (Outcome at 2 years was classified as normal, moderately impaired or severely impaired, based on clinical judgment.) Predicting severe impairment from abnormal jitter scores yielded sensitivity of 0.67, specificity of 0.83 and predictive value of 0.44. These indices appear promising for clinical use, but the prevalence of severe impairment is much lower than their sample rate of 0.17, so the predictive value of their jitter measure would be significantly lower in the general population. Nevertheless, the new acoustic measures will be worth investigating alongside the more 'classic' spectrographic and digital measures.

(6) If the clinical focus could be narrowed somewhat, the value of cry acoustics might also be enhanced. Here, one possibility lies in the detection of vocal tract pathology. Hirschberg (1990) summarizes the acoustic features (measured spectrographically) and auditory perceptions associated with various pathologies and noninflammatory diseases of the larynx. He suggests that acoustic analysis can augment traditional, invasive endoscopic methods of diagnosis. Further, he argues that acoustic analyses might be of particular value in tracing the course of the disease and/or in monitoring the results of drug treatment or surgery.

(7) In addition to the foregoing directions focusing on the value of cry acoustics, models of cry production should receive more attention. As we have noted, some key assumptions of these models are probably incorrect, and future investigations should be directed at the relationships among cry acoustics, heart rate, respiration, vagal tone and even brain activity. These efforts will probably require collaboration of neonatologists, speech pathologists, radiologists, psychologists and others. Incorporating new acoustic measures like jitter and shimmer into the cry production models should enhance our understanding of their promise for clinical use.

(8) New models should be borrowed from the developmental literature in order to better understand the uncertainties inherent in prediction of long-term outcomes from neonatal measures. A traditional linear model that assumes direct cause and effect from some indicator

to later difficulty has been noted by Sameroff and Chandler (1975) to be insufficient for predicting the outcomes of hypoxia, preterm birth and infant temperament. Social factors such as the parents' level of education and socioeconomic status were identified as the best predictors of later intellectual development by Sameroff and Chandler. Even our best measures of cognitive functioning early in infancy account for only a small amount of the variance of later functioning (*e.g.* Thompson *et al.* 1991). Moreover, it appears that our acoustic measures of crying are not as reliable as our measures of information processing skills (*e.g.* habituation and attention to novelty).

The exciting possibility is that the study of crying will take a central place in broader theories of infant adaptation and development. Cry analysis, broadly conceived, could play a key role in the measurement of constructs like irritability, temperament and adaptability. Current theories of temperament, for example, suggest that a broad array of physiological measures should be integrated with more traditional measures (Rothbart and Bates 1998). In addition to its potential role in social and personality development, cry research could address issues related to general communication skills and prelinguistic development. Infant crying, and the social interactions it engenders, are hypothesized to foster the development of pragmatic language skills prior to the appearance of first words (Gustafson and Green 1991). Indeed, there are few behaviors as ubiquitous, and long lasting, in the course of human development as crying. It is time to capitalize on this fact and ask cry researchers both to help us understand basic developmental processes and to address clinical issues.

ACKNOWLEDGEMENTS

We thank Ron Barr for his comments on an earlier draft. Work on the manuscript was supported by a grant from the University of Connecticut Research Foundation to the first author.

REFERENCES

Barr, R.G. (1990) 'The normal crying curve: what do we really know?' *Developmental Medicine and Child Neurology*, **32**, 356–362.

Bayley, N. (1969) *Bayley Scales of Infant Development*. San Antonio, TX: Psychological Corporation.

Brazelton, T.B. (1973) *Neonatal Behavioral Assessment Scale. Clinics in Developmental Medicine No. 50*. London: Spastics International Medical Publications.

Colton, R. H., Steinschneider, A. (1980) 'Acoustic relationships of infant cries to sudden infant death syndrome.' *In:* Murry, T., Murry, J. (Eds.) *Infant Communication: Cry and Early Speech*. Houston: College-Hill, pp. 183–208.

Corwin, M.J., Lester, B.M., Sepkoski, C., Peucker, M., Kayne, H., Golub, H.L. (1995) 'Newborn acoustic cry characteristics of infants subsequently dying of sudden infant death syndrome.' *Pediatrics*, **96**, 73–77.

—— —— Golub, H.L. (1996) 'The infant cry: What can it tell us?' *Current Problems in Pediatrics*, **26**, 325–334.

Denes, P.B., Pinson, E.N. (1973) *The Speech Chain: The Physics and Biology of Spoken Language*. Garden City, NY: Anchor Press.

Droussard-Roosevelt, J.A., Porges, S.W., Scanlon, J.W., Alemi, B., Scanlon, K.B. (1997) 'Vagal regulation of heart rate in the prediction of developmental outcome for very low birthweight preterm infants.' *Child Development*, **68**, 173–186.

Fant, G. (1973) *Speech Sounds and Features*. Cambridge, MA: MIT Press.

Flanagan, J.L. (1965) *Speech Analysis, Synthesis, and Perception*. New York: Academic Press.

Fuller, B.F., Keefe, M.R., Curtin, M. (1994) 'Acoustic analysis of cries from "normal" and "irritable" infants.' *Western Journal of Nursing Research*, **16**, 243–253.

Golub, H.L. (1980) 'A physioacoustic model of the infant cry and its use for medical diagnosis and prognosis.' Doctoral dissertation, Massachusetts Institute of Technology, Boston.

—— Corwin, M.J. (1982) 'Infant cry: A clue to diagnosis.' *Pediatrics*, **69**, 197–201.

—— —— (1985) 'A physioacoustic model of the infant cry.' *In:* Lester, B.M., Boukydis, C.F.Z. (Eds.) *Infant Crying: Theoretical and Research Models.* New York: Plenum, pp. 59–82.

Grauel, E.L., Höck, S., Rothgänger, H. (1990) 'Jitter-index of the fundamental frequency of infant cry as a possible diagnostic tool to predict future developmental problems. Part 2: Clinical considerations.' *Early Child Development and Care*, **65**, 23–30

Green, J.A., Gustafson, G.E. (1990) 'Interrelations among the acoustic features of cries: How many features do we need?' *Early Child Development and Care*, **65**, 31–44.

—— —— Irwin, J.R., Kalinowski, L.L., Wood, R.M. (1995) 'Infant crying: Acoustics, perception, and communication.' *Early Development and Parenting*, **4**, 161–175.

—— —— McGhie, A.C. (1998) 'Changes in infants' cries as a function of time in a cry bout.' *Child Development*, **69**, 271–279.

Gustafson, G.E., Green, J.A. (1989) 'On the importance of fundamental frequency and other acoustic features in cry perception and infant development.' *Child Development*, **60**, 772–780.

—— —— (1991) 'Developmental coordination of cry sounds with visual regard and gestures.' *Infant Behavior and Development*, **15**, 51–57.

—— —— Cleland, J.W. (1994) 'Robustness of individual identity in the cries of human infants.' *Developmental Psychobiology*, **27**, 1–9.

Hirschberg, J. (1990) 'The values of the acoustic analysis of pathological infant cry and breathing noise in everyday practice.' *Early Child Development and Care*, **65**, 57–70.

Illingworth, R.S. (1955) 'Crying in infants and children.' *British Medical Journal*, **75**, 75–78

Irwin, J., Gustafson, G.E., Green, J.A. (1997) 'Age changes in relation to facial and vocal cues to distress.' *Paper presented at the 6th International Workshop on Infant Cry Research, Bowness-on-Windermere, July 4, 1997.*

Karelitz, S., Fisichelli, V.R. (1962) 'The cry thresholds of normal infants and those with brain damage.' *Journal of Pediatrics*, **61**, 679685.

Lester, B.M. (1987) 'Developmental outcome prediction from acoustic cry analysis in term and preterm infants.' *Pediatrics*, **80**, 529–534.

—— Zeskind, P.S. (1982) 'A biobehavioral perspective on crying in early infancy.' *In:* Fitzgerald, H.E., Lester, B.M., Yogman, M.W. (Eds.), Theory and research in behavioral pediatrics, 1. (pp.133180) New York: Plenum Press.

Lind, J. (Ed.) (1965) 'Newborn infant cry.' *Acta Paediatrica Scandinavica*, Suppl. 163, 1–132.

Lüdge, W., Rothgänger, H. (1990) 'Early diagnosis of CNS disturbance from computer analysis of infant cries: A new method of fundamental frequency jitter computation with high resolution in frequency and time.' *Early Child Development and Care*, **65**, 83–90.

McCarthy, D. (1972) *McCarthy Scales of Children's Abilities.* San Antonio, TX: Psychological Corporation.

Michelsson, K. (1971) 'Cry analyses of symptomless low birth weight neonates and of asphyxiated newborn infants.' *Acta Paediatrica Scandinavica*, Suppl. 216, 11–40.

—— (1980) 'Cry characteristics in sound spectrographic analysis.' *In:* Murry, T., Murry, J. (Eds.) *Infant Communication: Cry and Early Speech.* Houston: College-Hill, pp. 85–105.

—— Sirviö, P., Wasz-Höckert, O. (1977) 'Pain cry in fullterm asphyxiated newborn infants correlated with late findings.' *Acta Paediatrica Scandinavica*, **66**, 611–616.

—— Raes, J., Rinne, A. (1984) 'Cry score—an aid in infant diagnosis.' *Folia Phoniatrica*, **36**, 219–224.

Nowicki, S., Nelson, D.A. (1990) 'Defining natural categories in acoustic signals: Comparison of three methods applied to 'chick-a-dee' call notes.' *Ethology*, **86**, 89–101.

Porges, S.W., Doussard-Roosevelt, J.A. (1997) 'Early physiological patterns and later behavior.' *In:* Reese, H.W., Franzen, M.D. (Eds.) *Biological and Neuropsychological Mechanisms: Life-span Developmental Psychology.* Mahwah, NJ: Erlbaum, pp. 163–179.

—— —— Maita, A.K. (1994) *Vagal Tone and the Physiological Regulation of Emotion. Monographs of the Society for Research in Child Development, Vol. 59, Nos. 2–3.* Chicago: University of Chicago Press.

—— —— Portales, L.A., Suess, P.E. (1995) 'Cardiac vagal tone: Stability and relation to difficultness in infants and 3-year-olds.' *Developmental Psychobiology*, **27**, 289–300.

—— —— —— Greenspan, S.I. (1996) 'Infant regulation of the vagal 'brake' predicts child behavior problems: A psychobiological model of social behavior.' *Developmental Psychobiology*, **29**, 697–712.

Porter, F.L., Porges, S.W., Marshall, R. (1988) 'Newborn pain cries and vagal tone: Parallel changes in response to circumcision.' *Child Development*, **59**, 495–505.

Potter, R., Kopp, G.A., Gren, H.C. (1947) *Visible Speech*. New York: Van Nostrand.

Raes, J., Dehaen, F., Despontin, M. (1990) 'Towards a standardized terminology and methodology for the measurement of durational pain cry characteristics.' *Early Child Development and Care*, **65**, 127–138.

Rothbart, M.K., Bates, J.E. (1998) 'Temperament.' *In:* Eisenberg, N. (Ed.) *The Handbook of Child Psychology. 5th Edn. Vol. 3. Social, Emotional and Personality Development*. New York: Wiley, pp. 105–176.

Rothenberg, S.J., Cansino, S., Sepkoski, C., Torres, L.M., Medina, S., Schnaas, L., Poblano, A., Karchmer, S. (1995) 'Prenatal and perinatal lead exposures alter acoustic cry parameters of neonate.' *Neurotoxicology and Teratology*, **17**, 151–160.

Sameroff, A.J., Chandler, M. (1975) 'Reproductive risk and the continuum of caretaking casualty.' *In:* Horowitz, F.D., Hetherington, M., Scarr-Salapatek, S., Siegel, G. (Eds.) *Review of Child Development Research. Vol. IV*. Chicago: University of Chicago Press, pp. 187–244.

Stark, R.E., Nathanson, S. (1975) 'Unusual features of cry in an infant dying suddenly and unexpectedly.' *In:* Bosma, J.F., Showacre, J. (Eds.) *Development of Upper Respiratory Anatomy and Function*. U.S. Department of Health and Welfare Publication No. NIH 75-941, pp. 233–249.

Stevens, K.N. (1998) *Acoustic Phonetics*. Cambridge, MA: MIT Press.

Thodén, C-J., Koivisto, M. (1980) 'Acoustic analyses of the normal pain cry.' *In:* Murry, T., Murry, J. (Eds.) *Infant Communication: Cry and Early Speech*. Houston: College-Hill, pp. 124–151.

Thompson, L.A. , Fagan, J.F., Walker, D.W. (1991) 'Longitudinal predictions of specific cognitive abilities from infant novelty preference.' *Child Development*, **62**, 503–538.

Truby, H., Lind, J. (1965) 'Cry sounds of the newborn infant.' *Acta Paediatrica Scandinavica*, **163**, 7–59.

Wasz-Höckert, O., Valanne, E., Vuorenkoski, V., Michelsson, K. Sovijärvi, A. (1963) 'Analysis of some types of vocalization in the newborn and in early infancy.' *Annales Paediatriae Fenniae*, **9**, 1–10.

—— Partanen, T.J., Vuorenkoski, V., Michelsson, K, Valanne, E. (1964a) 'The identification of some specific meanings in infant vocalization.' *Experientia*, **20**, 154.

—— —— —— Valanne, E., Michelsson, K. (1964b) 'Effect of training on ability to identify preverbal vocalizations.' *Developmental Medicine and Child Neurology*, **6**, 393–396.

—— Lind, J., Vuorenkoski, V., Partanen, T., Valanne, E. (1968) *The Infant Cry: A Spectrographic and Auditory Analysis. Clinics in Developmental Medicine No. 29*. London: Spastics International Medical Publications.

Zeskind, P.S. (1983) 'Production and spectral analysis of neonatal crying and its relation to other biobehavioral systems in the infant at risk.' *In:* Field, T., Sostek, A. (Eds.) *Infants Born at Risk*. New York: Grune & Stratton, pp. 23–43.

—— Barr, R.G. (1997) 'Acoustic characteristics of naturally-occurring cries of infants with 'colic'.' *Child Development*, **68**, 394–403.

—— Marshall, T.R., Goff, D.M. (1996) 'Cry threshold predicts regulatory disorder in newborn infants.' *Journal of Pediatric Psychology*, **21**, 803–819.

10
CRYING IN INFANT PRIMATES: INSIGHTS INTO THE DEVELOPMENT OF CRYING IN CHIMPANZEES

Kim A. Bard

'Crying' is a common feature of infants among most primate species (Newman 1985). Or, to be more accurate, most primate infants emit some specific types of vocalizations upon separation from their mother, or upon physical discomfort and/or injury. We might say that some species of nonhuman primate infants emit pain cries and discomfort cries, much like human infants.

Crying in nonhuman primates is often thought of differently than crying in human infants. Recent books that include references to infant crying do not focus on crying *per se* but rather discuss crying in the context of aspects of nonverbal vocal communication. These other aspects include developmental and comparative approaches to the study of vocal communication (Papousek *et al.* 1992), the evolution of communication (Hauser 1996), social influences on vocal development (Snowdon and Hausberger 1997), and the influence of nature and culture on nonverbal communication (Segerstrale and Molnar 1997). One theme of importance in regard to primate vocalizations is the link with language in humans. This focus on discovering parallels between primate vocalizations and human verbalization includes research on the referential nature of certain vocalizations, such as calls to recruit help during agonistic encounters (*e.g.* Gouzoules *et al.* 1984) and alarm calls emitted by vervet monkeys to specific predators (Seyfarth *et al.* 1980). Another theme within the area of primate vocalization is flexibility in the development of calls (*e.g.* Hopkins and Savage-Rumbaugh 1991). This includes research on cross-fostering experiments (*e.g.* Owren *et al.* 1993), operant conditioning of calls (*e.g.* Owren and Rendall 1997), and individual differences in calls (Mitani *et al.* 1996) and in 'dialects' (*e.g.* Mitani *et al.* 1992).

In reviewing the literature on primate vocal communication, however, it is often difficult to ascertain the meaning or function served by a vocalization because researchers avoid the use of functional terms, and do so for a variety of reasons. In some cases, only the *acoustic structure* of the vocalization is used as an identifier. For example, 'smooth early high' and 'smooth late high' are two types of 'coos' emitted by Japanese macaques that are distinguished by when the peak fundamental frequency occurs during the course of the cry (Green 1975). Others label the vocalization by the *distinctive context* in which it occurs. For example, 'isolation calls' are those produced by infant squirrel monkeys when put in a room alone after being separated from the mother (Newman 1985). Many studies of primate vocalizations are focused on identifying the *evolutionary foundations of language*. These tend to focus on aspects of the vocalization that have implications for the evolution of linguistics, such as the question of categorical versus graded signals, and whether primate communication is referential. Finally, some researchers study facial and vocal expressions as ways to convey the *emotional and/or motivational aspects* of the behavior (*e.g.* Goodall 1986: Masataka and Kohda 1988).

Problems when studying nonhuman primates

My interest in crying stems from studies that I conducted from 1983 to 1995 on emotional development and intentional communication in nonhuman primates, specifically chimpanzees and orangutans, two species of great ape. I admit to being frustrated by those accounts of primate vocal communication that omit the context(s) in which the vocalization naturally occurs, and/or do not describe the social/communicative function(s) typical of the calls. (Note that this is also true of some ethological accounts of primate behavior in general, in which the form of the action is described in detail, but the reader has little idea of the 'meaning' of the behavior.) For example, you need to be an experienced chimpanzee observer to know that, if a chimpanzee is described as displaying extreme piloerection while its lips are bulging and compressed and it is running, this represents an angry facial expression, and probably an aggressive, charging behavioral display. Helpfully, some of the early ethograms of chimpanzee communicative behaviors combined approaches and gave both spectrographic analysis and detailed behavioral accounts of the context and typical social outcomes associated with vocalizations (*e.g.* van Hooff 1973).

There are many good reasons why researchers have been cautious about attributing mental processes, emotions or intentions to nonverbal primates (this applies to both nonhuman and very young human infants). First, emotional states are given different labels in nonhuman primates to clearly distinguish them from their human counterparts until clear evidence is found of comparability. Second, we sometimes give them different labels because there are some distinguishing characteristics. However, from my perspective of studying the development of emotions, the term used to describe a vocalization or facial expression should be one that describes the emotional meaning, so that it is easier to understand the underlying emotional nature of the expressive behavior. My preference is to give the functional nature precedence, rather than relying on morphological similarities.

This can be illustrated by the continuing controversy concerning 'smiles'. In chimpanzees, the facial expression that accompanies play-chasing, tickling and laughing is sometimes called a 'relaxed open mouth display' (van Hooff 1973), a 'playface full' or 'playface half' (Plooij 1984), or a smile (Yerkes and Yerkes 1929, van Lawick-Goodall 1968, Bard 1998). The chimpanzee smile, however, does not look like a human smile (Fig. 10.1). In chimpanzees, the jaw is dropped open, the lower teeth are exposed, the upper teeth are covered, and the lip corners may be retracted. I choose to call this facial expression a smile for three reasons: first, it occurs in relaxed social contexts accompanying 'happiness'; second, it is the facial expression that accompanies the vocalization 'laughter', and both the facial expression and the vocalization can reliably be elicited by tickling; and third, it is species-typical, *i.e.* evident in all chimpanzees in the wild and in captivity, and in chimpanzees of all ages (for more details on the development of emotions and the influence of rearing environments,

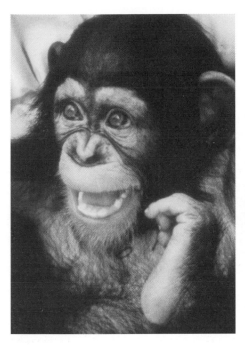

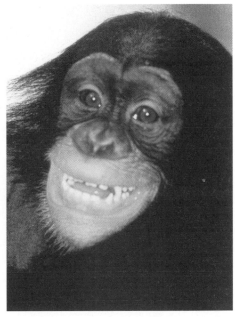

Fig. 10.1. A prototypic species-typical chimpanzee smile, the facial expression accompanying 'laughter' in play and tickling. (Photo by K.A. Bard.)

Fig. 10.2. The 'fear grimace' is an expression indicative of extreme excitement, in which the context determines the positive or negative valence. (Photo by E. Ferorelli.)

see Bard and Gardner 1996, Bard 1998). The chimpanzee facial expression that is more morphologically (but not functionally) similar to a human smile is called the 'fear grimace' (Fig. 10.2), an expression that is indicative of extreme excitement (with either a positive or negative valence). A chimpanzee may 'fear grimace' at the sight of a bunch of bananas and at the sight of an approaching aggressive rival. This comparison of function and morphology with regard to the smile and fear grimace respectively serves as an excellent example of why I describe facial and vocal expressions with the appropriate emotional term rather than by means of terms that may describe similar morphology.

Distress vocalizations and parenting in chimpanzees
In chimpanzee infants, distress vocalizations can occur from birth and are accompanied by facial expressions. Different expressions are indicative of different degrees of distress. Mild distress can be exhibited with "hoo" vocalizations and/or a 'pout face' (Fig. 10.3). Moderate distress is expressed with "hoo" whimpers and a 'whimper face' (Fig. 10.4). Severe distress is expressed with a scream face and crying (Fig. 10.5). I call the mild and moderate distress, 'fussing', and the severe distress, 'crying'. The pout face typically accompanies discrete hoos whereas the more continuous whimpering hoos accompany the facial expression seen in Figure 10.4. In contrast, cries (often called screams) are shrill and loud, with a more

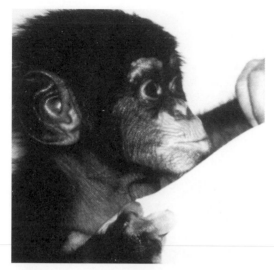

Fig. 10.3. The pout face is indicative of mild distress and accompanies fussy "hoo" vocalizations. (Photo by K.A. Bard.)

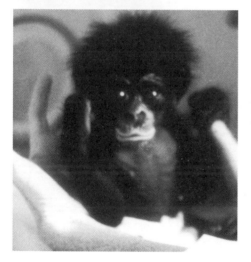

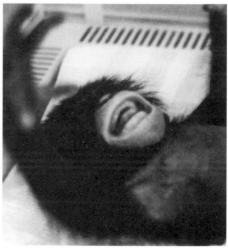

Fig. 10.4. The whimper face is indicative of moderate distress and accompanies fussy "hoo" whimpers. (Photo by K.A. Bard.)

Fig. 10.5. The scream face is indicative of severe distress and accompanies crying in the very young chimpanzee. (Photo by J. Schneider.)

piercing quality than human baby cries, but easily discernable as distress cries by undergraduate psychology students. With crying, one of the most obvious dissimilarities between human and nonhuman primates is that humans produce tears while crying, whereas no other primate does.

In terms of parenting of infants, the most relevant distinction in crying behavior between chimpanzees and humans is very clearly illustrated by the experience of raising my own son. (Perhaps it should be noted that I have direct experience with the parenting of over 50 chimpanzee infants.) My son exhibited bouts of inconsolable crying from 6 to 18 weeks of age. Human infants often cry, sometimes with no discernable cause (see also Chapter 4). For some human babies, there are periods when there seems to be nothing that a caregiver can do to help them calm. Chimpanzee infants can cry, sometimes even for extended periods of time (minutes to hours), but only when they are out of physical contact with a caregiver. Chimpanzees, in contrast to many human infants, rarely cry while being cradled or carried in the arms of their primary caregiver. If they cry because they are not in physical contact with the caregiver, then crying stops within seconds when the caregiver picks up the chimpanzee infant.

In instances of inadequate maternal caregiving, infant chimpanzees can fuss and cry for most or all of an hour-long observation period. I observed a mother chimpanzee nurse her infant and then gently place her on the floor and move to the other side of the enclosure. The infant fussed and then cried, and propelled herself across the floor with reflexive crawling movements that amounted to rather jerky lurches. Finally, after minutes of crying and moving, the infant would be in close proximity to the mother, who would then get up and move away. After two or three of these cycles, the infants' cries would become more intense. The mother would pick up the infant when she arrived close by, let her nurse, and then gently remove her and place her on the floor again. When the infant was about 3 months old, she was severely injured with a bite to her thigh and placed in the nursery. Although none of the research observers wished her to be injured, we were all relieved to have this baby removed from the very stressful situation caused by inadequate maternal care (for more details about parenting in chimpanzees, see Bard 1994a, 1995). It is worth noting that this chimpanzee was successfully integrated into a chimpanzee social group when she was approximately 4 years old.

The point of this story is that very young infant chimpanzees do have the capacity for sustained crying, but I have observed it only in situations of inadequate care, when the infant is out of physical contact with the mother, or when the mother is engaging in atypical behavior (such as overgrooming the infant). When young infant chimpanzees are placed in the nursery (usually when the mother has no maternal skills and does not even pick up the infant after it is born), infants fuss and cry when they are hungry, are in pain, or need physical contact. Once they are picked up, however, they do not continue to cry. Fussiness may continue until they are fed if they are hungry, but otherwise nursery-raised infant chimpanzees do not continue to fuss once they are picked up and held. In human infants, crying can continue after picking up, even after the infant is swaddled, rocked and given something to suck, and when the infant is not hungry. When crying continues for long periods of time and parental behaviors do not consistently calm the infant, we label this behavior 'colic'. Colic seems to be exceedingly rare in chimpanzees. Note that I am referring to crying in very young infant chimpanzees before the onset of separation anxiety (that occurs in chimpanzees between 6 and 8 months and is manifest in similar types of behavioral distress as seen in human infants between 7 and 9 months).

Chimpanzees and emotional development
Chimpanzees are the most emotionally expressive of the nonhuman primates, and therefore

are good models for the study of the development of emotional expressions. Chimpanzees have expressions that parallel those in humans, including smiling, laughter, anger, pouting, surprise, excitement and crying (van Lawick-Goodall 1968). Chimpanzees negotiate social interactions with emotional displays of the face and body posture (Goodall 1986). In the neonatal period, we can identify smiles, laughter, anger, pouting, threat, greetings and crying with and without vocalizations (Bard 1998). In addition, one can identify a characteristic emotional mood of a chimpanzee (*i.e.* temperament). 'Temperament' can also be identified in rhesus monkeys (Stevenson-Hinde and Zunz 1978). In the chimpanzee at least, it is flexible early in life; that is, an individual's characteristic mood is modifiable as a result of differential rearing within the first year of life (Bard and Gardner 1996). This flexibility is important because, like the flexibility in vocal expression, it is a demonstration that emotional expression in chimpanzees, as in human infants, is the result of the interaction between inborn characteristics and the environment.

The 'normal curve' and crying in chimpanzee infants

Other chapters in this volume attest to the widespread interest in crying in human infants. Particularly fascinating is the period between birth and 3 months of age when many normally developing infants have periods of inconsolable crying, particularly in the evening hours (Barr 1990; see also Chapter 4). These periods of fussiness and crying show a developmental pattern with a peak around 6 weeks of age and a noticeable decrease by 12 weeks. Caregiving regimes may affect the length of crying within a bout but appear not to affect the number of crying bouts in a day (Hunziker and Barr 1986, Barr *et al.* 1991). For example, in the !Kung San who practice caregiving regimes consisting of almost continuous physical contact and carrying, infants typically cry for only seconds to a few minutes at a time. In contrast, in many middle class communities in North America with caregiver regimes consisting of less carrying, infants typically cry for many minutes at a time in prolonged bouts. In addition, Barr *et al.* (1989) suggest that type of feeding may contribute to some aspects of crying (switching from breast to bottle-feeding may decrease the amount of night-time crying). Regardless of feeding type and environment, however, the basic finding is that human infants cry for many minutes (up to hours) per day when very young, and exhibit a peak in cry bout duration and total crying at around 6 weeks of age.

In the remainder of this chapter, I report results of my studies into the developmental pattern of crying behavior in chimpanzees. In general, the goal was to compare the development of crying across the first 12 weeks of life in chimpanzees with that of humans. In addition, I studied young chimpanzees raised under different caregiving regimes, to explore the effect of differential rearing environments on their crying. Finally, I wanted to establish objectively whether or not 'colic' (*i.e.* inconsolable crying) occurs in chimpanzee infants.

The chimpanzee studies

Chimpanzees born and raised at the Yerkes Regional Primate Research Center of Emory University were the subjects for my studies. I wanted to observe infants who were living with their mothers in order to gain a perspective on more naturally occurring interactions. I also wanted to observe infants who were living in the nursery environment (that is,

TABLE 10.1
Maternal parity, behaviors coded, and cagemates of mother–infant chimpanzee subjects

Mother–infant	Live births	Behaviors coded		Cagemates*
		State	Soothing	
Joice–Olin	2	√	√	1 A♀, 1 A♂
Leslie–Dara	1	√	√	1 A♀, 1 J, 1 inf
Vivienne–Wilma	1	√	√	3 A♀, 1 A♂, 1 inf
Barbi–Elvira	0	√	√	3 A♀, 1 A♂, 1 inf
Lil'One–Pollyanna	3	√	√	4 A♀, 1 A♂, 1 J, 2 inf
Cynthia–Alicia	0		√	4 A♀, 1 A♂, 1 J, 2 inf
Cissie–Travis	0		√	2 A♀, 1 A♂, 2 adol♀, 1 inf
Banana–Ronald	2	√		Temporarily alone
Barbara–Kevin	1		√	2 A♀, 1 A♂, 1 adol♀, 1 adol♂
Erica–Virginia	2		√	4 A♀, 1 A♂, 1 J, 2 inf
Tai–Daisey	4		√	4 A♀, 1 A♂, 1 J, 2 inf

*A = adult; adol = adolescent; J = juvenile; inf = infant.

separated from their mothers) because, in the nursery, I was able to conduct standard behavioral tests by means of the Neonatal Behavioral Assessment Scale (NBAS) devised by Brazelton (1984). Note that infants were placed in the nursery only when their mothers did not exhibit adequate maternal care, a condition that I suggest is due to limited experience with infants during pre-adulthood (for further discussion of parenting in primates, see Bard 1995). In contrast, those chimpanzees who were raised by their biological mother were observed with naturalistic methods because handling by humans puts the infant at risk for at least two reasons. First, anaesthesia would be required to remove the infant from the mother which carries a risk. Second, once the infant is removed there is an additional risk that the mother would not take the infant back at all even upon recovery from the anaesthesia.

MATERNAL SOOTHING AND INFANT STATE OBSERVATIONS

Ten infants were raised by their biological mothers who exhibited adequate maternal care (Bard 1994a). The mother–infant pairs were housed with other chimpanzees in indoor–outdoor enclosures [the indoor area was either 8 ft × 8 ft × 8 ft (2.4 m × 2.4 m × 2.4 m) or 8 ft × 10 ft × 10 ft (2.4 m × 3.0 m × 3.0 m); the outdoor area was either 8 ft × 14 ft × 8 ft (2.4 m × 3.6 m × 2.4 m) or 10 ft × 10 ft × 15 ft (3.6 m × 3.6 m × 3.8 m)]. The subject names, maternal parity, and composition of cagemates are listed in Table 10.1. From the mother-raised infants, hour-long observations were conducted during the first months of life. These observations involved no manipulation of the mother–infant pair, the subjects were not separated from their cagemates, and they were not constrained in movement or influenced in any way by the observer. In short, these were observations of behavior occurring naturally in this setting. Although these observations were videotaped daily (during the morning hours), only a subset was analyzed. Infant state was coded in six individuals during the infants' first 30 days of life, and maternal soothing was coded in 10 individuals during selected periods within the first three months of life.

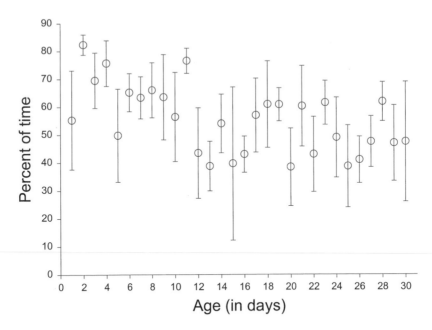

Fig. 10.6. Daily average (with SE) amounts of time spent sleeping by chimpanzees in the first 30 days of life (n=5).

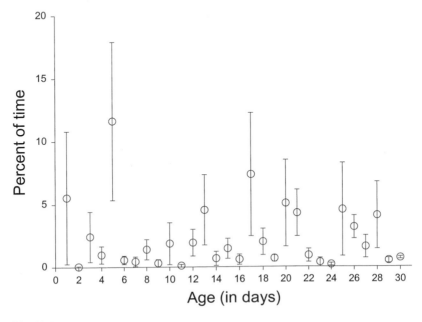

Fig. 10.7. Daily average (with SE) amounts of time spent fussing and crying (combined) by chimpanzees in the first 30 days of life (n=5).

Infant state was continuously coded into one of eight mutually exclusive and exhaustive behavioral categories (sleep, quiet–awake, active–awake, fussy, crying, nuzzling, nursing, not visible). The average (percentage) times spent by the neonatal chimpanzee in sleeping, and in fussing/crying states, during daily one-hour observations are illustrated in Figures 10.6 and 10.7 respectively (personal data, unpublished). Interobserver reliability was assessed among the four primary coders. We found that it was not possible to reliably distinguish REM sleep from deep sleep and that chimpanzees rarely spent time in a drowsy state, so these three categories were combined. Reliability was good to excellent (Bakeman and Gottman 1997), with kappa values (a statistic that corrects for chance agreement) of ≥0.69 (0.71, 0.69, 0.83, 0.79 and 0.78 among the pairs of coders) and percentage agreement ≥79% (79%, 85%, 90%, 93% and 85% respectively).

Fussiness was defined as comprising brief fussy vocalizations and considerable motor activity in an awake infant, comparable to State 5 as described by Brazelton (1984). Fussiness was distinct from the behavior of an active awake infant: distress facial and/or vocal expressions were required to score the state as fussy. Fussiness could be exhibited with a distress face (either the hoo or the whimper type: see Figures 10.3, 10.4) with or without a distress vocalization (single hoos or whimpers). The fussy vocalization, sounding like "hoo, hoo, hoo", is the one that accompanies the popular image of sound-making in 'monkeys' in which they scratch their armpits and hunch their shoulders. Crying was defined as a scream face (Fig. 10.5) with or without scream vocalizations in an awake infant, similar to State 6 as described for human infants (Brazelton and Nugent 1995). In general, scream vocalizations sound considerably higher pitched and louder than hoos and hoo whimpers.

The amount of time that mother-raised infant chimpanzees spent fussing and crying is depicted in Figures 10.8 and 10.9 respectively. The average fussiness was approximately 2 per cent of an hour-long observation during each week of the first month of life (*i.e.* a rate of approximately 1 minute 12 seconds per hour). The average amount of crying was less than 0.1 per cent (less than four seconds per hour). Note that three subjects, half of the sample, did not exhibit any bouts of crying during any of the observation periods.

Observations of maternal parenting were coded in 10 individuals (Bard 1994a) at three points during the first three months of life (*i.e.* the day that was the most prototypic of each mother–infant during each of three age periods, *viz.* 2–4 weeks, 6–8 weeks and 10–12 weeks). Continuous coding of maternal parenting (with 13 mutually exclusive and exhaustive codes) permitted us to calculate the percentage of time mothers engaged in *soothing* their distressed infant. Soothing was defined as any maternal behavior shown when the infant was fussing or crying that resulted in the infant returning to a calmer behavioral state (*i.e.* quiet–alert was the typical calm behavioral state of infant chimpanzees). Interobserver agreement was good with a kappa of 0.60 and percentage agreement of 83% between the primary coders (for more details, see Bard 1994a).

Maternal soothing typically occurred after the infant had cried following a period of fussiness. Infant fussiness was typically associated with infant nuzzling (reflexive 'searching' for the nipple) that remained unsuccessful in obtaining the nipple over a period of time. Infant fussiness was often accompanied by considerable motor activity that typically resulted

165

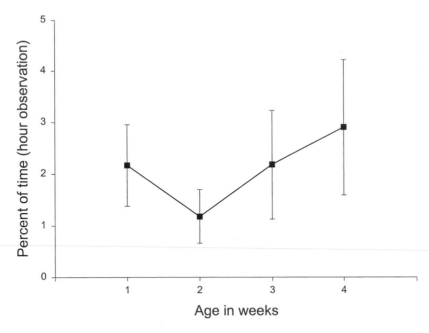

Fig. 10.8. Fussiness in mother-reared chimpanzees (mean ± SE for six infants) measured during a 60-minute naturalistic observation.

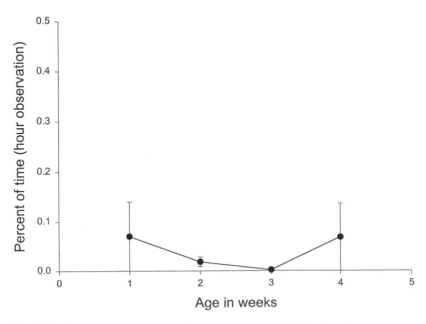

Fig. 10.9. Crying in mother-reared chimpanzees (mean ± SE for six infants) measured during a 60-minute naturalistic observation.

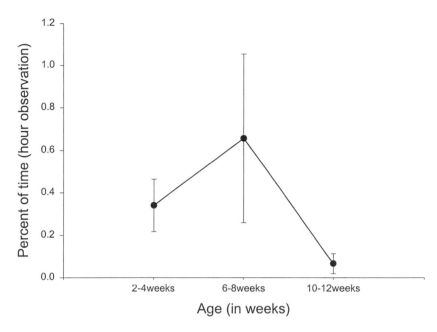

Fig. 10.10. Maternal soothing in mother-reared chimpanzees (mean ± SE for 10 infants) measured during a 60-minute naturalistic observation.

in the infant reaching the nipple and suckling. Mothers only occasionally facilitated the process by repositioning the infant or moving it closer to the nipple. Maternal repositioning seemed to be a response to the level of infant distress rather than an interpretation of the infant's nuzzling as a communication of the infant's desire to nurse. This assumption is based on the fact that repositioning tended to occur following distress vocalizations rather than following silent nuzzling behavior. Maternal repositioning did not necessarily result in prolonged infant calming. In contrast, maternal soothing was almost always effective in quieting the infant. Very occasionally, infants cried in response to a painful stimulus (such as the mother sitting on the infant's foot). In these cases, maternal soothing (including repositioning the infant) was the immediate response to the infant's cry and immediately resulted in the cessation of the cry.

As illustrated in Figure 10.10, maternal soothing occurred infrequently and for relatively short duration [0.3% of the time (approximately 10 seconds per hour) when infants were 2–4 weeks of age; 0.6% of the time (20 seconds per hour) when infants were 6–8 weeks; and 0.05% of the time (2 seconds per hour) when infants were 10–12 weeks of age]. Soothing occurred for about 10 seconds when infants were 2–4 weeks of age; and when direct observations of infant crying were made, crying occurred for approximately 3 seconds per hour when the infant was 1–4 weeks of age. Thus, given that maternal soothing is an adequate marker of infant crying, this suggests that crying peaks at 6–8 weeks in mother-raised infant chimpanzees.

NURSERY-RAISED CHIMPANZEES: CRYING AND FUSSING AS A FUNCTION OF
REARING

Twenty infants raised in the Great Ape Nursery under one of two different human caregiving routines (Standard Nursery Care or Responsive Nursery Care) were sampled (for details, see Bard and Gardner 1996). Standard Care consisted of scheduled feedings and diaper changes and regular interactions with human caregivers. As early as 30 days of age, peer groups were formed of between four and six individuals. Standard Care philosophy was that the chimpanzees would learn how to interact properly with all chimpanzees through interaction with same-aged peers. People did interact with the chimpanzees, but the purpose was to socialize the chimpanzees and for the people to have fun while tickling and playing chase with the chimpanzees.

Responsive Care consisted of four hours per day for five days per week of interactions designed to meet the needs of infant chimpanzees in a developmentally appropriate manner akin to that of chimpanzee mothers. Bottle feedings were on demand and diapers were changed as needed (with lots of opportunities to be 'diaperless'). Chimpanzees were held in an upright posture and were encouraged to support their own weight. From about 5 months of age, species-typical communicative and social behaviors were nurtured. The Responsive Care philosophy was that a competent adult was needed in addition to peers to provide the social context in which to learn chimpanzee species-typical communicative and social behaviors.

For the nursery-raised infants (n=20), the NBAS was administered (lasting 20–30 minutes per assessment) at the same time each day, midway between feedings, in a dimly lit room by a certified examiner (for details of NBAS performance by newborn chimpanzees, see Bard 1994b). The NBAS provided the data to calculate the percentages of time that the infant spent in a fussy and crying state during the assessment. The percentage of time in each behavioral state was estimated by the examiner at the completion of the test. This was a way to compare chimpanzee infant state organization (assessed by noting the two predominant states as recommended by Brazelton 1984) to that of human infants. In addition, the items of the NBAS pertaining to behavioral state and state regulation were used to compare the neonatal fussy and crying behaviors of 37 nursery-raised chimpanzees with those of 42 human newborns (Bard 1994b).

In the nursery-raised chimpanzees, the amount of fussing and crying was examined during the NBAS examination. Results for *fussing* are shown in Figure 10.11 (A—males *vs* females; B—Standard Care *vs* Responsive Care). Overall (collapsing across sex and care modalities), the infants typically fussed during 6 per cent of the examination (approximately 1 minute 15 seconds) in the first three weeks. In the fourth and sixth weeks, fussiness peaked at 9 and 8 per cent respectively (approximately two minutes). By nine weeks, fussiness leveled off to approximately 2 per cent (approximately 30 seconds), and it continued at this low level through 12 weeks of age.

Repeated measures analysis of variance (group—Standard Care *vs* Responsive Care; sex—male *vs* female; and age in monthly segments) were conducted on the percentage of time spent fussing during the NBAS test. During the first four weeks, there was no significant change in the amount of fussing, and no differences between the care groups or between

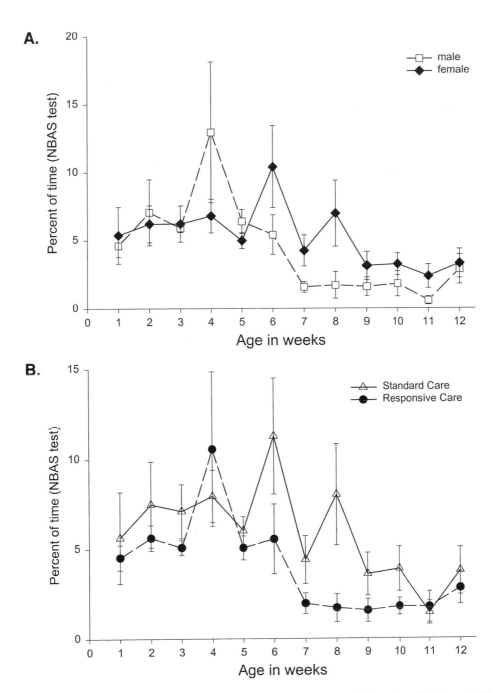

Fig. 10.11. Fussiness in nursery-raised chimpanzees (mean ± SE for 20 infants from birth through 12 weeks of age) measured during a 20-minute NBAS test. (A) Comparison between male (n=8) and female (n=12) chimpanzees. (B) Comparison between two types of rearing environment, standard care (n=10) and responsive care (n=10).

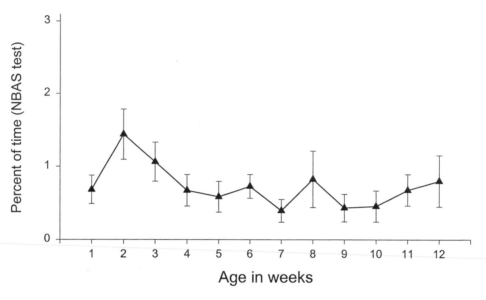

Fig. 10.12. Crying in nursery-raised chimpanzees (mean ± SE for 20 infants) measured during a 20-minute NBAS test.

males and females. During the second four weeks (weeks 5–8) there was a significant change [F(3, 45) = 3.92, p<0.05]. *Post hoc* contrasts revealed that fussing decreased at 7 weeks [F(1, 15) = 9.04, p<0.01]. During this time, females fussed more than males [F(1, 15) = 5.02, p<0.05] (Fig. 10.11A) and Standard Care infants fussed more than Responsive Care infants [F(1, 15) = 7.41, p<0.02] (Fig. 10.11B). In the third month, fussing was significantly lower than during the first week of life [F(1, 10) = 9.11, p<0.02] but not lower that the level of fussing at 7 weeks of age [F(1,10) = 0.87, ns]. There was a trend for the Responsive Care infants to fuss less than those in Standard Care during the third month, but, because there were fewer subjects in the sample, I would be cautious in the interpretation of this finding.

Crying during administration of the NBAS occurred rather consistently during less than 1 per cent of the test (*i.e.* approximately 15 seconds: Fig. 10.12). Note that the NBAS protocol involves at least two instances when the infant is laid down and removed from physical contact with the examiner. This is the most reliable means of eliciting fussiness or crying in infant chimpanzees (whether mother-raised or nursery-raised, although nursery-raised infants do adjust to this regularly occurring event). The examiner intervened after 15 seconds of infant distress in order to assess the extent of help needed by the infant to return to a calm behavioral state. Thus, the amount of crying may appear to be determined by the protocol of the NBAS. It is illuminating, however, to use the same procedures with chimpanzees and humans, in order to specify similarities and differences.

In an attempt to see how chimpanzees and humans compared in crying patterns during the second and third months, two additional measures were obtained for each subject: (1)

the age (in days) at which they exhibited their highest percentage of crying and fussing during the NBAS examinations; and (2) the highest daily percentage, *i.e.* the percentage of time crying during the examination on the day that the peak frequency of crying occurred. The average age at which the *chimpanzees* exhibited peak crying was 19 days (range 3–84 days, median 12 days). The percentage time crying on the day of peak crying frequency averaged 4 per cent of the test (range 0–15%, median 3%). Four per cent time crying is approximately one minute of crying during the 25-minute NBAS test. For *fussiness* during the examination, the peak occurred in week six (at 12% of the time) in the Standard Care chimpanzee infants and in week four (at 10.5% of the time) in the Responsive Care chimpanzee infants. It is of interest that, in diary studies in human infants, the age of peak crying is around 35–42 days (the sixth week of life—Barr *et al.* 1989). Furthermore, it appears that human infants cry and/or fuss about 10 per cent of the time at the peak period around 6 weeks (not counting night-time between midnight and 6.00 a.m.—Barr *et al.* 1989). Note, however, that these human data are not from standardized testing situations, but rather from diaries in everyday life situations.

DIRECT COMPARISON OF HUMAN NEWBORNS AND CHIMPANZEE NEWBORNS

From the NBAS tests, we are able to compare chimpanzee and human newborns on the same measures, Range of State and State Regulation. When the baby cries, how often the baby cries, how many items cause the baby to fuss, and how many times the baby moves from one state to another are measured in Range of State. In all these areas, there are significant differences. Human infants cry more than twice during the examination, whereas chimpanzees are predominantly fussy (Peak of Excitement: human 6.6±0.9, chimpanzee 4.7±0.8). Human infants are likely to cry when undressed (within the first five minutes of the test), whereas chimpanzee infants are likely to cry at the end of the test (Rapidity of Buildup: human 5.2±1.5, chimpanzee 2.2±1.4). Human infants, on average, exhibit a range of six to eight state changes during the course of the test compared to three to five state changes by chimpanzee infants. The smallest difference (although still statistically significant) is in the number of items to which the infant fusses. Humans fuss to three or four items whereas chimpanzees fuss to two items.

Previous analysis of the State Regulation cluster of the NBAS (Bard 1994b) revealed that neonatal chimpanzees cry/fuss later in the test compared with human infants and that they maintain a quieter (*i.e.* less aroused) behavioral state. In the first 30 days of life, there was no difference in the consolability of human and chimpanzee infants if consolability was measured from crying to calm for humans and from fussing to calm for chimpanzees (Consolability: human 6.1±1.7, chimpanzees 5.7±0.6—note that a score of 5 represents "Calms when picked up and held", and 6 is "Calms with examiner's hand on belly and restraining one or both arms"). It is revealing, however, that there is quite a bit more variance in the human infant scores than in the chimpanzee infant scores. Chimpanzee neonates almost always quiet when they are picked up, whereas some human newborns remain inconsolable with rocking, swaddling and a pacifier even after they are picked up. Chimpanzee infants were also more able to comfort themselves compared with human infants (Self-quiet: human 5.9±1.9, chimpanzee 7.5±2.0—note that a score of 6 represents "One successful attempt to maintain a quiet state after crying", and 7 is "One sustained self-quieting bout and several brief successes"). In fact, the items that required the baby to be in State 6 (crying) were typically not given a score during infant chimpanzee examinations, because they did not maintain a crying state for the required 15 seconds. For this reason, consolability and self-quieting were scored from a fussy state in infant chimpanzees. With this revision, chimpanzees and humans scored similarly. Therefore, it seems that the stronger parallel to human crying is chimpanzee fussiness, rather than chimpanzee crying (van Hooff 1967).

Discussion

Fussiness and crying occur in infant chimpanzees from the first day of life, regardless of whether the infant is raised with the biological mother or by humans in different types of nursery environments. Fussiness increases in occurrence during the second month of life, and decreases in the third month to levels lower than during the first month. This pattern of fussing parallels that found for crying in human infants. It seems clear, however, that there are lower absolute levels of both crying and fussiness in the chimpanzee compared with the human. Rearing environment seems to influence the amount of fussiness and crying in chimpanzees as in human infants. Much lower levels were found in mother-raised infants than in either group of nursery-raised infants. Quality of caregiving is also important. Nursery-raised infants who received responsive caregiving in the afternoon were less fussy during standardized tests given in the morning than infants raised under standard nursery care. Infants raised by mothers who were inadequate in their caregiving (often indicated by a lack of physical contact) were noticeably more fussy and could cry for the majority of an hour-long observation period if they remained out of physical contact with the mother. The amount of infant crying was used informally by staff as a measure of the quality of maternal care.

Species differences were notable. Chimpanzees quiet when picked up, and crying is very rare when the chimpanzee infant is in physical contact with the caregiver. Moreover, chimpanzees very rarely exhibit inconsolable crying. Inconsolable crying was not exhibited during the neonatal period, during NBAS testing, or in any mother-raised chimpanzee who was in physical contact with the mother.

Three of 20 infants raised under responsive care exhibited short periods of inconsolable fussiness. One of these was approximately 1 month of age when the crying episodes occurred, while the other two were older (3 and 6 months respectively). In the Responsive Care nursery, there were many caregivers (two full-time research assistants and up to five work-study students). One of the goals of Responsive Care was to have each infant be equally comfortable with each caregiver, and so different caregivers were assigned different infants on different days. In the 1-month-old infant, the crying seemed to be alleviated by changing the human caregiver. Occasionally, specific caregiver–infant mismatches occurred, and occasionally caregivers formed special attachments to specific infants (or vice versa). These were the types of occasions during which we found the older two infants exhibited distress, sometimes for 10–20 minutes. In the 3-month-old infant, the crying was probably related to parenting style issues. In the 6-month-old, the crying was probably related to attachment issues (Bard, unpublished data). For one infant, however, distress bouts lasted several minutes and recurred daily for approximately 7–10 days without the cause of distress being readily identifiable. These bouts caused the caregiver considerable discomfort and frustration. In addition, this caregiver stated that she was very concerned about the well-being of the infant, similar to the parenting response to colic. In the chimpanzees, however, all cases resolved within a short period of time either without special interventions, or with an intervention consisting of changing caregiver–infant pairings.

Mother-raised chimpanzees exhibit extended periods of fussing when they begin to crawl and climb at around 3 months of age. Mothers allow their infants to move about but always maintain a firm grasp on one of their limbs. The mother may hold the infant's leg in her hand, and then not pay any visual attention to the infant as s/he pulls up on the cage mesh or locomotes around on the floor. In the Bard (1994a) paper, I label this maternal behavior 'restrain', and it peaks when the infant is 10–12 weeks old. Infants may exhibit an increase in fussiness during this period, but the cause seems clear ('distress to limitations': Rothbart 1986) and the dynamics quite different from the fussing/crying of colicky human babies.

Comparisons of range of behavioral state and behavioral state regulation during a standardized test revealed that human infants cried more often, cried at the beginning of the test, and were more irritable compared with chimpanzees. Chimpanzees rarely cried, but if they did, it was at the end of the examination. Chimpanzees were more responsive to the examiner's soothing interventions and were more able to comfort themselves compared with human infants.

These results suggest that there may be a common biobehavioral shift in fussiness and crying that occurs in the second month of life in both human and chimpanzee infants (St.James-Roberts and Plewis 1996). When born, chimpanzees are as helpless to survive as human infants, but they develop motor skills more quickly. Chimpanzees hold their head erect in the pull-to-sit by 30 days of age, and sit with support shortly thereafter. Chimpanzees are able to locomote independently by 5 months (especially climbing, although their judgment is not very good with regard to their ability to climb back down, after successfully climbing up). However, in terms of emotional development, it appears that chimpanzees develop at a rate much more comparable to human infants (Bard 1998, Bard and Russell 1999). Smiles begin around 4 weeks of age, wariness of strangers occurs around 5–7 months (mean = 6.2 months, range 3.7–9.9 months, N=16—personal data, unpublished). At the earliest age tested (14 months), chimpanzees are able to use caregivers' emotional reaction to evaluate novel objects (Russell *et al.* 1997). In addition, the Ainsworth Strange Situation (Ainsworth *et al.* 1978) conducted at 12–14 months of age elicits the full range of attachment classifications seen in humans (Bard 1991). The fact that preterm human infants show a peak in crying at 6 weeks corrected age suggests that there is a strong maturational component to crying behavior that is probably unrelated to motoric development (Barr *et al.* 1996). Comparing these data with those from the chimpanzee, I suggest that a biobehavioral shift may occur in the second month of life in both chimpanzees and humans, which may be related to the fact that emotional development in these species is extremely flexible (*i.e.* strongly influenced by environmental factors early in development). The comparison of crying and fussing across caregiving regimes in human cultures and chimpanzee rearing environments suggests that the occurrence of fussiness and crying may be related to the physiological status of the infant (*e.g.* endogenous arousal levels), and the duration of crying and fussiness may be modifiable based on the emotional responsiveness of the environment—that is, arousal modulation that occurs in the second month of life as a result of the interaction of the developing self-regulatory system with the responsiveness of the environment.

ACKNOWLEDGEMENTS

This chapter would not have been possible without the exceptional assistance of Kelly McDonald, Kathy Gardner, Josh Schneider, Carolyn Fort and Yvette Veira in conducting the chimpanzee studies and compiling the data for analysis. The state data were collected, analyzed and graphed with the assistance of Howard Coffman and Tim Groh. For help in keeping my scientific perspective sharply focused, I thank David Leavens; and for help in clarifying the distinct differences and clear similarities between human and chimpanzee infants, I acknowledge my son, Nicholas Leavens. Funding was provided by NIH grants RR-00165, RR-03591, RR-06158, HD-07105 and HD-08274.

REFERENCES

Ainsworth, M.D.S., Blehar, M.C., Waters, E., Wall, S. (1978) *Patterns of Attachment: A Psychological Study of the Strange Situation.* Hillsdale, NJ: Erlbaum.

Bakeman, R., Gottman, J. (1997) *Observing Interaction: An Introduction to Sequential Analysis. 2nd Edn.* Cambridge: Cambridge University Press.

Bard, K.A. (1991) 'Distribution of attachment classifications in nursery chimpanzees.' *American Journal of Primatology*, **24**, 88.

—— (1994a) 'Evolutionary roots of intuitive parenting: Maternal competence in chimpanzees.' *Early Development and Parenting*, **3**, 19–28.

—— (1994b) 'Similarities and differences in the neonatal behavior of chimpanzee and human infants.' *In:* Eder, G., Kaiser, E., King, F.A. (Eds.) *The Role of the Chimpanzee in Research.* Basel: Karger, pp. 43–55.

—— (1995) 'Parenting in primates.' *In:* Bornstein, M. (Ed.) *Handbook of Parenting. Vol. 2. Biology and Ecology of Parenting.* Mahwah, NJ: Erlbaum, pp. 27–57.

—— (1999) 'Social–experiential contributions to imitation and emotion in chimpanzees.' *In:* Braten, S. (Ed.) *Intersubjective Communication and Emotion in Early Ontogeny: A Source Book.* Cambridge: Cambridge University Press, pp. 208–227.

—— Gardner, K.H. (1996) 'Influences on development in infant chimpanzees: Enculturation, temperament, and cognition.' *In:* Russon, A., Bard, K.A., Parker, S.T. (Eds.) *Reaching into Thought: The Minds of the Great Apes.* Cambridge: Cambridge University Press, pp. 235–256.

—— Russell, C.L. (1999) 'Evolutionary foundations of imitation: social, cognitive, and developmental aspects of imitative processes in non-human primates.' *In:* Nadel, J., Butterworth, G. (Eds.) *Imitation in Infancy.* Cambridge: Cambridge University Press, pp. 89–123.

Barr, R. (1990) 'The normal crying curve: what do we really know?' *Developmental Medicine and Child Neurology*, **32**, 356–362.

—— Kramer, M.S., Pless, I.B., Boisjoly, C., Leduc, D. (1989) 'Feeding and temperament as determinants of early infant crying/fussing behavior.' *Pediatrics*, **84**, 514–521.

—— Konner, M., Bakeman, R., Adamson, L. (1991) 'Crying in !Kung San infants: a test of the cultural specificity hypothesis.' *Developmental Medicine and Child Neurology*, **33**, 601–610.

—— Chen, S., Hopkins, B., Westra, T. (1996) 'Crying patterns in preterm infants.' *Developmental Medicine and Child Neurology*, **38**, 345–355.

Brazelton, T.B. (1984) *Neonatal Behavioral Assessment Scale. 2nd Edn.* Clinics in Developmental Medicine No. 88. London: Spastics International Medical Publications.

— Nugent, J.K. (1995) *Neonatal Behavioral Assessment Scale. 3rd Edn.* Clinics in Developmental Medicine No. 137. London: Mac Keith Press.

Goodall, J. (1986) *The Chimpanzees of Gombe: Patterns of Behavior.* Cambridge: Belknap Press.

Gouzoules, S., Gouzoules, H., Marler, P. (1984) 'Rhesus monkey (*Maccaca mulatta*) screams: Representational signaling in the recruitment of agonistic aid.' *Animal Behaviour*, **32**, 182–193.

Green, S. (1975) 'The variation of vocal pattern with social situation in the Japanese monkey (*Macaca fuscata*): A field study.' *In:* Rosenblum, L. (Ed.) *Primate Behavior. Vol 4.* New York: Academic Press, pp. 1–102.

Hauser, M. (1996) *The Evolution of Communication.* Cambridge, MA: MIT Press.

Hopkins, W.D., Savage-Rumbaugh, E.S. (1991) 'Vocal communication as a function of differential rearing experiences in *Pan paniscus*: A preliminary report.' *International Journal of Primatology*, **12**, 559–583.

Hunziker, L.A., Barr, R. (1986) 'Increased carrying reduces infant crying: A randomized controlled trial.' *Pediatrics*, **77**, 641–648.

Masataka, N., Kohda, M. (1988) 'Primate play vocalizations and their functional significance.' *Folia Primatologica*, **50**, 152–156.

Mitani, J., Hasegawa, T., Gros-Louis, J., Marler, P., Byrne, R. (1992) 'Dialects in wild chimpanzees?' *American Journal of Primatology*, **27**, 233–244.

—— Gros-Louis, J., Macedonia, J.M. (1996) 'Selection for acoustic individuality within the vocal repertoire of wild chimpanzees.' *International Journal of Primatology*, **17**, 569–583.

Newman, J. (1985) 'The infant cry of primates: An evolutionary perspective.' *In:* Lester, B.M., Boukydis, C.F.Z. (Eds.) *Infant Crying: Theoretical and Research Perspectives.* New York: Plenum Press, pp. 307–323.

Owren, M., Rendall, D. (1997) 'An affect-conditioning model of nonhuman primate vocal signaling.' *In:* Owings, D., Beecher, M., Thompson, N. (Eds.) *Perspectives in Ethology. Vol. 12. Communication.* New York: Plenum Press, pp. 299–346.

—— Dieter, J.A., Seyfarth, R.M., Cheney, D.L. (1993) 'Vocalizations of rhesus (*Macaque mulatta*) and Japanese (*M. fuscata*) macaques cross-fostered between species show evidence of only limited modification.' *Developmental Psychobiology*, **26**, 389–406.

Papousek, H., Jurgens, U., Papousek, M. (1992) *Nonverbal Vocal Communication: Comparative and Developmental Approaches.* Cambridge: Cambridge University Press.

Plooij, F.X. (1984) *The Behavioral Development of Free-living Chimpanzee Babies and Infants. Monographs on Infancy, Vol. 3.* Norwood, NJ: Ablex.

Rothbart, M. (1986) 'Longitudinal observation of infant temperament.' *Developmental Psychology*, **22**, 356–365.

Russell, C.L., Baird, K.A., Adamson, L.A. (1997) 'Social referencing by young chimpanzees (*Pan troglodytes*).' *Journal of Comparative Psychology*, **111**, 185–193.

Segerstrale, U.C., Molnar, P. (Eds.) (1997) *Nonverbal Communication: Where Nature Meets Culture.* Mahwah, NJ: Erlbaum.

Seyfarth, R., Cheney, D., Marler, P. (1980) 'Monkey responses to three different alarm calls: Evidence of predator classification and semantic communication.' *Science*, **210**, 801–803.

Snowdon, C.T., Hausberger, M. (Eds.) (1997) *Social Influences on Vocal Development.* Cambridge: Cambridge University Press.

St James-Roberts, I., Plewis, I. (1996) 'Individual differences, daily fluctuations, and developmental changes in amounts of infant waking, fussing, crying, feeding, and sleeping.' *Child Development*, **67**, 2527–2540.

Stevenson-Hinde, J., Zunz, M (1978) 'Subjective assessment of individual rhesus monkeys.' *Primates*, **19**, 473–482.

van Hooff, J.A.R.A.M. (1967) 'The facial displays of the catarrhine monkeys and apes.' *In:* Morris, D. (Ed.) *Primate Ethology.* London: Weidenfeld & Nicolson, pp. 7–68.

—— (1973) 'A structural analysis of the social behavior of a semi-captive group of chimpanzees.' *In:* Cranach, M.V, Vine, I. (Eds.) *Social Communication and Movement: Studies of Interaction and Expression in Man and Chimpanzee.* New York: Academic Press, pp. 75–162.

van Lawick-Goodall, J. (1968) 'A preliminary report on expressive movements and communication in the Gombe Stream chimpanzees.' *In:* Jay, P.C. (Ed.) *Primates: Studies in Adaptation and Variability.* New York: Holt, Rinehart & Winston, pp. 313–374.

Yerkes, R.M., Yerkes, A.W. (1929) *The Great Apes.* New Haven, CT: Yale University Press.

11
DEVELOPMENT OF CRYING IN NORMAL INFANTS: METHOD, THEORY AND SOME SPECULATIONS

Brian Hopkins

Section 1: Introduction

In ancient Greece, crying was interpreted by adults that an infant needed something. Thus, in Aeschylus' *Libation Bearers*, we can read that when the young Orestes cried, his nurse Cilissa assumed that it indicated he was hungry, thirsty or needed to urinate (French 1995). Some two thousand years later, we continue to be intrigued by the communicative capacities of newborn crying, how they develop, and their ramifications for other aspects of development. This abiding interest has culminated in a multifaceted approach to the scientific study of crying during infancy, involving, for example, developmental psychologists, ethologists, paediatricians and those in the speech sciences.

The outcome of all this activity is a set of fragmented insights into the phenomenon of infant crying. On the one hand, we now know much about how the newborn controls voicing during crying, the diagnostic implications of variations in such voicing and the social significance of crying at various ages during early infancy. On the other hand, we continue to lack the broader canvas of how crying develops in normal infants, particularly in terms of qualitative changes. As Zeskind (1985) aptly put it, there is a need for teasing out the developmental processes involved together with their underlying determinants at the expense of further studies that provide yet more catalogues of their products. Such an endeavor raises methodological and definitional issues that are pertinent to studies on the development of crying and which will be dealt with in Sections 2 and 3 respectively.

Ultimately, issues relating to definitions and methodology cannot be divorced from the research questions one is asking and the theoretical background that should guide their formulation. In order to ask the right questions, we need to recognize that there are two major problems about development in general, namely, origin and change (Section 4). Of these, the problem of change is perhaps the one that has been most neglected in the study of infant crying. Thus, what is required is a theoretical scenario on the development of crying that can account for the fact it is an expression of a number of mechanisms that undergo transformations as a result of interrelated changes at many different levels of organization. As we shall see, theories or models of infant cry production are restricted as they do not address the other major developmental problem, namely, the ontogenetic origins of crying. They are also restricted in that they do not go beyond the newborn period and tend to seek their explanations at the level of neural or neuromuscular constraints. Thus, other mainly non-neural constraints are evaluated that have to be 'broken' and 're-made' if developmental change is to be realized (Section 5).

Two other topics are not treated thematically, but course throughout the contribution. One concerns the distinction between quantitative and qualitative change and what it means for research on the development of crying (mainly featured in Section 4). The second is what has been termed the two-to-three month transformation in developmental functions (Hopkins and Prechtl 1984). It is asked how the well-documented peak in crying occurring around age 6 weeks (an example of quantitative change) partakes of this transformation (see especially Section 4). Finally, I conclude with an overview of the main issues raised and elaborate on them as a means of highlighting future directions of research on the development of crying in normal infants (Section 6).

Section 2: Some methodological issues relevant to a developmental perspective

ACOUSTIC ANALYSIS VERSUS PHONETIC TRANSCRIPTION

Computer-aided analyses of cry recordings provide accurate, quantitative data about duration, frequency, amplitude and spectrum of the sound. The main analytical tool has been some variant of the standard waveform analysis such as the fast Fourier transform. This algorithm has at least two shortcomings. First, in order to analyze frequencies up to 5000 Hz, it requires a sampling rate of about 10,000 data points per second. Second, it cannot adequately identify the dimensionality of a system such as whether it is a chaotic system or one consisting of random noise (Bergé *et al.* 1984)—an important consideration if one is interested in identifying any qualitative changes in the dynamics of cry sound production during development.

Auditory-based assessments of cry sounds typically use predefined categories and sometimes rating scales. Most systems for classifying infant cries discussed in the next section are based on this approach. It assumes that human listeners are capable of converting audible sound waves into discrete acoustic parameters. Unfortunately, the human auditory system does not function quite like a digital computer as it is poor in isolating individual acoustic parameters. Thus, one should not expect consistent relationships between auditory assessments and digital analyses of infant crying. Judgments of fundamental frequency, for example, are affected by a host of other factors including the distribution of energy across the spectrum (Laver 1980). Nevertheless, one of the commendable features of the human auditory system is its ability to integrate diverse sources of information such as the loudness, pitch and amplitude of voicing. In this respect, auditory assessments have an undoubted value in research concerned with how listeners recognize individual differences in the crying sounds of infants. The problem that still remains is how to convert an auditory impression of a cry into a quantitative judgment on some rating scale.

In the past, auditory-based assessments of infant crying involved the use of phonetic transcription, which attempts to describe the segmental or suprasegmental categories of vocal sounds. It was used, for example, by Irwin and Curry (1941) in their study of newborn cries, motivated by the claim of learning theory that prelinguistic vocalizations are selectively reinforced to become meaningful speech. Since then, transcribing the cries of infants by means of a phonetic alphabet steadily declined to the point where it is hardly ever used in cry research. One reason is that the use of phonetic transcription rests on the questionable assumption that infant sounds conform to the phonetic elements of adult speech, a criticism dating back to Jakobson's (1941) view of language development. This view will be challenged as we come across support for the claim that infant crying and subsequent speech development are functionally related. If such a developmental scenario is deemed to be credible, then something akin to phonetic transcription is still required in studying the development of crying. The solution could be a metaphonological or metaphonetic approach, which assumes a position somewhere between acoustic and phonetic assessments (Oller 1980). As such, it dwells on nonsegmental parameters common to all languages (*e.g.* pitch, voice quality or phonation type, resonance pattern, amplitude and timing). Together, these parameters enable the listener to identify a variety of phonological features, examples of which are plosives, fricatives, sibilants and distinctions between high, stressed and unstressed vowels. While the metaphonological approach has limited applications in the analysis of newborn cries, it will assume more validity as crying becomes increasingly modified by improvements in the voluntary control of respiratory and articulatory movements.

If most of our current knowledge about newborn cry production stems from acoustic analyses based on spectrography and high-speed digital computation, then information about subsequent development rests largely on what has been gleaned from parental diaries. What are the pitfalls associated with the diary method and how well do the data derived from it compare to those obtained from a less subjective approach?

PARENTAL DIARIES VERSUS AUDIO RECORDINGS
Parental diaries rely on complex judgments about the daily activities of infants. Thus, they are not necessarily a true reflection of, for example, the amount and patterning of infant crying within and across days or weeks. What parents report are not individual cry vocalizations, but bouts of crying that discount any short pauses between cries (Barr 1990a). It is pertinent to ask, therefore, if findings derived from diaries are comparable to those obtained by means of concurrent audio recordings.

In a home-based study, the diaries of 10 mothers were compared to voice-activated radio-telemetric tape recordings of vocalizations made by their 6-week-old infants over a period of 24 hours (Barr *et al.* 1988). An interesting feature of this study was the request made by mothers that the diary include a way of distinguishing between crying and fussing. The audio recordings were transcribed for infant sounds in terms of 'negative' and 'non-negative' vocalizations. There are three relevant findings. First, while there was the expectable difference between the mean duration of combined crying and fussing (2 hr. 3 min.) computed from the diaries and that obtained for recorded negative vocalizations (29 min.), the mean frequency for the former (9.5 in 24 hours) was similar to that for the latter (10.5 in 24 hours). Second, the correlations between the frequency and duration measures obtained from the two methods of recording were as follows: moderate and positive for the former in the case of crying/fussing and negative vocalizations ($r = 0.64$, $p = 0.03$) and best for the latter when it involved only crying ($r = 0.67$, $p = 0.02$). Excluding an inadequately completed diary boosted the correlation for both measures. Finally, when diaries were checked with their corresponding recorded episodes, it appeared that mothers omitted on average 20 per cent of the total duration of negative vocalization episodes and 14 per cent of their total number. Reassuring was the fact that missing episodes were not more frequent during the six hours of night-time (midnight to 6.00 a.m.). These outcomes led the authors to conclude that the parental diary is a valid method of recording crying and fussing in the short term.

In another study, 24-hour maternal diaries and voice-activated audio recordings obtained from 16 infants considered by their mothers to be excessive criers were compared (St James-Roberts *et al.* 1993). In brief, there were moderate to strong correlations between the diary and audiotaped recordings for both the frequency and duration of crying. Thus, the findings and conclusions of this study were in good correspondence with those of Barr *et al.* (1988) (see also Barr *et al.* 1989).

A related method to parental diaries for measuring maternal perception of infant crying and fussing is the Crying Patterns Questionnaire (CPQ) devised by St James-Roberts and Halil (1991). In a recent cross-cultural comparison, it was pitted against audio recordings of crying in a sample of infants from the town of Manali in the Himalayan region of northern India (n=107) and another recruited from three London hospitals (n=30). CPQ reports showed that Manali mothers perceived about 10–20 per cent less crying in their 2- to 6-week-old infants than those in the London sample (St James-Roberts *et al.* 1994). In contrast, the audio recordings revealed that the Manali infants cried as much as their counterparts in London. This set of findings reiterates the point that parental perceptions of crying do not necessarily tally with more objective measures of duration and warns us that the interpretation of crying may vary across different sociocultural settings.

None of the methods we have considered can adequately deal with qualitative changes in the development of crying. By these, I mean not just changes in the quality of voicing during crying, but more importantly, in the accompanying facial and limb movements. In my opinion, changes in the patterning of such movements as well as posture are cardinal features of developmental transformations in crying. Thus, while Ostwald (1972) may be right in contending that ". . machines will never completely replace the human ear in listening for the intriguing and informative sounds of infancy", I would add that neither can judgments made by the human eye. Certainly, machines are of little help in demarcating crying from fussing, a distinction that surfaces in attempts at defining and classifying the sounds of infancy.

Section 3: Defining and classifying crying

DEFINITIONS

There is little consensus on how crying and fussing should be operationally defined, and many studies simply avoid the task, especially those founded on the diary method. Perhaps it is not avoidance as such, but a belief that crying and fussing are phenomenologically so self-evident that they do not need to be defined. Given the circumstances, we can justifiably ask what it is that changes during the development of crying. Table 11.1, which includes only studies that attempted to define crying or fussing or both, illustrates the nature of the problem.

TABLE 11.1
Definitions of crying and fussing derived from selected studies on infant crying

Author(s)	Method(s)/ design*	Infant age(s)	Crying	Fussing
1. Aldrich et al. (1945)	DM	Newborn	Crying spells longer than 3 min.	Not defined
2. Barr et al. (1988)	DM	6 w	Complex including movement elements, facial expresssion and voice, and is usually interpreted as expressing negative emotion	Not quite crying, but not awake and content either
3. St James-Roberts et al. (1995)	DM	5–6 w	Periods of prolonged distressed vocalizations	Baby unsettled and irritable and may be vocalizing, but not continuosly crying
4. Truby and Lind (1965)	AR	Newborn	Sequence of motor performances and associated acoustic manifestations including vocalizing, constricted silence, coughing, interruptions or various combinations of such performances	Not defined
5. Rebelsky and Black (1972)	AR/L	1–13 w	Rhythmic and arhythmic cry: five consecutives and similar unhappy sounds with strained quality	Arhythmic sound with pauses and strained quality, but less unhappy impression than crying
6. Stark et al. (1975, 1978)	AR + DO	1–8 w	Series of sounds[1] due to acute distress to hunger, pain, temporary parental absence, etc. Accompanied by cry face[2], stiffness of trunk and limbs, some apparently random limb movements— all of which sustained for long periods, often up to 30 s	Discomfort sounds: produced in distress, of lesser degree than crying, e.g. due to inability to reach a toy, protest at being given unwanted spoonful of food. Accompanied by cry face, less stiffness and more trunk and limb movements than for crying—none of which sustained as long as in crying
7. Gustafson et al. (1984)	AR	30 d	Wails (typical crying sounds) and of longer duration and higher amplitude than other sounds. Most contain rising–falling or falling intonation contour	All other cry sounds
8. D'Odorico et al. (1985)	AR + DO	4–8 mo	Cry vocalizations include **fussy** sounds and moans as they are accompanied by the same facial expressions as cries (frowning, trembling of chin, etc.) and similar acoustic features	—
9. Wolff (1987)	AR + DO/L	Newborn to 6 mo	Five or more distinct cycles and individual utterances not separated by more than 3 s. Accompanied by cry grimace and vigorous limb activity	Intermittent moaning or crylike sounds which conform to no distinct temporal pattern, and separated by periods of silence lasting 3 s or more

TABLE 11.1
(cont'd)

Author(s)	Method(s)/ design*	Infant age(s)	Crying	Fussing
10. Simner (1971)	DO	Newborn	An audible, intermittment vocalization accompanied by facial grimaces and increased motor activity lasting at least 1–2 s	Not defined
11. Bell and Ainsworth (1972)	DO/L	3–54 w	All vocal protests from unhappy noises to **fusses** to full-blown cries	—
12. Moss (1974)	DO	1 + 3 mo	Intense, shrill and blatant vocalizations reflecting distress	Low-level, intermittment protest vocalizations similar to a whimper or whine
13. Roe (1975)	DO/L	3–9 mo + 9–15 mo	Include intermittment gasps of air in soblike vocalization	Vocalizations definitely unpleasant and whiny, but not reached point of crying
14. Landau (1982)	DO	2–11 mo	High-pitched vocalization of a whiny nature accompanied by tears	Similar to crying, but not accompanied by tears
15. Hopkins et al. (1987)	DO/L	3–18 w	High-intensity loudness and accompanied by eye closure and cry face. Arms flexed and adducted with rigid trunk posture in partial extension	Moderate loudness, made on expiration with a glottal stop and accompanied by cry face, but with eyes remaining open
16. Barr and Elias (1988)	DO	2 + 4 mo	Repeated rhythmic whining with duration throughout time	Nearly rhythmic whining vocalization associated with fret or pucker face
17. Papousek (1989)	DO	2 mo	Indicated by jerky proximal movements of all limbs and cry face	Discomfort indicated by squirming or jerky irregular movements of one or more limbs, closed fists, frown, facial expressions of distress or yawn
18. Barr et al. (1991)	DO	1–99 w	Repeated rhythmic whining vocalizaton with duration	Nonrhythmic whining vocalization associated with fret or pucker face
19. Gustafson and Green (1991)	DO/L	3–12 mo	What others described as crying, howling, weeping, grizzling, **fussing**, nonverbal griping and negative vocalizations	—
20. Barr et al. (1992)	DO/L	3–12 mo	What others described as consecutive inspiratory–expiratory negative vocalizations	Not defined

*DM = diary method; AR = audio recording; DO = direct observation; L = longitudinal design (absence of L indicates a focus on one age, a cross-sectional design involving different infants at different ages, or fewer than 10 infants seen only at two or more consecutive ages).

[1]A series of sounds is a group of vocalization segments separated from all other groups by more than two inspiratory sounds, but in which no segment is separated from any other by more than two inspiratory sounds. A segment is a vocalization unit separated from all others by at least 50 ms of silence.

[2]Mouth open, eyes closed at least some of the time and frowning.

A perusal of this table reveals that crying is defined and delineated from fussing in a variety of ways. Some of the definitions simply offer synonyms for crying, a few refer to accompanying nonvocal behaviours, and still fewer to the temporal organization or respiratory-based nature of crying. If there is any commonality, then it resides in the attempt to capture the quality of voicing, which is then treated as differing from fussing in intensity of expression or as something distinctively different. More specifically, this array of definitions leads to the following points about how infant crying is studied:

- The majority of studies (14/20) are focused on the first three to four months after birth. Few are truly longitudinal in design (6/20), with a follow-up of at least 10 infants at more than two consecutive ages. Furthermore, no single definition accounts for any possible developmental changes or age-related differences in crying.

- Crying consists of a sequence or series of sounds in most studies using audio recordings (4,5,6,9). Employment of this method not only reflects an interest in crying as sound with certain acoustic features, but also as an act or motor phenomenon involving complex coordinations between respiration and movements of the vocal tract, the face and the articulators. Following Stetson (1951), and linking this double-edged interest, we might say that crying is movement made audible.

- Excluding reference to just motor activity (10), almost half of the studies using direct observation (mainly with the aid of video recordings) incorporate accompanying nonvocal behaviors into their definitions. These include the cry face/grimace or limb movements or both (6,8,9,14,15,17). Only two studies (6,15) refer to any postural accompaniments—in my opinion, unavoidable components if crying is to be treated as a phenomenon involving a complex set of motor coordinations.

- Attempts at distinguishing crying from fussing (or fret/discomfort sounds) give rise to the following comments:

  (a) Only 7/20 studies do not make this distinction, omissions that embrace just the newborn period. According to Wolff (1969), fussing does not emerge until some time after 3 weeks of age, which possibly represents the first major developmental transformation in the control and regulation of vocal output.

  (b) Some studies make the distinction in terms of rhythmic (crying) and nonrhythmic (fussing) sounds (4,9,16,18). Wolff (1967) was perhaps the first to portray crying as a rhythmic repetition consisting of an expiratory sound, a brief pause and an inspiratory sound followed by another pause prior to the next sound made on expiration. Only one study appears to have examined this portrayal using an appropriate statistical technique (Zeskind et al. 1993). Based on spectral analyses of 90 s of spontaneous crying in 1-month-old infants, the main finding was that the power spectra of all cries revealed dominant frequencies at one cycle about every 30, 15 and 1 s. This suggests that crying in young infants has a complex rhythmic structure. Such rhythmicity in crying may facilitate the development of coordination within and between motor systems involved in sound production (Kent 1984).

  (c) A few studies appear to treat crying and fussing as being both quantitatively and qualitatively different from each other (6,9,14,15). Qualitative distinctions include differences in facial expression, limb movements and posture. The study (14) by Landau

(1982) is unusual in that it makes the distinction on the basis of the presence (crying) or absence (fussing) of tears. Touwen (1976) reported that lacrimation during crying becomes evident only at around 2–3 months—an age, as we shall see, that heralds other more significant changes in the development of crying. Whether differences between crying and fussing and within crying itself are quantitative or qualitative distinctions continues to be a major theoretical debate (Barr 1995a). The issue at large is whether the differences represent continuous, but graded, signals along some arousal continuum or discontinuous state-like distinctions. With regard to the comparison between crying and fussing, Wolff (1987) has taken a clear stance on this issue: crying is a distinct behavioural state, while fussing is a transitional period between crying and other states.

(d) Finally, few studies using the diary method incorporate a definition of crying or fussing. However, as Barr *et al.* (1988) discovered, parents do not regard crying and fussing as synonymous. It is probably the case that they code fussing in terms of behaviors other than vocalization. Thus, if parents are not required to record both crying and fussing, then salient signs of distress may be missed. When both are included, it appears that fussing accounts for 60–70 per cent of diary-recorded distress vocalization in infants with or without colic (Hunziker and Barr 1986, St James-Roberts *et al.* 1995). This finding has implications for our understanding of the 6-week 'peak' in crying (Section 4).

CLASSIFICATIONS

Moving from the problem of defining crying and distinguishing it from fussing, we turn next to attempts at classifying categorical differences within crying. Once again, it proves to be an enterprise fraught with problems and shortcomings. Table 11.2 presents some of the classifications that have been devised as a means of identifying different categories of infant crying.

The classification made by Truby and Lind (1965) refers only to pain cries elicited in newborns by means of pinching. That provided by Wasz-Höckert *et al.* (1968) is derived primarily from the cries of newborns obtained by various different methods of elicitation. The three remaining classifications involve both elicited and spontaneous crying (Wolff 1969, 1987) or only the latter (Stark and Nathanson 1974, Gustafson and Green 1991). The classification devised by Gustafson and Green is unique in having an explicit developmental perspective. These similarities and differences between the five systems of classification lead to the following remarks:

• The spontaneous–elicited distinction is important to bear in mind when considering developmental changes in the acoustic properties of crying. It has been estimated that the mean F_0 of cries in healthy term newborns falls somewhere in the range of 425–600 Hz (Ostwald and Peltzman 1974). Within that range, the mean value for pain cries is typically higher than for hunger cries with the former being 510 Hz and the latter 450 Hz (Murry *et al.* 1977, Thodén and Koivisto 1980). This difference in pitch could be due to greater tension in the intrinsic muscles of the larynx during pain-induced crying (Wasz-Höckert *et al.* 1968) or to changes in subglottal air pressure within a respiratory cycle (Lieberman

1967). Given that, in adults, subglottal pressure only influences F_0 at frequencies of less than 100 Hz (Atkinson 1978), increased laryngeal tension resulting in tauter vocal folds would seem to be the favoured explanation for the higher pitch of pain cries. Whatever the case, the pain cry of the healthy newborn achieves a remarkable level of loudness, *viz.* about 80 dB at a distance of 30.5 cm from the mouth (Ringel and Kluppel 1964). According to Ostwald (1972), it is one of the loudest sounds that humans ever emit, being 20 dB louder than normal adult speech and equivalent to the noise of an unmuffled truck engine. As such, this feature undoubtedly contributes to the sense of urgency that caregivers experience on hearing the pain cry of a newborn.

TABLE 11.2
Five systems for classifying different types of infant crying

Author(s)	Type of cry: definitions		
	Phonated/basic cry	*Dysphonated/turbulent cry*	*Hyperphonated cry/shift*
1. Truby and Lind (1965)	Smooth, symmetrical harmonic structure and intensity pattern with pitch range of 200–600 Hz. Regular opening and closing of vocal folds. No indication of great stress or discomfort	Aperiodic sound or turbulence overriding all or most of basic cry harmonics. Irregular movement of vocal folds. Sounds harsh, raucous or rough	Very high pitch of 1000–2000 Hz with sudden shift to lower or higher F_0. Not clear how this cry produced.[1] Whistle-like sound in response to great stress
	Phonated cry	*Dysphonated cry*	*Hyperphonated cry*
2. Wasz-Höckert et al. (1968)[2]	Same as Truby and Lind (1965)	Same as Truby and Lind (1965)	Same as Truby and Lind (1965). Also: often occurs together with dysphonation
	Basic/hunger cry	*Angry/mad cry*	*Pain cry*
3. Wolff (1969; 1987)[3]	Similar to phonated cry of Truby and Lind (1965). Pitch range of 250–450 Hz, but mainly 350–400 Hz. Expiration lasts 0.6–1.4 s. Followed by: brief silence of about 0.2 s, then sometimes brief inspiratory whistle of 0.1–0.2 s and another brief rest of about 0.2 s before next expiration. Sound similar to /a/ ("ah") vowel. Occurs about 30 min. after birth and then remains constant up to about 2 months	Similar to dysphonated cry of Truby and Lind (1965) in containing turbulence due to excess air being forced through vocal folds. Parents infer it to mean exasperation or rage	Sudden onset of loud crying without initial moaning sound. Mean duration about 3 s with first unit longest (4.1–5.2 s). Subsequent units decrease in duration. Extended period of breath holding of up to 7 s after first unit

TABLE 11.2
(cont'd)

Author(s)	Type of cry: definitions			
	Low intensity cry	*Regular cry*	*Low, non-intensity cry*	*Other cries*
4. Stark and Nathanson (1974)	Cry units[4] less loud (at least 10dB lower in peak intensity) than in sustained crying	Inspiration and expiration follow each other without a marked pause. Cry units not broken by silence or marked decrease in loudness in mid-cry	Breath unit[4] length greater than longest cries classed as regular and not low intensity cries	Shorter duration than long cries and not classed as regular or low intensity
	Simple cry	*Uncoordinated crying*	*Coordinated crying*	*Elaborated crying*
5. Gustafson and Green (1991)	Crying in absence of looking at mother or gesturing	Crying accompanied by looking, but onsets of two behaviours separated by at least 10 s	Onset of crying accompanied by looking, but not by any other infant behaviour	Onset of crying accompanied by gesture (*e.g.* reaching for or pulling at mother or pointing) or by gesture and looking

[1]There are at least five hypotheses to account for the mechanisms of hyperphonation: (a) due to marked constriction of the vocal folds (Wasz-Höckert *et al.* 1968); (b) produced by open glottis as a result of losing control over laryngeal resistance to subglottal air pressure such that vocal folds blown apart (Lieberman *et al.* 1971, Ostwald 1972); (c) newborns control tension of laryngeal muscles in a discontinuous fashion, which can result in a sudden shift in pitch (Golub and Corwin 1985); (d) increased parasympathetic activity and reduced vagal tone leading to increased laryngeal contractions (Lester 1984); (e) combination of increased tension in muscles of larynx and blowing apart vocal folds (Lester 1984).

[2]These authors also distinguished birth, pain and hunger cries. *Birth cry:* rising–falling repetitive contour with relatively high mean F_0, and which involves brief inspirations and longer expirations accompanied by coughing (see also Bosma *et al.* 1965). *Pain cry:* rising–falling contour, can be dysphonated or hyperphonated and tends to having longer duration than other cries. *Hunger cry:* most have rising/falling contour, glottal plosives and maximum pitch lower than pain cry. Unlike pain cry, pitch shift and subharmonic break rarely present. Occurs four hours (±20 min.) after previous feed. The Helsinki group identified two additional spectrographic features of crying in later publications (Michelsson 1980): *double harmonic break* or harmonic doubling and *biphonation*. Biphonation is very uncommon in healthy infants, but found in those with metabolic or neurologic disorders.

[3]This classification has a number of essential differences from that of Wasz-Höckert *et al.* (1968). To begin with, hunger cries do not necessarily have any causal relationship to hunger—hence the label 'basic'. In fact, angry and pain cries are variations on this basic type. A hunger cry is made up of a series of 1 s pulses separated by brief pauses. While hunger and pain cries begin to resemble each other over measurement time, the former are more stable and rhythmic and the latter are usually much tenser as well as having a different rhythm (see also Rosenhouse 1977, 1980). Finally, Wolff identified pain cries not on the basis of acoustic features, but rather by means of the temporal patterning of the first two or three expiratory sounds.

[4]*Breath unit:* time between beginning of one inspiration and that of the next. *Cry unit:* time between beginning and end of an expiratory cry within a breath unit.

- If hunger cries are not responded to for a protracted period of time, they become acoustically similar to those elicited by a painful stimulus (Wolff 1969). This finding supports the claim that spontaneous and elicited crying do not have unique determinants, but rather reflect differences in the degree of discomfort experienced by the infant (Murray 1979, Porter *et al.* 1986, Barr 1995b).
- Beyond the newborn period, findings on the acoustic properties of spontaneous and elicited crying have to be treated with caution as there are few relevant studies, most with very small sample sizes. Fairbanks (1942) reported that the F_0 increased only slightly during the first two to three months and thereafter—a finding subsequently replicated by others who also studied spontaneous crying (Sheppard and Lane 1968, Prescott 1975). Between 1 and 6 months, the pitch of hunger crying rose by about eight semitones and then began to assume a bimodal distribution. The latter dovetails with more recent evidence that the typical falling or rising–falling melody type, found for both spontaneous crying (Michelsson 1980) and elicited crying (Lieberman 1967) in the newborn, becomes increasingly more complex with development (Prescott 1975). Such findings suggest not only increases in lung strength, but also improvements enabling the flexible control of the vocal tract (Zeskind 1985).
- At least one study made direct comparisons between spontaneous and elicited crying derived from age-sectioned samples of recordings. Fuller and Horii (1988) investigated the distribution of spectral energy in pain and hunger cries as well as for fussing and cooing vocalizations at the ages of 2, 4 and 6 months. Regardless of age, they found that pain cries differed from the other sorts of vocalizations in having not only a higher mean F_0, but also greater amplitudes in the high frequency components and overall spectral energy levels. Moreover, the mean spectral energy was highest in pain cries and was lower in the 6-month-old infants than in the younger infants for all vocalization types. While these findings support the claim that pain cries are more tense than other forms of vocal output, all vocalizations show a reduction in tenseness with age. Here we find another indication that control over the striated muscles of the vocal tract such as the cricothyroid has a rapid rate of development after birth.
- Other acoustic parameters related to F_0 include jitter, shimmer and formants. Jitter or fundamental frequency perturbation represents cycle-to-cycle variations in F_0 and thus irregular vibrations of the vocal folds. Shimmer reflects fluctuations in the amplitude of vibrations and has been shown to be related to hoarseness in adults with vocal pathologies (Haji *et al.* 1986). Peaks of acoustic energy in a sound spectrum are referred to as formants and they are numbered from the lowest to the highest (F_1, F_2 etc). Formants, determined by the contour and cross-sectional area of the supraglottal airway, have higher frequencies in infants due to the shorter supralaryngeal tract in infants relative to adults (Lester 1987). As with shimmer, formants have rarely been a focus in studies of infant vocalizations, perhaps because their structure is a feature of all vowels and some consonants. However, the higher formants (F_4 to F_6) appear to indicate individual differences in the resonance of the vocal tract and not differences between vowels (Fant 1960). Given that formants cannot be manipulated as actively as F_0, they may be sensitive to the emotional contents of communication. Thus, formants could be useful in detecting infant-specific characteristics

186

of crying and in understanding developmental changes in the emotional signals conveyed by distress vocalizations.

Jitter has been the subject of at least one study involving infants. Fuller and Horii (1987) reported that it did not differ between pain cries, hunger cries, fussing and cooing in 2-, 4- and 6-month-old infants. They found the F_0 for pain cries to be significantly higher than for hunger cries and cooing (but not compared to fussing)—a surprising finding in that jitter is assumed to be related to emotional arousal (Lieberman and Michaels 1962).

- Finally, most measures of both spontaneous and elicited crying display a marked degree of intraindividual variability regardless of such factors as gender and age. While making it difficult to find significant sex- and age-related differences, at least with regard to acoustic parameters, the magnitude of such within-subject variation probably serves to characterize the development of crying in healthy infants. Following Touwen (1976) on the broader context of neurological development, persistent stereotypies in cry production may serve to identify the compromised infant. Once again, we are faced with the dilemma of finding a quantitatively derived cut-off point for distinguishing between 'normal' and 'abnormal' crying.

In this section, consideration of different systems for classifying infant crying led us to consider evidence for developmental changes in the acoustic features of both spontaneous and elicited crying in infants. While these two general types of crying have undoubted, but not very striking, differences across ontogenetic time, acoustic analyses remain uninformative about the mechanisms of developmental change beyond the newborn period. This brings us to the problems concerning change and the origins of infant crying. More importantly, it confronts us with the outstanding issue of providing a theoretical perspective that goes beyond depicting crying as a motor phenomenon in accounting for the problem of change.

Section 4: Two problems and their theoretical implications

The origin problem refers to events that predispose or prepare a developing organism to achieve a particular developmental outcome (*e.g.* the ability to emit cry vocalizations). Each event is a necessary, but not sufficient, condition for the emergence of a new ability with a readily ascribable function (*viz.* when that ability emerges, the infant can perform functions that were previously not possible). For example, the human fetus begins to display breathing movements at a gestational age of about 10 weeks (de Vries *et al.* 1982). First described by Ahlfeld in 1888, these movements do not become functional in the sense of gas exchange in and out of the lungs until after birth and with the accompanying change from fetal to neonatal circulation. Antenatal breathing movements can therefore be regarded as a necessary exercise that prepares the developing fetus to achieve the act of taking in and expelling air from the lungs as required by the transition to the extrauterine environment.

Does crying have its origins in prenatal life? If so, what events in fetal development may serve as preparations for the postnatal act of crying? Such questions are hardly ever posed by students of infant crying, perhaps because its definitions mandate a vocal component. As pointed out previously, this requirement leads to an overly narrow view of what constitutes crying and as such depicts it as originating with the birth cry of the newborn. Consequently, systematic research on the prenatal origins of crying has been effectively excluded.

The change problem involves both description and explanation. The descriptive task is to answer the question, "How does change in a developing system occur?" Put another way, it becomes, "What are the dynamics of change?" In the past, such questions have been embroiled in debates about the nature of developmental change, which have impinged on theorizing about infant crying. One debate revolves around the issue of whether developmental change is quantitative or qualitative in nature. Thus, does the development of crying consist of a continuous and gradual accumulation of small changes (quantitative change) or of abrupt and discontinuous reorganizations resulting in the emergence of novel patterns of behaviour (qualitative change)?

Explanation consists of two entities: the explanandum (what it is that has to be explained) and the explanans (an answer to the question why something behaved or changed in the way it did). The main implication of this distinction is that description (*i.e.* of the explanandum) has logical priority over the actual explanation (*i.e.* the explanans). Crying has a multitude of descriptions, but we lack developmentally based theories of crying that address the determinants or mechanisms of change. The study of infant crying to date can be characterized as a series of loosely formulated explananda in search of an elusive set of explanatia. Explaining the process by which crying develops requires teasing out the determinants or mechanisms of change. This can really only be achieved through experimental manipulations of theoretically justified parameters in and around previously identified transitions in the development of crying. What has to be explained is how the development of crying involves changes in various coordinations between, for example, the vocal tract, respiratory, articulatory and facial movements and other functions such as auditory perception and postural control.

To understand the change problem more fully, we need to consider empirical examples of quantitative and qualitative changes in crying and the ages at which they generally occur. In comparing the acoustic properties of spontaneous and elicited crying, we made a start on this task. With regard to the problem of change, it was not a particularly informative exercise. Before embarking on this task, however, it is necessary to return to the origin problem in order to exemplify what might be construed as prenatal precursors to the postnatal development of crying. While unavoidably speculative in nature, the motivation to do so is based on the premise that an understanding of the change problem requires a deeper appreciation of the origin problem. Both problems are inescapable components in any attempt at building a theory about the development of crying.

THE ORIGIN PROBLEM EXEMPLIFIED

Given what is known about prenatal development in the human and other species, it is highly improbable that crying appears *de novo* in its entirety only after birth. What is more probable is that some of the nonvocal accompaniments of crying are developed before birth with the transition to the extrauterine environment resulting in the establishment of the vocal component. What are these nonvocal behaviours developed prenatally that form part of the complex act of crying postnatally? Educated guesses include not only the previously mentioned breathing movements but also movements of the tongue and possibly the larynx, as well as of the mouth and other parts of the face.

As revealed by ultrasonography and other methods of recording fetal behaviour, breathing movements undergo salient changes during the first half of pregnancy (de Vries *et al.* 1984, 1985) and in the last trimester (Patrick *et al.* 1980, Trudinger *et al.* 1980, Nijhuis *et al.* 1983). They increase on average from 6 per cent of recording time at 20 weeks to 30 per cent after 30 weeks. The mean breath-to-breath interval has a complex pattern of decreasing, increasing and then decreasing again at 36 weeks. By the last four weeks, there are distinct periods in which the movements are either regular or irregular, thus reflecting the establishment of discrete behavioural states, which are discussed below. Such changes indicate increasing CNS control and regulation of the actions generated by the diaphragmatic, abdominal and intercostal muscles. In addition, they suggest that their actions would function sufficiently to force air from the lungs into the vocal tract so as to make the vocal folds vibrate some time after 20 weeks. This assumption is supported by a fact well known to paediatricians, namely, that the preterm infant of about 24 weeks gestational age is capable of producing crying sounds (Gesell and Amatruda 1945, Carmichael 1970). That the cry-related actions of the respiratory muscles still have some way to develop after this age is indicated by the observation that these sounds have a shorter duration and higher F_0 than in term newborns, in addition to possessing a 'mewing' quality (Michelsson 1971).

The notion of an archetypal unmarked or hypothetical referential 'breath group' (Lieberman 1967) also has implications for understanding the prenatal origins of crying. Organized so that expiratory length and inspiratory depth preceding an expiration are geared to the duration of a sentence before its utterance in adults, it is supposedly evident in newborn crying (Lieberman 1985). If innate is taken to mean nothing more than 'present at birth' then this form of respiratory control probably has its origins in the prenatal development of breathing movements. With it being hypothesized as a means by which adults augment the flow of speech into sentence-like units, there is a further far-reaching implication to be drawn. This is that at least one feature of newborn crying is continuous with later speech development. On this rendering, we might go on to conclude that one fundamental mechanism of speech production is established during prenatal life—a conclusion complementing the claim that the fetus is capable of speech perception (De Casper and Fifer 1980).

Another relevant, though less thoroughly investigated, finding is that fetal breathing movements sometimes co-occur with jaw openings and swallowing during the first 20 weeks (de Vries *et al.* 1984). It is not known if such co-occurrences develop systematically in the second half of pregnancy. Both jaw openings (sometimes with tongue movements) and swallowing (together with sucking) appear, like breathing movements, during the first trimester (de Vries *et al.* 1982). Initially appearing as isolated events, the jaw movements tend to occur repetitively by 20 weeks with openings varying in duration from less than 1 s to 5 s (de Vries *et al.* 1984). Sucking and swallowing resulting in the ingestion of amniotic fluid involve not only tongue movements but also displacements of the larynx. Thus, these movements that serve to modulate sounds after birth are established and subsequently exercised in a different functional context before birth (*i.e.* they undergo a functional shift). This supposition abides by the long-standing principle of preadaptation in evolutionary biology (Mayr 1976). According to this principle, a preadaptation is ". . a previously existing structure, physiological process, or behavior pattern which is already functional in another context and available as a stepping stone to the attainment of a new adaptation" (Wilson 1975). Developmentally, it has been taken to mean that a (prenatal) behaviour can markedly alter its function as a consequence of a (postnatal) change in context, but without any major alterations in its underlying mechanisms (Hopkins 1983). As such, it is a form of developmental opportunism devoid of mystifying concepts like 'foresight' and 'purposiveness'. The principle allows us to see a pre- to postnatal continuity in the development of crying from a different, and possibly fruitful, perspective than has hitherto been the case.*

Apart from jaw openings, the developmental course of facial movements in the fetus is not well documented. It is known, however, that the facial musculature and its innervations are evident by 8 weeks (Crelin 1969) and complete by 18–29 weeks of gestation (Gasser 1967). In addition, Oster (1978) reported that all but one of the discrete facial actions observable in adults can be identified in preterm newborns during the last trimester. Clearly, the development of facial expression must be rooted in prenatal life. But what about the expressive gestalt termed the 'cry face'? Birnholz (1986) demonstrated the rich potential of ultrasound recordings for monitoring facial expressions in the mid-third trimester fetus, including that resembling a 'cry face' (Birnholz and Farrell 1984).

Four behavioural states have been classified in the human fetus and shown to achieve a stable organization only in the last month of a term pregnancy (Nijhuis *et al.* 1982). Consisting of active and inactive sleep and wake states categorized on the basis of the presence or absence of body and eye movements and four heart rate patterns, the classification does not include a crying state. However, ultrasound recordings of orofacial movements subjected, for example, to the Neonatal Facial Coding System (Grunau and Craig 1987) could provide a first step in identifying the prenatal homologue of the crying state. Additional criteria might include hand movements (*e.g.* presence or absence of fisting) and the patterning of fetal heart rate. Noting the much lower incidence of wake compared to sleep states in the near-term fetus (Nijhuis *et al.* 1982), we would not expect crying to emerge as anything more than a fleeting state towards the end of pregnancy. Developmentally, we would expect evidence of cry acts before the last trimester which, as they become longer lasting, begin to assume state-like characteristics (*e.g.* simultaneous change in two or more criteria as proposed by Nijhuis *et al.* 1982).

In summary, it has been argued that the prerespiratory components of crying have their developmental origins in early prenatal life. Subsequently, they undergo developmental changes so that they become increasingly intercoordinated, which results in the emergence

*Other insights it provides into the prenatal origins of crying and its adaptive significance after birth derive from the fact that humans are born in a less advanced state than other primates. This outcome is thought to be due to a shortening of pregnancy during hominoid evolution (Washburn 1960). While the reasons for this shortening are not properly understood (see Prechtl 1984), the state of the human newborn represents a pre-adaptation in that it gives relatively more time for enculturation and learning (Dobzhansky *et al.* 1977). The downside is that our newborns are considerably more helpless, but with one notable exception: the ability to communicate their needs by means of crying. This emphasizes the point that the crucial mechanisms for cry production must be established during prenatal life. In addition, crying itself may be preadaptation for postnatal development in general in that it promotes the acquisition of social, perceptual and cognitive abilities (Gustafson and Green 1989).

of the crying state during the last few weeks of a term pregnancy. We now pursue the change problem further in considering the postnatal development of crying.

THE CHANGE PROBLEM EXEMPLIFIED

During the newborn period itself, both spontaneous and pain-elicited crying show quantitative changes: the duration of cries and the intervals between them become shorter over the first nine days (Prechtl *et al.* 1969). In addition, the number of pitch shifts decreases markedly (Wasz-Höckert *et al.* 1968). Such changes are indicative of a recovery in physiological stability following the stress of delivery. How does crying develop after the achievement of physiological stability? In the descriptive sense, what subsequent quantitative and qualitative changes does it undergo?

The most striking change of a quantitative nature concerns the so-called 6-week peak in crying. First documented systematically by Brazelton (1962), this phenomenon has been replicated many times in the ensuing decades, mainly on the basis of data obtained from daily diaries. Studies in the 1970s (Bell and Ainsworth 1972, Bernal 1972, Rebelsky and Black 1972, Roe 1975, Emde *et al.* 1976) through the 1980s (Snow *et al.* 1980; Hunziker and Barr 1986; Hubbard and Ijzendoorn 1987; Barr *et al.* 1988, 1989) and into the present decade (Michelsson *et al.* 1990, St James-Roberts and Halil 1991, Baildam *et al.* 1995) have consistently described a developmental function conforming to something like an inverted U or n-shaped curve: an increase in duration up to about 6 weeks of age followed by a gradual decrease until around 4 months. This modal trend seems to be quite robust and universal as it is evident across different methods of data collection (Barr 1990b) and variations in child-rearing practices to be found in both Western societies (Alvarez and St James-Roberts 1996) and non-Western cultures (Barr *et al.* 1991, St James-Roberts *et al.* 1994). Its universality is further attested to by the fact that it occurs in preterm infants after correcting postnatal age for degree of prematurity (Barr *et al.* 1996, Malone 1997). This developmental depiction turns out to be in need of the following qualifications, which illustrate well some of the complexities of dealing with the change problem:

• *Duration versus frequency.* Most studies have focused on the cumulative duration of crying per day (diaries) or per hour (audio recordings) to the exclusion of its relative frequency of occurrence. Thus, evidence for a developmental function that assumes an n-shaped curve with a peak at about 6 weeks stems largely from this measure of duration. Other measures of duration such as the length of cry bouts are rarely considered, despite the fact they are typical units of measurement in diary studies (Barr 1990a). From the few studies reporting measures of frequency, it appears that there is not an age-related peak (Bell and Ainsworth 1972, Landau 1982, Hubbard and Ijzendoorn 1987), or at least that it is only weakly present compared to that for the duration of crying (Barr *et al.* 1991, 1996). After the age of about 2 months, the frequency of crying does not decrease significantly up to the end of the first year, unlike its duration (Gustafson and Green 1991, Baildam *et al.* 1995). Finally, we should remember that what is comparable across studies is the peak-related patterning of crying over age and not absolute amounts at any one age (Barr 1990b).

• *Individual differences.* Between-subject variability in the amount of crying during the first year is perhaps the most common finding. It tends to be largest at the age of peak crying or during the first three months (Barr 1990a). A peak does not occur precisely at 6 weeks for all infants, with some never manifesting it at any age. Individual consistency (*i.e.* stability of ranking across age) seems to be present up to about 3 months of age for both the duration (Rebelsky and Black 1972) and frequency (Moss 1967) of crying. At least one study reported its persistence up to the end of the first year for frequency (Baildam *et al.* 1995). However, Bell and Ainsworth (1972) could find such consistency for both duration and frequency only during the second half of the first year. The amount of attention given to the issue of individual consistency has led to a neglect of intra-individual differences in the development of crying. One of the few studies to address this form of variability reported it to be only slightly less than that between subjects across the ages of 1–13 weeks for the duration of crying (Rebelsky and Black 1972). This finding reiterates the point that individual infants are unlikely to comply with the population-level pattern derived from group means in all its details.

- *Time of day.* Another common finding associated with diary studies is that within any one day, the amount of crying is greatest during the late afternoon and evening (16.00–24.00 hours). Apparent at 10 days of age (Bernal 1972), this diurnal peak becomes more evident by the age of peak crying and then lessens after 3 months (Hunziker and Barr 1986). Constituting about 40 per cent of the total amount of crying before 3 months (Barr *et al.* 1989), it remains unclear if this peak arises from the same processes as the age-related peak (Barr 1990b). The finding that supplementary carrying of infants by their parents removes the 6-week, but not the evening, peak (Hunziker and Barr 1986) suggests that they are based on different processes.

- *Crying versus fussing.* It is becoming clear that what most infants emit vocally at the 6-week peak is fussing or fretting rather than clear-cut crying (St James-Roberts *et al.* 1995). It can be concluded, therefore, that this peak mainly consists of fretful fussing during the evening hours (Barr *et al.* 1991). Even in 6-week-old infants considered to be persistent criers, maternal diaries reported that the majority had a predominance of this sort of fussing regardless of the time of day (St James-Roberts *et al.* 1995). Here again, we can appreciate the beneficial insights to be gained from including fussing in studying the development of crying.

- *The assumption of universality.* There is a strong case for treating the age-related peak in crying as a universal characteristic of infant development based on the cross-national/cultural comparisons and studies of preterm infants discussed previously. However, such examples of 'unity in diversity' should not lead us into the trap of regarding it as a maturationally determined phenomenon impervious to environmental influences. Returning to the effects of supplementary carrying, while it eliminated the 6-week peak, there was no difference between the experimental and control groups in the frequency of crying/fussing bouts at this age (Hunziker and Barr 1986). This finding brings us full circle back to the first qualification in that it suggests the duration and frequency of crying are founded on different processes. We should also bear in mind that English infants had high durations of crying at 2 and 6 weeks (St James-Roberts *et al.* 1995), which prompts us to acknowledge that the universality assumption is not such a simple one after all. The immediate reaction is perhaps to raise the (obvious) spectre of methodological differences, but it is equally plausible to suppose culturally specific variations in child-rearing practices as an explanation. Whatever the case, these exceptions, and other qualifications considered, should temper our awareness of the difficulties to be surmounted in dealing with the change problem—even in the case of quantitative changes in crying during early postnatal development.

What about other changes in the development of crying that are more qualitative in appearance? There are two studies that provide some relevant answers. The first considers crying in the context of the sweeping functional changes around 2–3 months after birth (Hopkins and van Wulfften Palthe 1987) while the other informs us about the nature of change after this age (Gustafson and Green 1991). Both are rare examples of studying the development of both the vocal and nonvocal components of crying longitudinally.

In the first study, 14 infants were observed every three weeks from 3 to 18 weeks by means of video recordings in their homes while they were alone or during interaction with the mother. In contrast to crying, fussing and cooing vocalizations were not present until 6 weeks of age. After this age, these vocalizations became intermingled in a state-like entity referred to as 'interrupted fussing' (rapid alternations between fussing and cooing). This new form of vocal output was associated with at least two nonvocal behaviours: the eyes remained open and the hands were involved in manipulatory activities. This suite of changes was only found in the alone situation.* Thus, at about 2–3 months of age, there is a major transformation in the crying state resulting from new coordinations between its component parts.

The study by Gustafson and Green (1991) involved home-based observations of a younger (n=12) and older (n=14) sample covering the age range of 3 to just after 12 months. Four patterns of crying were identified, with three of them accounting for nonvocal accompaniments (see Table 11.2, p. 185). Replicated in a later cross-sectional study using video recordings (Green and Gustafson 1997), a notable finding was the occurrence of the elaborated pattern in a small proportion of 6-month-olds and in the majority by the end of the first year. Consisting of the onset of a cry bout co-occurring with looking at the mother or a gesture or both, it reveals another qualitative change in crying subsequent to that apparent at 2–3 months. As with interrupted fussing, elaborated crying is achieved through the temporal coordination of behaviours previously performed independently of each other. Simple crying, by definition, excluded such an achievement. While it decreased significantly from 3 to 12 months, this form of crying involving only the vocal component was still more evident than the elaborated pattern by the end of the first year (Green and Gufstafson 1997). Such a finding led to the conclusion that ". . cry development reflects no single, all-or-none transition but, instead, increasing variability and sophistication in forms and functions" (Gustafson and Green 1991). Is this a justifiable conclusion? The answer is a qualified yes. The qualification arises from the fact that certain analytical tools are available for examining whether or not such a developmental scenario obtains, but were not applied in this study.

*Impressions not reported at the time for interrupted fussing included abrupt alternations between a cry face (together with a fussing vocalization) and smiling (together with a cooing vocalization), and coordinated movements of the head and eyes as if 'searching' the immediate environment.

Derived as a means of detecting qualitative change in time-evolving systems, it is generally referred to as a dynamic systems approach.

CONSIDERING THE CHANGE PROBLEM FROM A DYNAMIC SYSTEMS APPROACH (DSA)
According to a DSA, development can be portrayed as consisting of transitions between a succession of stable states or attractors (Fogel and Thelen 1987). Catastrophe theory, one variant of this approach, holds the promise of being able to detect whether any developmental transition is linear or nonlinear, and if nonlinear whether it involves quantitative or qualitative change. Detection is possible through applying so-called 'catastrophe flags' to the behavioral output of a system at its macrolevel of organization, at which level it is referred to as an order parameter or collective variable. Currently, there are eight such flags for detecting the onset and offset of a transition (Gilmore 1981; see also Hartelman *et al.* 1998). Three signal an upcoming transition (*e.g.* critical fluctuations in the order parameter) and the remaining five can become apparent during the transition (*e.g.* a sudden jump in the value of the order parameter).

Using these flags to detect developmental transitions and the sort of change involved is a far from easy task. To do so requires a combination of longitudinal research (to detect the timing of a transition by means of those flags associated with a system's spontaneous behaviour) and experimental studies in and around the age of a transition (to detect the nature of change). By itself, a sudden jump in an order parameter, which in essence is what Gustafson and Green (1991) referred to in their conclusion, cannot tell us unequivocally whether the change is really instantaneous or a continuous acceleration (van der Maas and Hopkins 1998). To make this distinction requires the presence of other flags such as critical fluctuations. The strongest evidence for qualitative change is not only when the system demonstrates critical fluctuations (as perhaps implied in the term 'increasing variability' used by Gustafson and Green), but more importantly when it reacts to a small perturbation with a divergent response.

Despite the considerable difficulties to be overcome, there is recent and encouraging evidence that the various catastrophe flags can be used to detect developmental transitions and to determine whether or not they represent qualitative change (*e.g.* van der Maas and Molenaar 1992, Wimmers *et al.* 1998). In terms of infant crying, they might be applied, for example, to examine whether the appearance of interrupted fussing represents a transition to a qualitatively different stable state. As with any other behaviour, their application depends on capturing an appropriate order parameter. This is by no means a trivial problem as it has to be a relational measure that is continuously scaled (*e.g.* the relative phase between limb movements as discussed in detail by Kelso 1995). A candidate order parameter for crying might include phase relationships between the respiratory movements of the diaphragm and intercostal muscles as recorded by surface EMG (Prechtl *et al.* 1977). Another could be based on the temporal relationships between brow and orofacial movements—assuming such movements can be measured in a continuous fashion.

Strictly speaking, a DSA to development does not provide us with a theory about infant crying. Its primary function is to expose the organizational principles, rather than the mechanisms, that concern the temporal evolution of an order parameter by means of the analytical tools it provides (Hopkins and Butterworth 1997). In this regard, it is completely neutral as to the domain-specific contents of an order parameter. The same neutrality obtains for the control parameter that may induce a particular developmental change in infant crying. Relative to development in general, it does, however, bring our attention to a theoretically important point: qualitative change in an order parameter may arise from the quantitative scaling-up of a control parameter beyond some critical value. On this view, the issue of whether development is a matter of qualitative or quantitative change becomes irrelevant. What is relevant is not only how we construe an order parameter for crying, but also how to do the same for a relevant control parameter at a more microlevel of organization.

The sort of control parameter responsible for change at the system's macrolevel may differ from one age to the next (Hopkins *et al.* 1993). The parameter for crying could reside at one age in the neural control of the vocal tract and at other ages in the control of respiration, the articulators, posture or perception. Developmentally, they may not only induce change, but also serve as constraints or rate-limiting factors (Soll 1979) on the attainment of a new developmental state. It is the maintenance, breaking and re-making of such constraints that are responsible for the stabilities (when a system is not undergoing a transition), instabilities (during a transition) and emergence of a new state (after a transition has been achieved) that typify a developmental process. What are the constraints that might operate on the development of crying?

Section 5: Constraints on the development of crying

The constraints to be considered represent a selection of sub-systems that become increasingly coordinated during the development of crying. The selection omits reference to potential neural constraints on the vocal tract as these receive considerable coverage in the richly formulated theories of Golub and Corwin (1982) and Lester (1984).*

RESPIRATION

More than 20 years ago, reference was made to the lack of knowledge about how the respiratory control of sound production develops (McNeilage and Ladfoged 1976). This situation has not changed much since then, particularly with respect to how respiratory muscles undergo changes in coordination during the development of sound production. Furthermore, what little we do know stems from findings derived from pain cries rather than spontaneous crying.

---

*There are similarities and differences between the two theories. Both assume that variations in the influence of the vagal (Xth cranial) nerve on the five intrinsic muscles of the larynx account for variations in the F_0 of the newborn cry. Vagal input achieves its effects mainly through activating contractions in the cricothyroid muscles. Both also assume that respiratory influences are indicated by the duration and intensity of a cry as well as by the ratio of phonation to dysphonation; laryngeal effects by the F_0 including hyperphonation; and those of the vocal tract by formant frequencies F_1 and F_2. A cardinal difference has to do with how the newborn might control tension in the laryngeal muscles. For Golub, who modifies the acoustic theory of sound production (Fant 1960) for the infant vocal tract, it is controlled in a quantal, discontinuous fashion. Lester, like Lieberman (1977), hypothesises a more continuous form of tension control due to increases or decreases in parasympathetic activity and vagal tone.

In the newborn, each cry cycle displays a consistent displacement of respiratory volume, which suggests a rather precise coordination between crying and respiration (Bosma *et al.* 1965). However, the newborn's cry contains evidence of inspiratory voicing, but some time between 1 and 3 months nearly all cries are produced in the expiratory phase of tidal breathing (Fischelli *et al.* 1966). This change can be explained by the observation that the duration of inspiration changes little while that for expiration increases markedly during the first eight months (Prescott 1980). More specifically, this reorganization in the inspiratory–expiratory cycle permitting prolonged voicing on expiration is present by 12 weeks and develops rapidly during the next month (Wilder and Baken 1978). By 1 year, the breathing rate during crying has decreased from 50 breaths per minute at 1 month to a mean of 19, which is very similar to the adult rate of 16 (Langlois *et al.* 1980). Thus, by the end of the first year, the infant when crying has acquired the (faster) inspiratory – (longer) expiratory pattern of respiration that characterizes adult breathing during speech production. Like the notion of an archetypal unmarked breath group, such a conclusion conforms to the claim that infant crying in some way functionally constrains the development of speech sounds.

What can account for the ability of the developing infant to prolong the expiratory phase during crying? What constrains the development of this ability? One suggestion hinges on the newborn's purported lack of a 'hold-back' mechanism (Wolff 1969, Lieberman 1975). This mechanism is deemed to be necessary for regulating subglottal air pressure so that long expirations can be produced. In the newborn, the rib cage is aligned almost perpendicularly to the spine (Langlois *et al.* 1980). As such, it imposes a mechanical constraint on the maintenance of a steady subglottal air pressure required for prolonging the expiratory phase. Due to the elastic recoil of the lungs being relatively low in the newborn, sufficient air pressure can be generated during short expirations for voicing to occur. Increases in lung volume during crying lead to an initial pressure that is too high for a long expiration to be sustained (Lieberman 1985). At about 3 months, a dramatic change occurs that removes constraints on long expirations: the rib cage begins to assume an adult-like configuration in which there is a downwards and outwards angle between it and the spine (Hixon 1973). As a consequence, the actions of the intercostal muscles can now complement those of the abdomen, which previously were the only ones available to assist in preserving a constant level of subglottal air pressure. The external (expiratory) intercostals perform the task of lifting and enlarging the rib cage. More crucially, the internal (inspiratory) intercostals can now act more fully to pull it down and decrease its size. This major restructuring of the rib cage enables greater control to be exercised over subglottal air pressure and thereby not only deeper and longer breathing, but also greater variations in the vocal output of crying.

In summary, the infant of about 3 months of age has acquired a rudimentary ability to hold back on the flow of subglottal air pressure—an essential achievement for the further development of crying. Some three months later, further improvements in the control of rib cage movements and increases in the elasticity of the costal cartilages result in the partitioning of lung volume and inspiratory/expiratory ratios with adult-like properties (Baken 1987). By about 6 months, and perhaps even earlier, there is clear evidence that the breathing cycle can be modified voluntarily in the service of crying and other vocalizations

(Oller 1980). If most of the constraints on the respiratory control of crying have been lifted during the first six months, what about those operating on the main sound producer (larynx) and its resonating chamber (pharynx)? Does the release of their rate-limiting factors codevelop with those identified for respiration?

LARYNX AND PHARYNX

The larynx not only is a sound producer in that it contains the glottis and vocal folds, but also serves as a valve to regulate air flow from the respiratory system. According to the myoelastic–aerodynamic theory (van den Berg 1958), it shifts from the valve-like function to being an organ of phonation with every closure of the glottis. This sort of functional switching is not well developed in the newborn. A possible constraint in this respect resides in the fact that the newborn's larynx is situated close to the base of the skull and thus has a high position relative to the adults of all primate species (Crelin 1969). Its high position, together with the velum and epiglottis forming a seal, allows the human newborn to breathe and ingest liquids at the same time (Laitman et al. 1977). However, this arrangement means that newborns are obligate nose breathers, which imposes severe constraints on the respiratory modulation of sound production. Starting at about 3 months, things begin to change in concert with the changes taking place in the rib cage.

What begins to happen around 3 months is the descent of the larynx to a position in the pharynx (George 1978). Due to the development of a system of suspension between the larynx, the mandible and the hyoid bone, it descends to a point resulting in the elimination of the seal between the velum and epiglottis, and thereby the opening of the airway to the nose. While the infant can no longer breathe and ingest simultaneously, breathing through the mouth becomes possible and with it an increased ability to regulate subglottal air pressure during crying. By about 6 months, this profound re-engineering of the laryngeal suspension system is almost complete (Sasaki et al. 1977).

The pharynx in adult humans is much longer than in other primates (Tzeng and Wang 1984) and provides us with the highest degree of vocal versatility in the primate order. However, it is much shorter in the human newborn relative to its size in adulthood (Lieberman 1998). Consequently the pharynx is a poor acoustic resonator, and there is little pharyngeal activity in the newborn. With changes in the size and geometry of the oropharyngeal tract occurring at or just before 3 months, vocalizations take on a fuller resonance (Hast 1970). An interesting observation is that newborns are capable of making clear resonant sounds when emitting cries that have a 'schwa-like' quality (Lieberman et al. 1971). As pointed out by Oller (1980), these cries have second and third formants with much higher frequencies than other sorts of vocalizations. The implication is that full resonance is developed first in crying and only later becomes a property of other forms of vocal output.

Some time around 3 months, the pharynx and larynx start to disengage in conjunction with the separation between the velum and epiglottis (Sasaki et al. 1977). The angle between the pharynx and larynx becomes increasingly rectangular, a uniquely human configuration that is strikingly evident by 6 months. The changing relationship between the two structures not only facilitates oral breathing, but also coordinates their respective actions with those of the thorax and the articulators of the oral cavity (Bosma et al. 1965). The net result is a significant contribution to control of sound production as witnessed by the emergence of babbling between 4 and 6 months and changes in the quality of crying across the same age range. This age range also encapsulates anatomical and other changes in the articulators.

ARTICULATORS

The upper teeth, the alveolar ridge behind them and the hard palate are classified as passive articulators. In addition to the pharynx, the velum, tongue, lips and jaw constitute the active articulators. Both sets of articulators constrain newborn vocalizations and both undergo change in concert.

With the restructuring of the basicranium around 3 months, the hard palate is shifted backwards along the base of the skull (Crelin 1969). In doing so, it enables the achievement of a uniquely human supralaryngeal tract. The roof of the mouth becomes reduced relative to that in nonhuman primates. Together with a reduction in the size of the lower jaw, it means that humans are relatively inefficient at chewing and that the teeth grow closely together, which increases the risk of impaction and thus infection. Set against these disadvantages is a marked improvement in the contribution of the supralaryngeal tract to phonation as the airway from the mouth to the nose can be sealed off. The infant is now able to produce consistent non-nasal sounds with readily identifiable patterns of formant frequencies (Lieberman 1977). Little attention has been given to whether changes in dentition accompany those in the quality of voicing during crying. Typically, the lower teeth are clearly apparent by about 3 months and the upper teeth some two to three months later. The most we can say is that both these first ages of appearance coincide with anatomical changes in the vocal tract and with significant alterations in sound production during crying.

Turning to the active articulators, we have already noted how the velum partakes in transforming the oropharyngeal system. Serving to direct the respiratory air stream, its movements in the newborn are constrained by the actions of two muscles (Kent 1981). One tenses the velum (musculus tensor veli palatini) while the other functions to raise or lower it (musculus levator veli palatini). Its direction of movement changes from cephalic to cephalodorsal with the establishment of the distinctively human craniovertebral angle (Kent 1981). Thus, by about 3 months, constraints on their functioning begin to diminish such that they become more actively involved in directing the flow of air through the oropharyngeal system. However, in terms of actual articulation, the tongue initially imposes perhaps even more severe constraints.

Due to the fact that the tongue almost fills the oral cavity of the newborn, its movements are markedly limited, making articulatory deformations more or less impossible. The best the newborn can do is to distort the tongue body in the oral cavity in order to obtain cross-sectional changes in the pharyngeal cavity required for articulation (Lieberman 1980). Another constraint on articulation has to do with the shape of the newborn's tongue, which is positioned entirely in the oral cavity due to the high position of the larynx. Lacking the circular shape of the adult tongue, it is long and slender with its dorsum almost in contact with the velum and epiglottis. In these respects, it is more like the tongue of the adult chimpanzee (Lieberman 1980). With the lowering of the base of the tongue and a reshaping of its fit within the oral cavity some time between 3 and 6 months, tongue movements acquire additional degrees of freedom and thus increased articulatory functions (Fletcher 1973, *cited in* Kent 1981). Added to these anatomical changes, the intrinsic and extrinsic muscles of the tongue gain increasing control over its movements—with the latter (*e.g.* the genioglossus that pulls the medial or pharyngeal portion in an anterior direction) being more important than the former (Kent 1981).

During crying and other vocalizations, there is little differentiation between the movements of the tongue, lips and jaw in the newborn (Wolff 1969). Moreover, the tongue and the jaw move out of phase with laryngeal action in both pain-elicited cries (Bosma *et al.* 1965) and spontaneous crying (Stark and Nathanson 1974). Between the ages of 3 and 9 months, movements of the jaw become increasingly independent from those of the tongue and lower lip, as reflected in the production of sounds such as r, s, z, th and w (Wolff 1969). Apart from this observation, we have little or no insight into the development of coordination between the various active articulators after the newborn period. In contrast to tongue movements, but similar to those of the face, the developmental problem is to reduce the large number of degrees of freedom in the articulatory muscles that have to be controlled to enable their coordination. For development in general, gaining control over the body's vast number of degrees of freedom in muscles (and joints) is facilitated by the development of postural control.

POSTURE

It has been noted that during crying, the supine newborn assumes an opisthotonic posture in which the arms are flexed and adducted with the trunk becoming rigid and partially extended (Wolff 1969, Hopkins and van Wulfften Palthe 1987). The suggestion has been made that this posture accounts for turbulence and pitch in the spontaneous crying of the newborn (Stark and Nathanson 1974). In preterm infants at 35–36 weeks gestation, there was greater variability in their cry spectra and more rapid variations in pitch compared to term newborns (Tenold *et al.* 1974). These differences were accredited to a poorer postural stabilization in the supine position for the preterm infants.

Another feature of the newborn's supine posture is that it is lateralized with the head typically maintained on the right side of the body (Hopkins and Rönnqvist 1998). In conjunction with flexion and adduction in the arms, it facilitates ipsilateral hand–mouth contact (Hopkins *et al.* 1987), which in turn should enable the newborn to self-regulate crying. This expectation was borne out: newborns could terminate a crying bout with hand–mouth contact, but never did so with contacts to other parts of the face (Hopkins *et al.* 1988). However, they were not very accurate in contacting the mouth with the hand during crying, possibly due to a lack of postural stability in the supine position.

All told, these observations vividly illustrate the constraints on crying imposed by the age-specific nature of postural control in the newborn. How then do changes in posture and crying co-develop after the newborn period? Unfortunately, there are only fragmentary pieces of evidence that can aid us in answering this neglected question.

To begin with, some of the anatomical changes considered previously alter important features of the infant's posture. One consequent alteration arises with the achievement of a vertical alignment between the head, neck and torso. With this alignment, the infant becomes capable of an adult-like control of respiration during sound production (Baken 1987). This form of developing control parallels the infant's ability to self-regulate the duration of crying. After the newborn period and up to the age of around 2 months, the ability to terminate a crying bout by means of hand–mouth contact disappears (Hopkins *et al.* 1988). The loss of this ability is associated with a change in posture, namely, the replacement of arm flexion in the newborn by one in which the arms become more extended and thus further away from the face. When able to alternate the arms between extension and flexion at about 3 months, hand–mouth contacting has clearly re-established itself as a means of ending a crying bout. What is intriguing about these findings is how closely they match the evidence for the 6-week peak in the duration of crying, especially that derived from samples of Western infants. In short, the peak coincides with an inability to terminate crying by way of hand–mouth contacting, and the subsequent decline with its reappearance. These co-developments in cry duration and an epiphenomenon of changes in postural control have so far not been incorporated into explanations for the n-shaped normal crying curve.

Over 40 years ago, it was suggested that the supine position exerts gravitational constraints on the sorts of vocalizations produced by infants (McCarthy 1952). In this position, the force of gravity should result in a closure of the velopharyngeal opening due to the velum falling backwards. Thus, vocal output should consist of non-nasal sounds. In the upright position, however, gravity would operate to prevent closure and thereby the production of nasal sounds. Unfortunately, this suggestion does not comply with the fact that young infants are obligate nasal breathers nor with the report that their crying contains nasality irrespective of posture (Stark and Nathanson 1974). It is further undermined by a study that found no differences in cooing between the supine and upright positions for infants of 1–4 months of age (Oller 1981). Nevertheless, in the light of interrupted fussing only being evident when the infant was supine (and alone) but not when upright (and faced with the mother) as found by Hopkins and van Wulfften Palthe (1987), this suggestion is worth pursuing further in the context of infant crying. Certainly, we know next to nothing about how the development of postural control may assist the infant in overcoming any constraints imposed by the force of gravity on the control and coordination of crying. What are also lacking are clear insights into the role of auditory perception during the development of crying.

AUDITORY PERCEPTION

The auditory system develops very rapidly during prenatal life. By 5 months gestation the sizes of the middle and inner structures are comparable to those of the adult (Northern and Downs 1974), and the auditory fibres begin to myelinate one month later (Tanner 1970). Do these developments enable the newborn to modulate crying by means of the auditory feedback they may provide? In other words, does the newborn use such feedback to control the actions of the larynx during crying? If not, when does this sort of coupling between perception and action become evident?

The notion of an inseparable coupling between perception and action stands central in the theory of ecological psychology advocated by Gibson (1979). Transported to the realm of crying, it would hold that, given the circular causality between perception and action, the cry act changes the properties of the acoustic field, which in turn changes the act and so on (R.G. Barr, personal communication 1994). How could such reciprocal interactions between (auditory) perception and (laryngeal) action during infant crying be investigated? One strategy could involve using the technique of delayed auditory feedback (DAF).

Widely used in research on adult speech production, DAF effects have been classified as either direct or indirect (Fairbanks 1955). Direct effects are signalled by prolongations in speech and an increase in the number of speech dysfluencies. Elevation of the F_0 and increased speech intensity are indicative of indirect effects. The most common finding is that the peak disturbance to speech occurs with a delay interval of 200 ms (Smith 1962), which corresponds to the mean syllabic length in nearly all languages (Lenneberg 1967). In seemingly the only study to have investigated DAF effects on newborn crying, this was precisely the delay interval that produced a noticeable disturbance (Cullen *et al.* 1968). The disturbance was restricted to the expiratory duration of cries elicited by snapping a rubber band against the sole of the foot, which was reduced by 100 ms. This single direct effect complies with Menyuk's (1971) claim that DAF results in only short-lasting cessations of crying in young infants.

The tentative conclusion from this sort of study is that some form of perception–action coupling found in adult speech is operative during crying after birth. How it subsequently develops is unknown. Animal studies have been used in this respect. For example, it has been shown that auditory feedback may exert some control over vocal tract configuration in the stress calls of kittens shortly after birth (Buchwald and Brown 1977). This would suggest that the loudness of the cry is being used as a feedback control as it is a function not only of pitch intensity, but also of the resonances produced by altering the internal configuration of the vocal tract. In experiments by Buchwald and Brown (1977), the destruction of both cochleae in 4-week-old kittens resulted in a striking disruption of the formant structure, but not of the F_0. Thus, by this age, formant frequency may rely more on auditory feedback than pitch. Lesions made in the central auditory pathway at the upper brainstem level in other kittens of the same age produced a more direct effect, namely, an increase in the duration of the stress call. These two sets of findings implicate the development of two kinds of auditory feedback: one controlling the duration of a call and the other its acoustic structure. Their development may be constrained by an auditory system that initially has a high threshold and poor transmission fidelity (Buchwald 1981).

In stressing that the development of crying involves changes in the coupling between perception and action (or rather movement), we should not forget that it also requires a reciprocal relationship between posture and movement. Thus, crying develops not only as a consequence of changes in perception–movement cycles, but also due to transformations in the coupling between movement and posture. With development, constraints on the couplings between perception, movement and posture diminish in such a way that the act of crying becomes increasingly task-specific (*e.g.* as a means of communicating a particular need).

Section 6: Conclusions
This contribution has addressed a variety of largely unresolved issues concerning the

development of crying. At least four of them merit further attention. First, there is the issue of how we define and classify crying and whether or not we should distinguish it from fussing. Second, our limited knowledge about the postnatal development of crying derives from a heterogeneous set of data collection methods, which focus on either its spontaneous or elicited forms of generation. Third, concerning spontaneous crying, we know next to nothing about its prenatal origins. And fourth, there has been a serious neglect of how the development of crying may undergo organizational change and of the constraint-breaking mechanisms that may account for such change.

In defining what is meant by crying, we need to account more fully for its nonvocal accompaniments in terms of movement and posture. In doing so, we may accrue a double-edged benefit: the possibility of being able to make clearer distinctions between crying and fussing as well as between different types of crying, and the provision of a descriptive framework more likely to capture significant developmental changes. Deriving such a framework should be motivated by the obvious fact that crying is a complex act requiring the formation of coordinations or functional synergies between a number of subsystems. In treating crying this way, the task of description can be guided by theoretical considerations arising from a dynamic systems approach to the development of movement coordination and action as expounded, for example, by Thelen and Smith (1994) and Goldfield (1995). Examples of how it can be applied to the development of crying have been mentioned, and more thoroughgoing discussions can be found elsewhere (*e.g.* see Wolff 1987, Barr *et al.* 1999).

Why is our understanding of how crying develops postnatally so limited? Perhaps the main reason is that most relevant studies are founded on the use of the diary method. This method has provided a number of valuable insights into the development of spontaneous crying, but it is ill-equipped for the purpose of describing qualitative change. That purpose, at least in the first instance, is better served by an approach that endeavors to capture the natural history of crying along the lines originally pioneered by Wolff (1969). The acoustic analysis of elicited pain cries is, like the diary method, restricted in its applications. While it has limited use in promoting insights into the normal development of crying, it continues to be pursued as a standardized method for the early detection of CNS disturbances. However, it could be the case that spontaneous crying is a more sensitive indicator of nervous system integrity than elicited crying. This assumption has been supported by animal experiments. If one looks across the history of such experiments (*e.g.* those where animals have been asphyxiated), there is a consistent, but neglected, finding: while responses can still be elicited from animals in a terminal condition, the quality rather than the quantity of their spontaneous movements is noticeably different from that of intact animals. Here again, we find another compelling argument for a closer study of the nonvocal accompaniments of infant crying and for continuing with attempts to delineate the more qualitative features of its voicing.

We have noted the paucity of theorizing about the development of crying outside the context of the newborn period. A major theoretical contribution would be made if more attention was given to the origin problem. Despite the considerable technical difficulties to be overcome, much would be gained from fetal ultrasound recordings focused on one or more of the suggested prerespiratory components of crying prior to the last trimester of pregnancy. Recordings made in the third trimester could be compared with observations on the spontaneous crying of healthy preterm infants before term age using the same or similar measures. Such comparisons, consisting of matched gestational ages, would provide a means for validating which behavioural expressions in the fetus are indicative of crying. In passing, and as noted by others, it is unknown if the additional extrauterine experience of preterm infants results in a crying peak before term age (Barr *et al.* 1996). If so, this would undermine a maturational account as to why the timing of peak crying occurs at around the post-term age of 6 weeks. Comparisons with fetuses of the same gestational ages could help in resolving this challenge to what has become a widely accepted account.

The change problem is the other outstanding issue in theorizing about the development of infant crying. More specifically, it boils down to detecting and explaining developmental transitions in crying. Detecting, for example, whether crying undergoes a qualitative change at 2 to 3 months along with a host of other functions is possible in principle through the application of catastrophe flags to appropriate development data. By appropriate, we mean appropriate order parameters. Identifying these parameters is stymied by the lack of a developmental theory with respect to crying. As suggested in this contribution, a key to unlocking this particular problem might be to treat the development of crying as a process of establishing temporal coordinations between two or more cry-related behaviours. The study by Gustafson and Green (1991) is an excellent example of progress in this direction.

Explaining or accounting for the mechanisms of change in crying requires specifying the initial constraints on its development. To regard them as being only neural in origin commits the Fallacy of Misplaced Concreteness (Bullock and Grossberg 1991). With this pitfall in mind, I have attempted to broaden the scope of potential constraints to include, for example, anatomical and biomechanical limitations on the development of crying. The ultimate goal is to identify those constraints amenable to some form of experimental manipulation as control parameters. Assuming that a developmental transition has been detected at a particular age, infants of this age can be subjected to changes in control parameter values. If the order parameter becomes reorganized at some value of the control parameter, then we have probably found an agent of change in the development of crying. For the transition at 2–3 months, postural control was offered as a potential control parameter. At this age, it undergoes a change from a lateralized, body-referenced posture to a more symmetrical, spatially oriented posture (Geerdink *et al.* 1994). An appropriate manipulation might be to shift a crying 2-month-old back and forth between the two postures scaled along some continuous dimension. The question to be answered is whether it produces successive reorganizations in crying at different values of the control parameter.

By way of a final comment on future directions, it may prove profitable for clinically based studies on infant crying to include some consideration of developmental transitions. If, as argued, the crying of compromised infants lacks in some way the normal variability of expression, then their capacity to embark upon and complete a developmental transition to a new mode of crying may be severely impaired. This impairment could be manifest by a marked delay or a different way in achieving the transition. In the worst case, the infant may never make the transition (*e.g.* to the elaborated crying described by Gustafson and

Green 1991). The clinical relevance of this recommendation will depend on detecting the timing and organizational features of developmental transitions in the crying of healthy infants. To achieve such a 'gold standard' requires a strategy of research that is conspicuously different from the ways in which we have studied infant crying in the past. Hopefully, this contribution has conveyed the rudiments of this strategy, and convincing evidence that the changes taking place in crying at about 2–3 months are such as to merit its initial application to infants of this age.

REFERENCES

Ahlfeld, D. (1888) 'Uber bisher noch nicht beschriebene Bewegungen des Kindes.' *Verhandlungen der Deutschen Gesellschaft für Gynäkologie*, **2**, 203–210.
Aldrich, C.A., Sung, C., Knop, C. (1945) 'The crying of newly born babies. I. The community phase.' *Journal of Pediatrics*, **26**, 313–326.
Alvarez, M., St James-Roberts, I. (1996) 'Infant fussing and crying patterns in the first year in an urban community in Denmark.' *Acta Paediatrica*, **85**, 463–466.
Atkinson, J.E. (1978) 'Correlation analysis of the physiological factors controlling fundamental voice frequency.' *Journal of the Acoustical Society of America*, **63**, 211–220.
Baildam, E.M., Hillier, V.F., Ward, B.S., Bannister, R.P., Bamford, F.N., Moore, W.M.O. (1995) 'Duration and pattern of crying in the first year of life.' *Developmental Medicine and Child Neurology*, **37**, 345–353.
Baken, R.J. (1987) *Clinical Measurement of Speech and Voice*. Boston: Little, Brown.
Barr, R.G. (1990a) 'The early crying paradox: A modest proposal.' *Human Nature*, **1**, 355–389.
—— (1990b) 'The normal crying curve: What do we really know?' *Developmental Medicine and Child Neurology*, **32**, 356–362.
—— (1995a) 'Introduction: Crying in context.' *Early Development and Parenting*, **4**, 157–159.
—— (1995b) 'The enigma of infant crying: The emergence of defining dimensions.' *Early Development and Parenting*, **4**, 225–232.
—— Elias, M.F. (1998) 'Nursing interval and maternal responsivity: Effect on early infant crying.' *Pediatrics*, **81**, 529–536.
—— Kramer, M.S., Boisjoly, C., McVey-White, L., Pless, I.B. (1988) 'Parental diary of infant cry and fuss behaviour.' *Archives of Disease in Childhood*, **63**, 380–387.
—— —— Pless, I.B., Boisjoly, C., Leduc, D. (1989) 'Feeding and temperament as determinants of early infant crying/fussing behavior.' *Pediatrics*, **84**, 514–521.
—— Konner, M., Bakeman, R., Adamson, L. (1991) 'Crying in !Kung San infants: a test of the cultural specificity hypothesis.' *Developmental Medicine and Child Neurology*, **33**, 601–610.
—— Richards, A., Yaremko, J., Leduc, D., Francoeur, T.E. (1992) 'The crying of infants with colic: A controlled empirical description.' *Pediatrics*, **90**, 12–21.
—— Chen, S.J., Hopkins, B., Westra, T. (1996) 'Crying patterns in preterm infants.' *Developmental Medicine and Child Neurology*, **38**, 345–355.
—— Beek, P.J., Calinoiu, N. (1999) 'Challenges to nonlinear modelling of infant emotion regulation in real and developmental time.' *In:* Savelsbergh, G.J.P., van der Maas, H.L.J., van Geert, P.L.C. (Eds.) *Nonlinear Developmental Processes*. Amsterdam: Royal Netherlands Academy of Arts and Sciences, pp. 15–37.
Bell, S.M., Ainsworth, M.S. (1972) 'Infant crying and maternal responsiveness.' *Child Development*, **43**, 1171–1190.
Bergé, P., Pomeau, Y., Vidal, C. (1984) *Order Within Chaos: Towards a Deterministic Approach to Turbulence*. New York: Wiley.
Bernal, J. (1972) 'Crying during the first ten days of life and the maternal responses.' *Developmental Medicine and Child Neurology*, **14**, 362–372.
Birnholz, J.C. (1986) 'Ultrasonic studies of human fetal brain development.' *Trends in Neurosciences*, **9**, 329–333.
—— Farrell, E.E. (1984) 'Ultrasound images of human fetal development.' *American Scientist*, **72**, 608–613.
Bosma, J.F., Truby, H.M., Lind, J. (1965) 'Cry motions of the newborn infant.' *Acta Paediatrica Scandinavica*, Suppl. 163, 61–92.

Brazelton, T.G. (1962) 'Crying in infancy.' *Pediatrics*, **29**, 40–47.

Buchwald, J.S. (1981) 'Development of vocal communication in an experimental model.' *In:* Friedman, S.L., Sigman, M. (Eds.) *Preterm Birth and Psychological Development.* New York: Academic Press, pp. 107–126.

—— Brown, K.A. (1977) 'The role of acoustic flow in the development of adaptive behavior.' *Annals of the New York Academy of Sciences*, **290**, 270–284.

Bullock, D., Grossberg, S. (1991) 'Adaptive neural networks for control of movement trajectories invariant under speed and force rescaling.' *Human Movement Science*, **10**, 3–53.

Carmichael, L. (1970) 'The onset and early development of behavior.' *In:* Mussen, P.H. (Ed.) *Carmichael's Manual of Child Psychology.* New York: Wiley, pp. 447–564.

Crelin, E.S. (1969) *Anatomy of the Newborn: An Atlas.* Philadelphia: Lea & Febiger.

Cullen, J.K., Fargo, N., Chase, R.A., Baker, P. (1968) 'The development of auditory feedback monitoring. I. Delayed auditory feedback studies on infant cry.' *Journal of Hearing and Speech Research*, **11**, 85–93.

De Casper, A.J., Fifer, W. (1980) 'Of human bonding: Newborns prefer their mothers' voices.' *Science*, **208**, 1174–1176.

De Vries, J.I.P., Visser, G.H.A., Prechtl, H.F.R. (1982) 'The emergence of fetal behaviour. I. Qualitative aspects.' *Early Human Development*, **7**, 301–322.

—— Visser, G.H.A., Prechtl, H.F.R. (1984) 'Fetal motility in the first half of pregnancy.' *In:* Prechtl, H.F.R. (Ed.) *Continuity of Neural Functions from Prenatal to Postnatal Life. Clinics in Developmental Medicine No. 94.* London: Spastics International Medical Publications, pp. 46–64.

—— —— —— (1985) 'The emergence of fetal behavior. II. Quantitative aspects.' *Early Human Development*, **12**, 99–120.

Dobzhansky, T., Ayala, F.J., Stebbins, G.L., Valentine, J.W. (1977) *Evolution.* San Francisco: Freeman.

D'Odorico, L., Franco, F., Vidotto, G. (1985) 'Temporal characteristics in infant cry and non-cry vocalizations.' *Language and Speech*, **28**, 29–46.

Emde, R., Gaensbauer, T., Harmon, R. (1976) *Emotional Expression in Infancy: A Biobehavioral Study.* New York: International Universities Press.

Fairbanks, G. (1942) 'An acoustical study of the pitch of infant hunger wails.' *Child Development*, **13**, 227–232.

—— (1955) 'Selective vocal effects of delayed auditory feedback on speech and key tapping.' *Journal of Speech and Hearing Disorders*, **20**, 333–346.

Fant, G. (1960) *Acoustic Theory of Speech Perception.* The Hague: Mouton.

Fischelli, V.R., Haber, A., Davis, J., Karelitz, S. (1966) 'Audible characteristics of the cries of normal infants and those with Down's syndrome.' *Perceptual and Motor Skills*, **23**, 744–746.

Fogel, A., Thelen, E. (1987) 'Development of early expressive and communicative action: Reinterpreting evidence from a dynamic perspective.' *Developmental Psychology*, **23**, 747–761.

French, V. (1995) 'History of parenting: The Ancient Mediterranean world.' *In:* Bornstein, M.H. (Ed.) *Handbook of Parenting: Biology and Ecology of Parenting. Vol. 2.* Mahwah, NJ: Erlbaum, pp. 263–284.

Fuller, B.F., Horii, Y. (1987) 'Differences in fundamental frequency, jitter and shimmer among four types of infant vocalizations.' *Journal of Communication Disorders*, **19**, 111–117.

—— —— (1988) 'Spectral energy distribution in four types of infant vocalizations.' *Journal of Communication Disorders*, **21**, 251–261.

Gasser, R.F. (1967) 'The development of the facial muscles in man.' *American Journal of Anatomy*, **120**, 357–375.

Geerdink, J.J., Hopkins, B., Hoeksma, J.B. (1994) 'The development of head position preference in preterm infants beyond term age.' *Developmental Psychobiology*, **27**, 153–168.

George, S.L. (1978) 'A longitudinal and cross-sectional analysis of the growth of the postnatal cranial base angle.' *American Journal of Physical Anthropology*, **49**, 171–178.

Gesell A., Amatruda C.S. (1945) *The Embryology of Behavior.* New York: Harper.

Gibson, J.J. (1979) *The Ecological Approach to Visual Perception.* Boston: Houghton-Mifflin.

Gilmore, R. (1981) *Catastrophe Theory for Scientists and Engineers.* New York: Wiley.

Goldfield, E.C. (1995) *Emergent Forms: Origins and Early Development of Human Action and Perception.* Oxford: Oxford University Press.

Golub, H.L., Corwin, M.J. (1982) 'Infant cry: A clue to diagnosis.' *Pediatrics*, **69**, 197–201.

—— (1985) 'A physioacoustic model of the infant cry.' *In:* Lester, B.M., Boukdyis, C.F. (Eds.) *Infant Crying: Theoretcal and Research Perspectives.* New York: Plenum Press, pp. 59–82.

Green, J.A., Gustafson, G.E. (1997) 'Perspectives on an ecological approach to social communicative development in infancy.' *In:* Dent-Read, C., Zukow-Goldring, P. (Eds.) *Evolving Explanations of Development.* Washington, DC: American Psychological Association, pp. 515–546.

Grunau, R.V.E., Craig, K.D. (1987) 'Pain expression in neonates: Facial action and cry.' *Pain*, **28**, 395–410.

Gustafson, G.E., Green, J.A. (1989) 'On the importance of fundamental frequency and other acoustic features in cry perception and infant development.' *Child Development*, **60**, 772–780.

—— —— (1991) 'Developmental coordination of cry sounds with visual regard and gestures.' *Infant Behavior and Development*, **14**, 51–57.

—— —— Tomic, T. (1984) 'Acoustic correlates of individuality in the cries of human infants.' *Developmental Psychobiology*, **17**, 311–324.

Haji, T., Horiguchi, S., Baer, T., Gould, W.J. (1986) 'Frequency and amplitude perturbation analysis of electro-glottograph during sustained attention.' *Journal of the Acoustical Society of America*, **80**, 58–62.

Hartelman, P.A.I., van der Maas, H.L.J., Molenaar, P.C.M. (1998) 'Detecting and modelling developmental transitions.' *British Journal of Developmental Psychology*, **16**, 97–122.

Hast, M.H. (1970) 'The developmental anatomy of the larynx.' *Otolaryngology Clinics of North America*, **3**, 413–439.

Hixon, T.J. (1973) 'Respiratory function in speech.' *In:* Minifie, F., Hixon, T.J., Williams, F. (Eds.) *Normal Aspects of Hearing, Speech and Language.* Englewood Cliffs, NJ: Prentice-Hall, pp. 73–125.

Hopkins, B. (1983) 'The development of early communication: An evaluation of its meaning.' *Journal of Child Psychology and Psychiatry*, **24**, 131–144.

—— Butterworth, G. (1997) 'Dynamical system approaches to the development of action.' *In:* Bremner, G., Slater, A., Butterworth, G. (Eds.) *Infant Development: Recent Advances.* Hove, Sussex: Psychology Press, pp. 75–100.

—— Prechtl, H.F.R. (1984) 'A qualitative approach to the development of movements during early infancy.' *In:* Prechtl, H.F.R. (Ed.) *Continuity of Neural Functions from Prenatal to Postnatal Life. Clinics in Developmental Medicine No. 94.* London: Spastics International Medical Publications, pp. 179–197.

—— Rönnqvist, L. (1998) 'Human handedness: developmental and evolutionary perspectives.' *In:* Simion, F., Butterworth, G. (Eds.) *The Development of Sensory, Motor and Cognitive Capacities in Early Infancy.* Hove, Sussex: Psychology Press, pp. 189–233.

—— van Wulfften Palthe, T. (1987) 'The development of the crying state.' *Developmental Psychobiology*, **20**, 165–175.

—— Lems, W., Janssen, B., Butterworth, G. (1987) 'Postural and motor asymmetries in newlyborns.' *Human Neurobiology*, **6**, 165–175.

—— Janssen, B., Kardoun, O., van der Schoot, T. (1988) 'Quieting during infancy: Evidence for a developmental change?' *Early Human Development*, **18**, 111–124.

—— Beek, P.J., Kalverboer, A.F. (1993) 'Theoretical issues in the longitudinal study of motor development.' *In:* Kalverboer, A.F., Hopkins, B., Geuze, R. (Eds.) *Motor Development in Early and Later Childhood : Longitudinal Approaches.* Cambridge: Cambridge University Press, pp. 343–371.

Hubbard, F.O.A., van Ijzendoorn, M. (1987) 'Maternal unresponsiveness and infant crying across the first 9 months: A naturalistic longitudinal study.' *Infant Behavior and Development*, **14**, 299–312.

Hunziker, U.A., Barr, R.G. (1986) 'Increased crying reduces infant crying: A randomized control trial.' *Pediatrics*, **77**, 641–648.

Irwin, O.C., Curry, T. (1941) 'Vowel elements in the crying vocalizations of infants under ten days of age.' *Child Development*, **12**, 99–109.

Jakobson, R. (1941) *Kindersprache, Aphasie und Allgemeine Lautgestetze.* Uppsala: Almqvist & Wiksell.

Kelso, J.A.S. (1995) *Dynamic Patterns: The Self-Organization of Brain and Behavior.* Cambridge: MA: MIT Press.

Kent, R.D. (1981) 'Articulatory–acoustic perspectives in speech development.' *In:* Stark, R.E. (Ed.) *Language Behavior in Infancy and Early Childhood.* Amsterdam: Elsevier, pp. 105–126.

—— (1984) 'The psychobiology of speech development: Co-emergence of language and a movement system.' *American Journal of Physiology*, **246**, 888–894.

Laitman, J.A., Crelin, E.S., Conologue, G.J. (1977) 'The function of the epiglottis in monkey and man.' *Yale Journal of Biology and Medicine*, **50**, 43–54.

Landau, R. (1982) 'Infant crying and fussing: Findings from a cross-cultural study.' *Journal of Cross-Cultural Psychology*, **13**, 427–444.

Langlois, A., Baken, R.J., Wilder, C.N. (1980) 'Pre-speech respiratory behavior during the first year of life.' *In:* Murry, T., Murry, J. (Eds.) *Infant Communication, Cry and Early Speech.* Houston: College Hill Press, pp. 56–84.

Laver, J. (1980) *The Phonetic Description of Voice Quality.* Cambridge: Cambridge University Press.

Lenneberg, E. H. (1967) *Biological Foundations of Language*. New York: Wiley.

Lester, B.M. (1984) 'A biosocial model of infant crying.' *In:* Lipsitt, L. (Ed.) *Advances in Infant Behavior and Development*. Norwood, NJ: Ablex, pp. 167–212.

—— (1987) 'Developmental outcome prediction from acoustic analysis in term and preterm infants.' *Pediatrics*, **80**, 529–534.

Lieberman, P. (1967) *Intonation, Perception and Language*. Cambridge, MA: MIT Press.

—— (1975) *On the Origins of Language: An Introduction to the Evolution of Speech*. New York: Macmillan.

—— (1977) *Speech, Physiology and Acoustic Phonetics: An Introduction*. New York: Macmillan.

—— (1980) 'On the development of vowel production in young children.' *In:* Yeni-Komishian, G.H., Kavanagh, J.F., Ferguson, C.A. (Eds.) *Child Phonology. Vol. 1. Production*. New York: Academic Press, pp. 113–142.

—— (1985) 'The physiology of cry and speech in relation to linguistic behavior.' *In:* Lester, B.M., Boukdyis, C.F. (Eds.) *Infant Crying: Theoretical and Research Perspectives*. New York: Plenum Press, pp. 29–57.

—— (1998) *Eve Spoke: Human Language and Human Evolution*. London: Picador.

—— Michaels, S.B. (1962) 'Some aspects of fundamental frequency and envelope amplitudes as related to the emotional content of speech.' *Journal of the Acoustical Society of America*, **34**, 922–927.

—— Harris, K.S., Wolff, P., Russell, L.H. (1971) 'Newborn infant cry and non-human primate vocalization.' *Journal of Speech and Hearing Research*, **14**, 718–727.

MacNeilage, P., Ladefoged, P. (1976) 'The production of speech and language.' *In:* Caterette, E.C., Friedman, M.P. (Eds.) *Handbook of Perception. Vol. 7. Language and Speech*. New York: Academic Press, pp. 75–120.

McCarthy, D. (1952) 'Organismic interpretation of infant vocalization.' *Child Development*, **23**, 273–280.

Malone, A. (1997) 'The crying pattern of preterm infants.' *Paper presented at the 6th International Workshop on Infant Cry Research, Bowness-on-Windermere, England, July 1–4.*

Mayr, E. (1976) *Evolution and the Diversity of Life: Selected Essays*. Cambridge, MA: Belknap Press.

Menyuk, P. (1971) *The Acquisition and Development of Language*. Englewood Cliffs, NJ: Prentice-Hall.

Michelsson, K. (1971) 'Cry analysis of symptomless low birth weight neonates and of asphyxiated newborn infants.' *Acta Paediatrica Scandinavica*, Suppl. 216, 1–45.

—— (1980) 'Cry characteristics in sound spectrographic cry analysis.' *In:* Murry, T., Murry, J. (Eds.) *Infant Communication, Cry and Early Speech*. Houston: College Hill Press, pp. 85–105.

—— Wasz-Höckert, O. (1980) 'The value of cry analysis in neonatology and early infancy.' *In:* Murry, T., Murry, J. (Eds.) *Infant Communication, Cry and Early Speech*. Houston: College Hill Press, pp. 152–182.

—— Rinne, A., Paajanen, S. (1990) 'Crying, feeding and sleeping patterns in 1- to 12-month-old infants.' *Child: Care, Health and Development*, **16**, 99–111.

Moss, H.A. (1967) 'Sex, age and state as determinants of mother–infant interaction.' *Merrill-Palmer Quarterly*, **13**, 19–36.

—— (1974) 'Communication in mother–infant interaction.' *In:* Krames, L., Pliner, P., Alloway, T. (Eds.) *Advances in the Study of Communication and Affect. Vol. 1. Nonverbal Communication*. New York: Plenum Press, pp. 171–191.

Murray, A.D. (1979) 'Infant crying as an elicitor of parental behavior: An examination of two models.' *Psychological Bulletin*, **86**, 191–215.

Murry, T., Amundson, P., Hollien, H. (1977) 'Acoustical characteristics of infant cries: Fundamental frequency.' *Journal of Child Language*, **4**, 321–328.

Nijhuis, J.G., Prechtl, H.F.R., Martin, C.B., Bots, R.S.G.M. (1982) 'Are there behavioural states in the human fetus?' *Early Human Development*, **6**, 177–195.

Northern, J., Downs, M. (1974) *Hearing in Children*. Baltimore: Williams & Wilkins.

Oller, D.K. (1980) 'The emergence of the sounds of speech in infancy.' *In:* Yeni-Komishian, G.H., Kavanagh, J.F., Ferguson, C.A. (Eds.) *Child Phonology. Vol. 1. Production*. New York: Academic Press, pp. 93–112.

—— (1981) 'Infant vocalizations: Exploration and reflexivity.' *In:* Stark, R.E. (Ed.) *Language Behavior in Infancy and Early Childhood*. Amsterdam: Elsevier, pp. 85–103.

Oster, H. (1978) 'Facial expression and affect development.' *In:* Lewis, M., Rosenblum, L.A. (Eds.) *The Development of Affect*. New York: Plenum Press, pp. 43–75.

Ostwald, P.F. (1972) 'The sounds of infancy.' *Developmental Medicine and Child Neurology*, **14**, 350–361.

—— Peltzman, P. (1974) 'The cry of the human infant.' *Scientific American*, **230**, 84–90.

Papousek, M. (1989) 'Determinants of responsiveness to infant vocal expression of emotional state.' *Infant Behavior and Development*, **12**, 507–524.

Patrick, J., Campbell, K., Carmichael, L., Natele, R., Richardson, B. (1980) 'Patterns of human fetal breathing and gross fetal body movements at 34 to 35 weeks of gestation.' *Obstetrics and Gynecology*, **56**, 24–30.

207

Porter, F.L., Miller, R.H., Marshall, R.E. (1986) 'Neonatal pain cries: Effect of circumcision on acoustic features and perceived urgency.' *Child Development*, **57**, 790–802.

Prechtl, H.F.R. (1984) 'Continuity and change in early neural development.' *In:* Prechtl, H.F.R. (Ed.) *Continuity of Neural Functions from Prenatal to Postnatal Life. Clinics in Developmental Medicine No. 94*. London: Spastics International Medical Publications, pp. 1–15.

—— Theorell, K., Gramsbergen, A., Lind, J. (1969) 'A statistical analysis of cry patterns in normal and abnormal infants.' *Developmental Medicine and Child Neurology*, **11**, 142–152.

—— van Eykern, L.A., O'Brien, M.J. (1977) 'Respiratory muscle EMG in newborns: A non-intrusive method.' *Early Human Development*, **1**, 265–283.

Prescott, R. (1975) 'Infant cry sound: Developmental features.' *Journal of the Acoustical Society of America*, **57**, 1186–1191.

—— (1980) 'Cry and maturation.' *In:* Murry, T., Murry, J. (Eds.) *Infant Communication, Cry and Early Speech*. Houston: College Hill Press, pp. 234–250.

Rebelsky, F., Black, R. (1972) 'Crying in infancy.' *Journal of Genetic Psychology*, **121**, 49–57.

Ringel, R.L., Kluppel, D.O. (1964) 'Neonatal crying—A normative study.' *Folia Phoniatrica*, **16**, 1–9.

Roe, K.V. (1975) 'Amount of infant vocalization as a function of age: Some cognitive implications.' *Child Development*, **46**, 936–941.

Rosenhouse, J. (1977) 'A preliminary report: An analysis of some types of a baby's cries.' *Journal of Phonetics*, **5**, 299–312.

—— (1980) 'Duration of infants' communication by cries.' *Journal of Phonetics*, **8**, 135–156.

Sasaki, C.T., Levine, P.A., Laitman, J.T., Crelin, E.S. (1977) 'Postnatal descent of the epiglottis in man.' *Archives of Otolaryngology*, **103**, 169–171.

Sheppard, W.C., Lane, H.L. (1968) 'Development of the prosodic features of infant vocalization.' *Journal of Speech and Hearing Research*, **11**, 94–108.

Simner, M.L. (1971) 'Newborn's response to the cry of another infant.' *Developmental Psychology*, **5**, 136–150.

Smith, K.U. (1962) *Delayed Sensory Feedback and Behavior*. Philadelphia: W.B. Saunders.

Snow, M.E., Jacklin, C.N., Maccoby, E.E. (1980) 'Crying episodes and sleep–wakefulness transitions in the first 26 months of life.' *Infant Behavior and Development*, **3**, 387–394.

Soll, D. (1979) 'Timers in developmental systems.' *Science*, **203**, 841–849.

St James-Roberts, I., Halil, T. (1991) 'Infant crying patterns in the first year: Normal community and clinical findings.' *Journal of Child Psychology and Psychiatry*, **32**, 951–968.

—— Hurry, J., Bowyer, J. (1993) 'Objective confirmation of crying in infants referred for excessive crying.' *Archives of Disease in Childhood*, **68**, 82–84.

—— Bowyer, J., Varghese, S., Sawdon, J. (1994) 'Infant crying patterns in Manali and London.' *Child: Care, Health and Development*, **20**, 323–337.

—— Conroy, S., Wilsher, K. (1995) 'Clinical, developmental and social aspects of infant crying and colic.' *Early Development and Parenting*, **4**, 177–189.

Stark, R.E., Nathanson, S.N. (1974) 'Spontaneous cry in the newborn infant: Sounds and facial gestures.' *In:* Bosma, J.F. (Ed.) *Fourth Symposium on Oral Sensation and Perception: Development in the Fetus and Infant*. Bethesda, MD: US Government Printing Press, pp. 323–347.

—— Rose, S.N., McLagen, M. (1975) 'Features of infant sounds: The first eight weeks of life.' *Journal of Child Language*, **2**, 205–221.

—— —— Benson, P.J. (1978) 'Classification of infant vocalization.' *British Journal of Disorders of Communication*, **13**, 41–47.

Stetson, R.H. (1951) *Motor Phonetics: A Study of Speech Movements*. Amsterdam: North-Holland.

Tanner, J.M. (1970) 'Physical growth.' *In:* Mussen, P.H. (Ed.) *Carmichael's Manual of Child Psychology*. New York: Wiley, pp. 77–156.

Tenold, J.L., Crowell, D.H., Jones, R.H., Daniel, T.H., McPherson, D.F., Popper, A.N. (1974) 'Cepstral and stationary analysis of full-term and premature infants' cries.' *Journal of the Acoustical Society of America*, **56**, 975–980.

Thelen, E., Smith, L.B. (1994) *A Dynamic Systems Approach to the Development of Cognition and Action*. Cambridge, MA: MIT Press.

Thodén, C.J., Koivisto, M. (1980) 'Acoustic analyses of the normal pain cry.' *In:* Murry, T., Murry, J. (Eds.) *Infant Communication, Cry and Early Speech*. Houston: College Hill Press, pp. 124–151.

Touwen, B.C.L. (1976) *Neurological Development in Infancy. Clinics in Developmental Medicine No. 58*. London: Spastics International Medical Publications.

Truby, H.M., Lind, J. (1965) 'Cry sounds of the newborn infant.' *Acta Paediatrica Scandinavica*, Suppl. 163, 7–59.

Trudinger, B.J., Aust, F., Knight, P.C. (1980) 'Fetal age and patterns of human fetal breathing movements.' *American Journal of Obstetrics and Gynecology*, **137**, 724–728.

Tzeng, O.J., Wang, S.Y. (1984) 'Search for a common neurocognitive mechanism for language and movements.' *American Journal of Physiology*, **246**, 868–883.

van den Berg, J. (1958) 'Myoelastic–aerodynamic theory of voice production.' *Journal of Hearing and Speech*, **1**, 227–244.

van der Maas, H.L.J., Hopkins, B. (1998) 'Dynamical systems theory: So what's new?' *British Journal of Developmental Psychology*, **16**, 1–13,

—— Molenaar, P.C.M. (1992) 'Cognitive development: An application of catastrophe theory.' *Psychological Review*, **99**, 395–417.

Washburn, S.L. (1960) 'Tools and human evolution.' *Scientific American*, **203**, 63–75.

Wasz-Höckert, O., Lind, J., Partanen, T., Valanne, E., Vuorenkoski, V. (1968) *The Infant Cry: A Spectrographic and Auditory Analysis. Clinics in Developmental Medicine No. 29*. London: Spastics International Medical Publications.

Wilder, C.N., Baken, R.J. (1978) 'Some developmental aspects of infant cry.' *Journal of Genetic Psychology*, **132**, 225–230.

Wilson, E.O. (1975) *Sociobiology: The New Synthesis*. Cambridge, MA: Belknap Press.

Wimmers, R.H., Savelsbergh, G.J.P, Beek, P.J., Hopkins, B. (1998) 'Evidence for a phase transition in the early development of prehension.' *Developmental Psychobiology*, **32**, 235–248.

Wolff, P.H. (1967) 'The role of biological rhythms in early psychological development.' *Bulletin of the Menninger Clinic*, **31**, 197–218.

—— (1969) 'The natural history of crying and other vocalizations in early infancy.' *In:* Foss, B.M. (Ed.) *Determinants of Infant Behaviour. Vol. 4*. London: Methuen, pp. 81–109.

—— (1987) *The Development of Behavioral States and the Expression of Emotions in Early Infancy: New Proposals for Investigation*. Chicago: University of Chicago Press.

Zeskind, P.S. (1985) 'A developmental perspective of infant crying.' *In:* Lester, B.M., Boukydis, C.F.Z. (Eds.) *Infant Crying: Theoretical and Research Perspectives*. New York: Plenum Press, pp. 159–186.

—— Parker-Price, S., Barr, R.G. (1993) 'Rhythmic organization of the sound of infant crying.' *Developmental Psychobiology*, **26**, 321–333.

12

THE CRYING INFANT AND TODDLER: CHALLENGES, EMERGENT THEMES AND PROMISSORY NOTES

Ronald G. Barr, Brian Hopkins and James A. Green

Challenges revisited

No-one ever said raising an infant, soon to become a toddler, would be easy. Mixed with the joys of the smiling and responsive infant are the frustrations of hearing her or his cry, becoming anxious about what the crying means, and being unable to soothe her/him. The previous chapters have been a testament to the complexity, salience and importance of crying in the early days, months and years of the life of infants and toddlers.

After the joy of the first 'birth cry' come the infant's responses to pain and situational challenges, followed by the first three or four months of increased crying, even in the face of optimal caregiving. Following the first four months, the crying—now quantitatively less but more intentional, communicative, complex, and still difficult to interpret—still raises anxieties and challenges parents. Even when language emerges in toddlers, crying continues to be manifest in enigmatic and difficult to explain temper tantrums, associated with signs of anger and physiological arousal manifested by flushing.

Although there are considerable individual differences in the amount, the timing and the manner in which they are manifest in each child, these are all normal phases of development and manifestations of crying. In infants and toddlers compromised since birth, these phases are often accentuated and prolonged, making their 'normative' interpretation more difficult for already concerned parents. Furthermore, these normative crying phases are supplemented by infections, illnesses, injuries and reactions to common environmental exposures on the one hand, and stressed and sometimes fragile family contexts on the other. As such, they generate countless visits to health services with concerns about what is causing the crying, what it means, and what one can do. There are many challenges that come with the joys and responsibilities of parenting. But when the infant or toddler is crying, it is the responsibilities rather than the joys that tend to come to the fore.

For those of us who experience crying as members of the helping professions or as researchers, there are also a number of challenges. Some of the challenges are the same (or at least similar) to those of parents. We, too, want to know what causes crying, what it means, and what one can do. But some of the challenges are different. For one, the priorities are different. Parents want to know about crying in their infant, while researchers want to know about crying in infants in general. Clinicians are somewhere in between; they want to know about crying in infants in general so that they can better understand, interpret and act on behalf of the infant for whom the parents sought out clinicians for care and advice. For another, the salience of the crying arises in a different context. Parents have to live with their infant (and the crying) for 24 hours a day, whereas clinicians are exposed to the infant's crying for only hours or even minutes at a time while they are trying to assess it. Researchers and their colleagues, depending on the methods they use, are likely to be even further removed from the crying experience, and may even want parents to 'let' their infants cry so they can obtain samples of behavior to measure and to study. In all cases, crying is a remarkably salient behavior, but for somewhat different reasons.

Occasionally (and helpfully), the contexts sometimes 'converge' and provide an important reminder of the commonality of our interests. In the laboratory of one of us (RGB), we had an experience that allowed us, as researchers, to appreciate to some extent what some parents are going through. When studying daily crying patterns recorded on audiotapes that used a voice-activating circuit, 24 hours of recording were 'compressed' into about one to three hours of recordings of almost nothing but cries (Barr *et al.* 1988). It is probably fair to say that the transcription of these tapes was the most stressful observational activity that we have ever undertaken in over 20 years of investigation.

A third difference is that parents know to what they are referring when talking about crying. Their anxiety stems from wanting to know what it means, or what their infants are 'saying'. Clinicians tend to find the phenomenon unambiguous too. Their anxiety is elevated if they have difficulty determining whether it is a sign of illness. Researchers, however, are not so certain they know what crying is, whether fussing is the same as or different than crying, and whether it is better understood, or in what way(s) it can be understood, as a sign or a signal.

In this volume, we have brought together a number of authors who have concerned themselves with crying behavior in both normative and clinical contexts, and for whom one or more of these challenges has been a focus in their own work. Primarily these have been clinicians and child developmentalists. As mentioned in Chapter 1, neither all professions nor all the challenges posed in the literature are represented. But even in this sample, some of the benefits of this juxtaposition have begun to emerge. In this epilogue, we would like to highlight just a few of what might be called 'emergent themes' from these contributions.

Emergent themes in research on crying

1. JUXTAPOSING CLINICAL (CRYING AS SYMPTOMS AND SIGNS) AND DEVELOPMENTAL (CRYING AS A SIGNAL) PERSPECTIVES

One emergent theme is that the juxtaposition of clinical and developmental perspectives appears to benefit both pediatric clinicians and child developmental researchers and, ultimately, parents and their infants. These juxtapositions have been reflected in a number of ways. Most obviously, some chapters have been written by clinicians and some by developmentalists. However, some chapters dealing with clinical issues have been written by developmentalists (Chapters 3, 8, 9), other chapters written by clinicians take a distinctly developmental perspective on the clinical problem (Chapters 4, 5, 7), and still others (Chapters 1, 4, 12) have been written by both. More important though is whether such a juxtaposition of clinical and developmental perspectives actually makes a difference for clinicians and developmentalists. We think it does, and in numerous ways, a few of which may serve as illustrations.

In a number of chapters, the benefits of seeing clinical symptoms and signs from a developmental perspective (as a signal) have some clear implications for our understanding, and often for our assessment, of clinical problems. The problem of colic—considered as a clinical syndrome (a clustering of symptoms and signs whose etiology is unclear)—can be redefined when considered from a developmental perspective. This is most clearly evident from the demonstration that the 'peak' pattern of crying in colic, considered one of the primary defining characteristics of the syndrome, is more accurately understood as a developmental crying pattern typical of normally developing infants, of whom the infants with colic are at the upper end of the spectrum (Chapter 4). This is also probably true of all of the other 'defining' characteristics of the syndrome (Chapter 4). In that light, it is less paradoxical, indeed more likely, that the outcomes for infants with colic should be good (as current evidence suggests—see Chapter 5), even though there may be persistent effects for the parents challenged to care for these infants. It also implies that textbook descriptions that define colic as a distinct, clinical entity due simply and unifactorily to a probable gastrointestinal pathophysiological process are at least misleading and probably wrong.

This developmental perspective also has implications for clinicians attempting to treat infants with colic. If an organic condition (say, cow's milk protein intolerance) is present concurrently with the normal crying peak, the crying induced by the organic condition is likely to be 'additive' to, or superimposed on, the crying curve that would be there anyway. This has two important consequences for clinicians and parents. One is that, if the wrong treatment (say, a switch to a lactose-free formula that does not remove the offending protein) is applied just when the crying would decline anyway, then the treatment might be considered 'effective' even though it did nothing for the real cause, the protein intolerance. Another is that, if the right treatment (say, a switch to a casein hydrolysate formula) is applied before the 'peak' crying occurs, then the treatment might be considered 'ineffective' because the partial relief due to removal of the offending protein was countered by the continuing developmental increase in crying.

For researchers, these sorts of scenarios have implications for the design and interpretation of clinical treatment trials in infants with colic, whether the treatments be formula interventions, medications, or parental advice and support. On the one hand, researchers must take into account the timing of the intervention. Interventions introduced prior to the peak are more likely to be good tests of their efficacy. If interventions are introduced after the peak, even efficacious interventions may be seen as nonefficacious (relative to the control group), resulting in a 'false negative' trial result (referred to in research design terminology as a 'Type II' error). On the other hand, researchers must take into account that even an efficacious intervention for an organic condition may not make all of the crying go away, but just that portion of it that is due to the condition over and above the normal rise in crying. Thus, the appropriate expected 'effect size' (on which the sizes of experimental and control samples are based) is much smaller than that which might be expected if 'all' early increased crying were assumed to be due to the organic condition. To compensate for this, the sizes of the samples of patients in studies of colic will need to be much bigger than those usually reported.

Alternatively, there is a long tradition of investigation in which 'pathological' or 'clinical' manifestations of a behavior are studied as a means of improving insights and knowledge about normal functioning. The juxtaposition of clinical and developmental perspectives brings these implications more clearly to the fore in regard to crying behavior as well. For example, the investigation of colic syndrome using developmental concepts from the fields of emotion regulation and temperament [and particularly, it is argued (Chapter 4), the core concepts of responsivity, reactivity and regulation] may teach us something important about the individual differences referred to as 'temperament'. For one, it provides a number of tests of whether earlier reported temperamental 'difficultness' is really a good predictor of later temperament (especially difficultness, but other dimensions as well), or whether something quite different is happening in the first three months of life. If the transient responsivity hypothesis turns out to be supported empirically, then the common assumption that increased difficultness (to the extent that it is equated with increased crying) is a way of assessing early temperament may be at least misleading, and possibly inappropriate.

Similar kinds of questions and insights can be raised in regard to other crying manifestations. From the developmental point of view, it is clear that the differential diagnosis that clinicians have to consider in the face of a complaint about persistent crying in the emergency room (Chapter 6) should be different depending on the age of the infant. 'Colic' is not an appropriate diagnosis if the crying is acute, if the infant has a fever, or after the age of 4 months. The very difficult problem of temper tantrums, when carefully documented through parental reports and considered as a 'window' on to underlying physiological systems rather than as a symptom, raises the possibility that they have two distinguishable anger and distress components (Chapter 8). Further, it is likely that sympathetic nervous system activity is more closely related to the anger component and withdrawal of parasympathetic system activity is more closely related to the distress component. Such careful delineation of the phenomenology of this anger–crying complex may lead to a different understanding of its psychobiological origins. Similarly, the intriguing possibility that there is an analogous distress 'curve' in nonhuman primates may provide opportunities for the investigation of psychobiological processes contributing to crying patterns (and emotion regulation) that are conserved across species (Chapter 10).

2. CRYING AS A GRADED SIGNAL

Another set of implications becomes apparent when comparing the senses in which crying is seen clinically as a sign or developmentally as a signal. Although there is still more important work to be done on this question, let us assume for the purposes of this discussion that crying is a graded signal, communicating in a graded fashion something about the degree of distress (sometimes called 'arousal') but not the source of the distress. Let us assume, too, that crying is more than just nonspecific 'noise', but that there are no 'cry types' (pain cries, hunger cries, etc.—see Chapters 2, 3). This does not mean, of course, that crying cannot also be useful as a sign in the clinical context (Chapter 3). Whether the graded signal of crying can also be useful as a clinical sign is an empirical question. However, if crying does not carry specific information that has 'sign' value (about pain or hunger or the 'integrity' of the central nervous system) but only relatively nonspecific information that has 'signal' value (about the current functioning of the nervous system), then it is not surprising that studies to answer the question "Is this infant in pain?" have been less promising than expected. However, it may still have some value as a sign in the more limited but still important sense of indicating degree of pain, in situations such as injection procedures in which it is unambiguous that pain is being experienced (Chapter 3).

Of course, even in diagnostically unambiguous situations, the question still remains unresolved as to whether the crying reflects specific pain experience or nonspecific stress (or arousal). This is just one illustration of the fact that our current neurophysiological models of cry production are not sufficiently precise about the determinants of the cry sound (Chapter 9). We are still far from clear about the extent to which 'arousal systems', 'pain systems' or 'hunger systems' relate to each other on the one hand and to cry production on the other. This may well have contributed to the limitations that have been documented when trying to use crying as a sign for diagnosis, and for prediction of developmental outcome (Chapter 9).

There is a third, very practical, implication if crying is a graded signal rather than a series of cry 'types'. Virtually every parenting magazine advises parents that they can become 'good' caregivers if only they would listen carefully to their infants' cries and learn to 'read' them to know whether the infant is hungry, cold, tired or in pain. If cries are graded signals (Chapters 2, 3), this well-intentioned advice is a recipe for caregiving failure rather than caregiving success. At the very least, the caregiver will need to take into account and judge whether other contextual information helps them to understand the reason for their infant's crying, a task made more difficult for infants with developmental challenges (Chapter 7). The focus on reading crying types probably contributes to the caregiver's frustration when the crying s/he thought s/he should know how to 'read' keeps increasing in the first two months (Chapter 4). The unquestioned assumption of 'cry types' is intuitively appealing, and dies hard. If we are to help parents, researchers have some work to do here. Both clinical texts and parenting magazines need to be more sensitized to these difficulties, if they want to do more good than harm.

3. Crying Measures of Continuous Versus Discontinuous Variables

A third emergent theme concerns the common question of whether behavioral phenomena are better understood and described in terms of continuous, dimensional variables or discontinuous, classificatory or categorical variables. To some extent, this distinction underlies the question of whether cries are graded signals or whether there are specific cry types. It is also generally true that developmentalists tend to be partial to continuous variables, while clinicians tend to be partial to discontinuous, classificatory ones. This is not because clinicians are unaware of the fact that many of the physiological and behavioral parameters they deal with on a daily basis are continuous rather than discontinuous. Rather, it is because, when faced with an individual patient, one has to have some guidelines to decide when to act to do an extra diagnostic procedure or to begin a specific treatment.

Defining the clinical condition we call 'hypertension' is a good analogue. Although blood pressure is a continuous variable and increased blood pressure itself is not a disease, a patient is considered to be 'hypertensive' when the blood pressure reaches a level at which the risk of negative consequences is increased or instituting an intervention significantly reduces the likelihood of negative consequences (strokes and heart attacks).

Similarly, the 'reinterpretation' of colic as the upper end of a continuous spectrum of amount, intensity, and increased presence of crying and associated behaviors is not antithetical to assigning some clinical crying presentations to a classificatory schema as Wessel's colic and some as non-Wessel's colic (Chapter 5), especially if there is reason to think that such a classification may be helpful in determining one's strategy toward the complaint (Gormally and Barr 1997). Imposing discontinuities on clinically significant variables is only problematic if the cut-off points (or 'slices' in the case of clinical pies) keep appropriate help from those who need it, or impose unnecessary interventions on those who do not. This requires more work, but it is a first step. Compared to the usual textbook description of colic as a relatively specific clinical entity that some infants 'have' and some do not, the proposed clinical pie is more responsive to the assumption of continuity in the distribution of crying behavior. This is achieved by including 'in' the pie the infants of parents who find one or more characteristics of the crying of their infants (represented in the different slices) to be a concern.

4. FROM JUXTAPOSITION TO INTEGRATION: THE IMPORTANCE OF BETTER MODELS
A fourth emergent theme concerns the importance, and the relative lack of, better theoretical models with which to approach crying phenomena. Good theories need to incorporate, account for, and predict crying behavior in its clinical and its nonclinical forms, in its various developmental transformations, and in its cross-species manifestations. They would need to be able to provide a meaningful answer to the question, "What is crying?" All of the chapters in this volume provide grist for the theoretical mill, and it is clear that there is much to be done. The previously mentioned limitations in our neurophysiological models of cry production (Chapter 9) are but one example. The semantic confusion with regard to what are the appropriate descriptors of crying phenomena (Chapter 11) is another. Adequate models will need to encompass crying not only as a sound, but also as a complex coordinated behavior of the infant. The complexity of this is well illustrated by attending to the prenatal precursors of crying behavior and the probable role of posture postnatally as a determinant of cry productions (Chapter 11).

Furthermore, crying studies, as is the case for many other areas of development, have limited themselves to applying models that assume linear relationships between relevant variables. The limitations of such models have always been problematic in the studies of developmental change, and this is no less true of crying phenomena. However, because of the complexity of crying, it seems clear that adequate models will require some form of systems thinking. Recent interest in the application of nonlinear dynamic systems theories (Wolff 1993, Thelen and Smith 1994, Wimmers *et al.* 1998, Barr *et al.* 1999) is one possibility that has yet to be explored in depth (Chapter 11).

Promissory notes
These four emergent themes (juxtaposing clinical and developmental perspectives; cries

as graded signals; continuous versus discontinuous variables; the need for adequate theoretical models) are only some of the ways in which the burgeoning interest in crying behavior has enriched and deepened our understanding of its clinical and developmental manifestations. On a historical note, it will come as no surprise that these themes also emerged at the International Cry Research Workshops, the first of which stimulated the previous 'Cry' volume (Wasz-Höckert *et al.* 1968) in the *Clinics in Developmental Medicine* series (of which the present volume is the second on this subject). That conference focused on spectrographic and auditory analyses of infant cries, and on the working assumption that, carefully studied, the infant's cry would yield specific 'sign' value. The conference (and the book) provided a significant impetus to further studies of infant crying.

This volume captures, at least to some extent, how far 'cry research' has come, and indicates at least some of the directions in which it needs to go. Interestingly, by the second Cry Research Workshop (in Lappnor, Finland, 1986), the topics had already widened to include discussions of, *inter alia*, clinical syndromes, developmental changes in cry sounds, vocalizations as one feature of infant behavioral states, and the value of crying as a signal to elicit caregiving responses. Indeed, the multitude of perspectives and disciplines for which crying behavior had become a significant subject was reflected in the introductions by the various participants. As many who attended remarked, the most repeated phrase of the meeting was: "I am not a 'cry researcher', but I am interested in crying because . . ." As those meetings have continued (in 1986, 1990, 1992, 1997, and one planned for July 2000), the range of interested disciplines and perspectives has continued to grow. So too have presentations and symposia in a wide range of specialty society meetings with an interest in the normative and clinical behavior of infants and children.

As this interest and (we believe) this volume attest, there is indeed good news to be found in the midst of these expressions of distress by infants and toddlers. Crying has provided a surprisingly fascinating window into how infants function, how they are organized, how they access resources, and how they develop increasingly complex and sophisticated modes of expression and interaction. We adults, whether as parents, clinicians or researchers, will continue to be drawn by this still enigmatic behavior to try to understand it as a sign, a symptom and a signal. In so doing, the findings in this volume and elsewhere suggest that we will come to know our infants and toddlers better, and ourselves as well.

REFERENCES

Barr, R.G., Kramer, M.S., Leduc, D.G., Boisjoly, C., McVey-White, L., Pless, I.B. (1988) 'Parental diary of infant cry and fuss behaviour.' *Archives of Disease of Childhood*, **63**, 380–387.
—— Beek, P., Calinoiu, N. (1999) 'Challenges to non-linear modelling of infant emotion regulation in real and developmental time.' *In:* Savelsbergh, G.J.P., van der Maas, H.L.J., van Geert, P.L.C. (Eds.) *Non-linear Developmental Processes.* Amsterdam: Royal Netherlands Academy of Arts and Sciences, pp. 15–37.
Gormally, S.M., Barr, R.G. (1997) 'Of clinical pies and clinical clues: proposal for a clinical approach to complaints of early crying and colic.' *Ambulatory Child Health*, **3**, 137–153.
Thelen, E., Smith, L.B. (1994) *A Dynamic Systems Approach to the Development of Cognition and Action.* Cambridge, MA: MIT Press.
Wasz-Höckert, O., Lind, J., Vuorenkoski, V., Partanen, T., Valanne, E. (1968) *The Infant Cry: a Spectrographic and Auditory Analysis. Clinics in Developmental Medicine No. 29.* London: Spastics International Medical Publications.

Wimmers, R.H., Savelsbergh, G.J.P., Beek, P.J., Hopkins, B. (1998) 'Evidence for a phase transition in the early development of prehension.' *Developmental Psychobiology*, **32**, 235–348.

Wolff, P.H. (1993) 'Behavioral and emotional states in infancy: A dynamic perspective.' *In:* Smith, L.B., Thelen, E. (Eds.) *A Dynamic Systems Approach to Development: Applications.* Cambridge, MA: MIT Press, pp. 189–208.

INDEX

(Page numbers in *italics* refer to figures/tables.)

A

Abdomen, in colic, 69
Abdominal examination, in excessive crying, 102
Abnormal cry
  prognostic value, 149, 150
  in sick infants, 100, 108, 148
Acoustic cry analysis, 137–154, 177–178
  basic acoustic principles, 138–139
  clinical value, 36
  cry gradations, 15–16
  cry types, 29–30
  digital frequency analysis, 142–143
  future directions, 152–154
  historical aspects, 139–141
  limitations, 202
  measures obtained, 141–143
  models of cry production and, 143–146
  in neonatal disease, 146–149
  neonatal outcome studies, 149–152, 153–154
  pain cries, 25–27, 186, 187
  in sick/disabled infants, 108–109, 110, 112–113
  see also Sound spectrography
Adaptive value, crying, 23–25
Adolescent mothers, 114
Adult crying, homeostatic theory, 24
Adverse consequences, crying, 24–25, 33
Age
  excessive crying complaints and, 74
  responsivity and, *49*, 51–52
  temper tantrums and, 126, 127, 128, 132–133
  see also Developmental changes
Age-related peak in crying, 3, 54, 162, 191
  in chimpanzee infants, 171
  in colic, 42, 68–69
  universality, 192–193
Aggression, temper tantrums and, 125–126, 134
Alarm value, crying, 33
Altruism, 24
Amplitude, acoustic, 138
Amygdala, 14, 145
Analgesia, outcome measures, 26, 32
Anger
  autonomic activation, 121–122, 130–131, 132
  cry, caregivers' responses, 20
  expression in tantrums, 124, 125–126
  flushing and, 131–132
Angry/mad cry, *184, 185*

Animals, nonhuman
  auditory perception–action coupling, 201
  discrete signals, 8–9
  sucrose taste responses, 58
  see also Chimpanzees; Primates, nonhuman
Anxiety
  excessive parental, 100, 113
  separation, 36, 161
Apnea
  in pain cries, 26
  pain-induced, 31
Arm restraint procedure, 56, 57
Arousability, 146, 149
Arousal, physiological, 20
Articulators, developmental changes, 198–199
Asphyxia, birth, *see* Birth asphyxia
Asthma, 85
Attachment
  in chimpanzee infants, 173
  problems
    in colic, 83, 88–89, 90–91
    in disabled children, 115
  theory, 111
Audio recordings, 178–179, 182
Auditory perception, development, 200–201
Autonomic nervous system, 14
  in cry production, 145, 149
  feedback effects on behavior, 132, 133–134
  response to pain, 32
  in temper tantrums, *see* Temper tantrums, visible
    autonomic activity
Aversive nature, crying of sick infants, 108

B

Babbling, 198
Bacteremia, occult, 104
Basic/hunger cry, *184, 185*
Bayley Scales of Infant Development, 85, 151–152
Behavior problems
  in disabled children, 114–115
  externalizing, 131, 132, 134
  in infants with colic, 85, 86
Behavioral states
  fetus, 190
  signaling, 25
Behavioral style, 45–46
Behavioral system, *45*, 47
Biobehavioral model (Lester and Zeskind), 145, 147
Biobehavioral shift, 53–55, 173–174

Bioevolutionary perspectives, pain signals, 23–25, 33
Biphonation, *185*
Birth asphyxia, 107
   acoustic cry analysis, 108, 146, 149–150
   behavior problems, 114
   infant–caregiver interaction, 113–114
Birth cry, 4, 9, *185*
Blood
   in stool, 100
   tests, 103
Blood pressure, in anger, 132
Blushing, 133
Body movements
   caregiver responses and, 18
   in definitions of crying, 182
   future research directions, 152–153
   in response to pain, 32
   see also Posture
Brain damage/injury, 107, 111, 116
   acoustic cry analysis, 147–148, 149–150
   latency to cry, 108
   minimal, 114
   see also Birth asphyxia
Brazelton, T. Berry, 3
Brazelton Neonatal Behavioral Assessment Scale
   (NBAS), 163, 168–170
Breast-fed infants, cow's milk protein intolerance, 75,
   77
Breath holding, 15
Breathing
   mouth, 197
   movements, fetal, 187, 189
   spasmodic, 15

C
Caregivers
   crying complaints, *see* Crying complaints
   discrimination of cry types, *see* Cry types, dis-
      crimination
   factors affecting colic, 72
   impact of colic on, 79, *80*, 82, 86, 88
   infant interaction, *see* Infant–caregiver interaction
   judging pain severity, 33–34
   pairings with chimpanzee infants, 172–173
   perceptions of excessive crying, 70–71
   physiological responses, 20
   see also Mothers
Caregiving regime
   effects on chimpanzee crying, 162–163, 168–171,
      172–173
   effects on human crying, 55, 162
Caregiving responses
   in colic, 82
   contextual factors, 18, 19
   to cry types, 9
   to graded signals, 17–18

   latency, 18
   persistent crying, 54
Carrying (picking up)
   chimpanzees *vs* humans, 161, 171, 172
   effect on frequency/duration of crying, 55
   infants with colic, 56
Catastrophe theory, 194
Causes of crying
   identifying, *see* Cry types, discrimination
   unknown, 19
Central nervous system abnormalities
   cry sounds, 108, 117
   presenting as colic, 76
Cerebral palsy, 107, 115, 150
Chest radiograph, 103
Chiari type 1 malformation, 76
Child abuse
   crying as risk factor, 25, 67
   in developmental disability, 117
   presenting as colic, 76, 88
   presenting as excessive crying, 100, 101, 104
Chimpanzees, 158–174
   crying in infants, 159–160, 161, 162–174
   effect of rearing method, 162–163, 168–171,
      172–173
   naturalistic observations, 163–167, 172, 173
   vs human infants, 171–172, 173–174
   distress vocalizations and parenting, 159–161
   emotional development, 161–162, 173
   problems in studying, 158–159
Circumcision surgery, 14–15, 26, 145, 152
Classification of crying, 183–187
   see also Cry types
Clinicians
   challenges to, 210–211
   clinical *vs* developmental approach, 211–212
Cocaine, *in utero* exposure, 111
Colic (syndrome), 3, 4, 41–61
   characteristics, 41–42, 68–69
   in chimpanzees, 161
   "clinical pies" approach, 67–91, 215
   clinical *vs* developmental approach, 212–213
   diagnostic criteria, 69–71, 96–97
   diagnostic pie, *70*, 71–73, 89, 91
   difficult temperament hypothesis, *see* Difficult
      temperament, hypothesis
   in emergency department, 96–97, 213
   etiology, 74–77
   follow-up guidelines, 91
   infants presenting with, 72
   management, 97, 104
   organic disease in, 72, 74–77, 88, 89
   prognosis, 77–87
      double hit hypothesis, 90–91
      in infants with diagnosed colic, 79–83
      longitudinal studies, 83–86

prognostic pie, 87–89, 90, 91
severe, 69–70
transient responsivity hypothesis, *see* Transient
    responsivity hypothesis
treatment trials, 212–213
as upper end of normal crying, 71–72, 215
use of word, 68
Wessel's criteria, *see* Wessel's rule of threes
Wessel's plus crying, 69–70, 73
Colicky crying, 69–70
Collier's sign, 75, 77
Communication
    by discrete signals, 8–9
    by graded signals, 13–14
    in nonhuman primates, 157–158
    role of crying, 2, 23–24
Complaints, crying, *see* Crying complaints
Computed tomography, 103
Consolability
    chimpanzee infants, 171, 172
    disabled infants, 116, 117
    infants with colic, 57
Consolation-seeking, in tantrums, 125
Constipation, 100, 102
Contextual factors
    cry type discrimination, 18, 19, 31, 35–36
    crying of disabled infants, 110
    judging child's pain, 34
    primate vocalizations, 158
Contractures, 107
Cooing, 29, 187
    developmental changes, 193
    see also Pleasure cry
Coordinated crying, *185*
Coping style, in temper tantrums, 126
Corneal abrasion, 101
Coronary artery, anomalous left, 76
Cortisol responses, 47–48
    in colic studies, 57
    developmental changes, 51–52, 54
Cough, 100
Counseling, parents of disabled children, 117
Cow's milk protein intolerance, 74–75, 77, 212
Cri-du-chat syndrome, 108, 113
Cricothyroid muscles, 195
Cross-cultural comparisons, early crying, 54
Cry modes, 26
Cry production
    developmental changes, 195–198
    models, 143–146, 149, 153, 214
Cry psychophysics, 28
Cry score system, 150
Cry types, 3, 19, 183–187
    acoustic/temporal characteristics, 29–30
    discrimination, 4, 8–21, 28–31, 214
        acoustic/temporal contrasts, 29–30

contextual factors, 18, 19, 31, 35–36
effects of experience, 10, 30–31, 111
in sick infants, 109–110, 112–113
subjective methods, 4, 8–21, 30–31
eliciting stimuli, 9, 11, 12–13
evidence against, 11–13
hypothesis, evidence for, 8–11
subjective analyses, 30–31, 36
use of exemplars, 9, 10
see also Hunger cry; Pain cry; *and other specific*
    types
Crying
    adverse consequences, 24–25, 33
    classification, 183–187
    definitions, 179–183, 202
    function, 23–25, 33
    meaning, 5
    in tantrums, 125
    vs fussing, 69, 178, 179, 182–183, 192
Crying bouts
    pain-induced, 26
    prolonged, 41, 69
    temporal changes, 17, 152
Crying complaints
    clinical approach, 67–91
    diagnostic pie, *70*, 71–73, 89, 91
    in emergency department, 96–105, 213
    etiology, 74–77
    prognosis, 77–87
    see also Colic (syndrome)
Crying Patterns Questionnaire (CPQ), 179
Cyproheptadine, 75–76

D
Dangers of crying, 24–25, 33
Darwin, Charles, 24
Delayed auditory feedback (DAF), 201
Depression, parental, 82, 86, 113
Development of crying, 176–204, 210
    change problem, *see* Developmental changes
    constraints on, 195–201, 203
    defining and classifying crying, 179–187
    methodological issues, 177–179
    origin problem, 187, 188–191, 202–203
Developmental changes, 54, 188, 191–194, 203
    articulators, 198–199
    auditory perception, 200–201
    biobehavioral shift concept, 53–55, 173–174
    in chimpanzee infants, 173–174
    cortisol responses, 51–52, 54
    in disabled children, 118
    dynamic systems approach, 194–195, 202
    future research needs, 153
    infant–caregiver interaction, 111–112
    larynx and pharynx, 197–198
    pain expression, 34–35

posture, 199–200, 203
respiration, 195–197
see also Age-related peak in crying; n-shaped curves
Developmental delay
  acoustic measures predicting, 151–152, 154
  behavioral problems, 115
  in colic, 85–86, 87
  screening for, in excessive crying, 102
Developmental disabilities, 106–107
  see also Disabled children
Diaries, parental, 178–179, 202
Diarrhea, 77, 100, 102
Difficult temperament, 41
  hypothesis, 41, 42–44, 60, 213
    evidence against, 56–57, 61
    evidence for, 42–44
    vs transient responsivity hypothesis, 49–51
  perceived, children with colic, 81, 86, 88
  reactivity and regulation of responses, 50–51
  vs colic, 58
Digital frequency analysis, 141, 142–143
Disabled children, 6, 106–118, 203
  behavior, 114–115
  case history, 107–108, 118
  causes of problems, 106–107
  clinical care, 117–118
  confusing signals from, 115–117
  crying and caregiver interactions, 111–114
  research on cry sounds, 108–111
Distress
  acoustic cry signal analysis, 26–27
  autonomic activation in, 130
  caregivers' responses, 17–18, 19
  in chimpanzee infants, 159–161
  cry gradation with, 14–15, 17
  expression in tantrums, 125
Diurnal pattern of crying, 192
  in colic, 68–69
Double harmonic break, *185*
Double hit hypothesis, outcome of colic, 90–91
Down syndrome
  crying behavior, 108, *109*, 114–115
  infant–caregiver interaction, 113, 114
Duration of crying, 141, 191
  after pain stimuli, 26
  in chimpanzee infants, 165
  in colic, 68–69, 71
  dissociation from frequency, 55–56
  in neonatal disease, 146, 149
  normal *vs* abnormal, 71
  in sick infants, 108
Dynamic systems approach (DSA), 215
  developmental change, 194–195, 202
Dysphonated/turbulent cry, *184*
Dysphonation, 141
  in non-Wessel's crying, 73

  in pain cries, 26
  in Wessel's crying (colic), 72

E
Ear infections, 101
Eczema, 85
Elaborated crying, *185*, 193
Elicited crying
  in colic studies, 56
  discrimination of cause, 9–10, 11–13
  in neonatal disease, 147
  vs spontaneous crying, 152, 183–186, 202
Emergency department, 96–105, 213
  febrile infant, 103–104
  medical evaluation in, 97–103
  treatment, 104
EMLA cream, 26, 32
Emotional development, chimpanzees, 161–162, 173
Emotional reactions
  autonomic reactivity mediating, 121–122
  graded signal view, 15
  vagal regulation, 14, 130, 144–146
Emotional states
  modalities of expression, 32–34
  in nonhuman primates, 158–159
  role of crying in signaling, 24
Esophagitis, reflux, 76
Excessive crying, 3, 41
  clinical algorithm, 98, 99
  complaints about, *see* Crying complaints
  diagnoses in infants presenting with, *98*
  future research, 104–105
  medical evaluation, 97–103
  in regulatory disorders, 110–111
  treatment, 104
  see also Colic
Experience, in identifying cry types, 10, 30–31, 111
Externalizing behavior disorders, 131, 132, 134
Eye
  examination, in excessive crying, 101
  pathology, 76
  tearing, *see* Lacrimation

F
F_0, *see* Fundamental frequency
Facial expressions
  adaptive value, 24
  caregiver responses and, 18
  in chimpanzees, 158–160, 162
  in definitions of crying, 182
  future research needs, 152–153
  information signaled by, 25
  of pain
    developmental changes, 34–35
    in infants, 31–32, 33–34
  prenatal development, 190

Facial flushing, *see* Flushing
Family function
  impact of colic, *80*, 81, 83, 84, 86, 87
  prepartum, infants with colic, 84, 90
Fast Fourier transform (FFT), 140, 141, 142, 177
Fathers, interactions with infants, 113
Fear
  cry, acoustic contrasts, 29
  display of, 24
  grimace, in chimpanzees, 159
Febrile infants, 74, 100, 103–104
Fetus
  behavioral indicators of crying, 189, 190, 202–203
  breathing movements, 187, 189
First-born infants, 73, 113
Fluoxetine hydrochloride (Prozac), 75
Flushing
  anatomical pathways, 122
  anger and, 131–132
  functional value, 133
  in temper tantrums, 121, 122, 127, 128
    age trends and individual differences, 132–133
    autonomic feedback effects, 132
    post-tantrum mood and, 131
    temporal locus, 129–130
Formants, 141, 186–187
  auditory feedback control, 201
  pain cries, 26
Frequency, acoustic, 138
  fundamental, *see* Fundamental frequency
  × amplitude plot, 138–139
Frequency of crying, 5, 191
  dissociation from duration, 55–56
Fretfulness
  unexplained, 19
  see also Fussing
Fructose intolerance, isolated, 75
Frustration, low tolerance, 114
Functional value of crying, 23–25, 33
Fundamental frequency (F_0), 141, 142–143
  developmental changes, 186
  in neonatal disease, 146, 149–150
  pain cries, 26, 183–184
  vagal control, 145
Fundoscopic examination, 101
Fussiness Rating Scale, 81
Fussing, 5
  acoustic discrimination, 29
  in chimpanzee infants, 159, *164*, 165–171, 172, 173
  definitions, 179–183
  developmental changes, 193
  interrupted, 193, 194, 200
  vs crying, 69, 178, 179, 182–183, 192

G
Gastroenteritis, 102

Gastroesophageal reflux, 76
Gender differences
  crying in chimpanzees, 170
  identifying causes of crying, 10
Glaucoma, congenital, 76
Gliding, in neonatal disease, 146
Glottal muscles, 143–144
Glottal rolls, in neonatal disease, 150
Goodness of fit concept, 113
Graded signals
  crying as, 13–18, 19–20, 30, 213–214
  identifying cause, 15–16, 109–110
  in nonhuman primates, 13–14, 18
Growth measures, in excessive crying, 100–101

H
Hair tourniquet syndrome, 101
Hand–mouth contact, 199–200
Heart, auscultation, 101
Heart rate
  in anger, 132
  in colic studies, 57
  in excessive crying, 100
  in externalizing disorders, 131, 132
  response to pain, 31, 32
  rhythms, poor arousability and, 149
  vagal control, 14, 130, 145
Heel lance, 32
Hitting, in temper tantrums, 125–126
Holaday's stages of parental responses, 111–112, 118
Homeostatic theory of adult crying, 24
Hunger cry, 183, *184*, *185*
  acoustic analysis, 29, 186, 187
  elicitation, 13
  gradations, 16–17
  subjective discrimination, 9, 12, 30
Hyperphonated cry/shift, *184*
Hyperphonation, *185*
Hypersensitivity, in disabled infants, 111, 116

I
Idiopathic crying of infancy, 97, 102, 104
Imaging studies, 103
Immunizations, 54
Individual differences
  in crying, 54, 55, 187, 191–192
  in temper tantrums, 132–133
Infant Behavior Questionnaire, 44
Infant Behavior Record, 85
Infant–caregiver interaction, 111
  adverse effects of crying, 25, 33
  outcome of colic, *80*, 81–83, 86, 88–89
  in sick/disabled children, 111–114
Infant Characteristics Questionnaire, 43
Infant Temperament Questionnaire, 42, 85

Infants
    expressions of pain, 31–32, 35
    outcome of colic, 80–81, 86, 87
Infections, 103
Injection, intramuscular, 32
Inspiratory–expiratory cycle, 196
Intensive care, infants in, 111
Intercostal muscles, 196
Internalizing disorder, 134
International Cry Research Workshops, 3, 137
Intestinal obstruction, 103
Intracranial pressure, in pain, 32
Intramuscular injection, 32
Intubation, 109, *110*, 116
Intussusception, 97
Irritability
    in disabled infants, 110–111, 114, 116, 117
    management, 118

J
Jaw movements, 189, 199
Jitter, 153, 186, 187
    in sick infants, 110
Joy, display of, 24

K
Kicking, in temper tantrums, 125–126
!Kung San hunter-gatherers, 54, 55, 162

L
Laboratory tests, 102, 103–104
Lacrimation, 100
    in chimpanzees, 160
    in crying, 183
    in temper tantrums, 121, 122
Lactose intolerance, 76
Language, expressing pain using, 35
Laryngeal muscles, 143, 195
Larynx
    developmental changes, 197–198
    pathology, detection, 153
    vagal control, 14, 130, 145
Latency
    caregiver responses, 18
    to cry, after pain stimuli, 26, 108
Lead exposure study, 85, 147–148
Likert scales, pain cries, 28
Limb movements, *see* Body movements
Loudness, 138
    feedback control, 201
Low birthweight infants, 146
Low intensity cry, *185*
Low non-intensity cry, *185*
Lumbar puncture, 103
Lung disease, chronic, 116
Lungs, auscultation, 101

M
McCarthy Scales of Children's Abilities, 151–152
McMaster Family Assessment Device, 81
Manali infants, 54, 178
Markov models, hidden, 26
Measurement methods
    crying, 5, 20–21, 214–215
    pain cries, 25
Medical conditions, *see* Organic disease
Medications, 100
Melody type, 141, 186
    in neonatal disease, 149
    in pain cries, 26
Metabolic disease, 100
Methadone-dependent mothers, infants of, 58
Migraine, infantile, 75–76
Models, theoretical, 215
Modified Behavioral Pain Scale (MBPS), 31
Momentary Poisson rates (MPRs), 124–125
Mood
    in nonhuman primates, 162
    post-tantrum, 131, 132
Mother–infant distress syndrome, persistent, 91
Mothers
    chimpanzee, naturalistic observations, 163–167,
        172, 173
    context-dependent responses, 18
    impact of colic on, 79, *80*, 82, 86, 88
    infant interaction, *see* Infant–caregiver interaction
    perceptions of child with colic, 81, 86, 88
    persistent criers, 54
    ratings of pain cries, 27, 28
    recognition of cry types, 9, 12, 15–16, 36
    see also Caregivers
Motivational state, 13
Multimethod, multimodal approaches, 3–4
Murphy Brown (television series), 4, 5, 8
Muscles, controling cry production, 143–144
Myoelastic–aerodynamic theory, 197

N
n-shaped curves, 53–54, 191
    colic syndrome, 49–50
    early crying, 54
    see also Developmental changes
Natural selection, 24–25
Needle sticking, 15
Neonatal Behavioral Assessment Scale (NBAS), 163,
    168–170
Neonatal Facial Coding System (NFCS), 31–32
Neonatal Infant Pain Scale (NIPS), 31
Neonates
    acoustic cry analysis
        in health and disease, 138, 146–149
        outcome studies, 149–152, 153–154
    developmental changes, 196, 197, 199

expressions of pain, 31–32, 35
vagal tone differences, 52
Neurological disease, 100, 117–118
Neurological examination, 102
Neuromuscular disease, 116
Night wakings, infants with colic, 43, 85
Noise, crying as undifferentiated, 11–13
Non-Wessel's crying, 73
Normal crying, 162
age-related peak, *see* Age-related peak in crying
colic as, 71–72, 215
infants presenting with, 73
vs abnormal, 187
Nose, runny, *see* Rhinorrhea
Nucleus ambiguus, 14, 130, 145
Nursing Child Assessment Feeding Scale (NCAFS),
81

O

Observation
in emergency department, 102–103
naturalistic, 3–4
chimpanzee study, 163–167
temper tantrums, 122–124, 134
Opioids, in sucrose taste responses, 58, 59
Organic disease
clinical clues, 77, 89
presenting as colic, 72, 74–77, 88, 89
presenting as excessive crying, 97–103
resembling colic, 96
undiagnosed, 73
Orogustatory calming, in colic studies, 58–59, *60*
Overstimulation, 100
Oxygen saturation, in pain, 32

P

Pacifier
calming, in colic, 58
withdrawal task, 56
Pain
colic presenting as, 69
crying as a sign, 1, 23–36
developmental changes in expression, 34–35
future research, 35–36
other signs, 31–32
physiological indicators, 32
sensation in infants, 1
severity
acoustic analysis, 14–15, 26–27
subjective assessment, 28, 33–34
Pain cry, 25–28, *184, 185*
acoustic and temporal analysis, 25–27, 186, 187
bioevolutionary view, 23–25
caregivers' responses, 20
dangers, 24–25
definition, 25

in disabled/sick infants, 116, 146
discrimination, 9, 12, 28–31
elicitation, 13
elicited *vs* spontaneous, 152, 183–184
gradations, 14–15, 16–17, 26–27
latency, 26, 108
subjective analyses, 27–28
vs other modalities of expression, 32–34
Palate, hard, 198
Palpation, in excessive crying, 101
Parasympathetic nervous system
in cry production, 145, 149
response to pain, 32
in temper tantrums, 122, 130–131
Parenting, in chimpanzees, 159–161, 165–167
Parents
challenges to, 210, 211
disabled/sick children, 113, 116, 117, 118
see also Caregivers; Mothers
Paroxysmal crying, 3
in colic, 41–42, 69
Peak pattern of early crying, *see* Age-related peak in
crying
Pediatric Diagnostic Service (PDS), 142, 148, 151
Perception–action coupling, 200–201
Perinatal difficulties, infants with colic, 84
Personality, mothers of infants with colic, 83
Pharynx, developmental changes, 197–198
Phonated/basic cry, *184*
Phonemes (cry modes), 26
Phonetic transcription, 177–178
Physical examination
in excessive crying, 101–102
mock, 57
Physioacoustic model of crying (Golub), 143–144, 149
Lester's modification, 144, 149
Physiological measures
in colic studies, 57
pain in infants, 32
Physiological system, *45*, 47
Picking up, *see* Carrying
Pitch, 138
Pitch of cry
in anger, 133
in hunger, 186
in pain, 26, 183–184
in sick/disabled infants, 100, 108, 113–114
vagal control, 130
Pleasure cry, 9, 30
see also Cooing
Polyvagal theory (Porges), 14, 130
Postmature infants, 58
Posture
developmental changes, 199–200, 203
in pain, 31
see also Body movements

Pout face, in chimpanzee infants, 159, *160*
Preadaptation, 189–190
Predators, 24–25, 33
Premature Infant Pain Profile (PIPP), 31
Prenatal difficulties, infants with colic, 84, 90
Prenatal origins of crying, 187, 188–191, 202–203
Preschool Behavior Questionnaire, 86
Preterm infants, 111, 189
    acoustic cry analysis, 150–151
    age-related pattern of crying, 54, 191, 203
    expressions of pain, 32, 34–35
    pain sensation, 1
    postural stabilization, 199
Primates, nonhuman, 157–174, 213
    graded signals, 13–14, 18
    problems in studying, 158–159
    see also Chimpanzees
Prolonged crying
    in colic, 41, 69
    see also Colic (syndrome); Excessive crying
Prozac (fluoxetine hydrochloride), 75
Psychopathology, temper tantrums and, 134
Psychophysics, cry, 28
Pulse oximetry, 103

R
Reactivity
    in colic studies, 56–59, 83
    concept, 44–48
    in difficult infants, 50–51
    dynamic parameters, 46
    limitations to concept, 47–48
    measures, 47–48
    transient changes, in colic, 50
Rearing method, *see* Caregiving regime
Rectal examination, in excessive crying, 102
Reflux esophagitis, 76
Regular cry, *185*
Regulation of responses
in colic studies, 55, 56–59, 61
    concept, 44–48
    in difficult infants, 50–51, 52
    dynamics, 46
    limitations to concept, 47–48
    measures, 47–48
    transient changes, in colic, 50, 51
Regulatory disorders, 110–111, 117–118
Regurgitation, 76, 77
Research, cry
    future directions, 210–211
    historical aspects, 3–4
Respiratory distress, in temper tantrums, 127
Respiratory muscles, 143
    developmental changes, 195–197
Respiratory rate
    in crying, 100, 196

in pain, 32
Respiratory symptoms, upper, 100
Responsivity
    age-related changes, *49*, 51–52
    in colic studies, 56–59
    components, 44–45
    concept, 44–48
    in difficult temperament hypothesis, 60
    dynamic parameters, 46
    limitations to concept, 47–48
    transient, *see* Transient responsivity hypothesis
Rhinorrhea (runny nose), 100
    in temper tantrums, 122, 127
Rhythmicity of crying, 182
Rib cage development, 196
Rigidity, body, 31, 199
Rubberband snap, 13, 20, 147

S
Salivation, in temper tantrums, 122, 127
Scandinavian research group, 3, 9–11, 141
Screaming, 5
    in chimpanzee infants, 159–160, 165
    in temper tantrums, 125, 126
Sedatives, in colic, 97
Self-quieting
    in chimpanzee infants, 171–172
    development, 200
Semantic differential scales
    cry types, 30–31
    pain cries, 27–28
Separation anxiety, 36, 161
Shaken baby syndrome, 76, 101
Sherman, M., 10, 11–12, 15, 19
Shimmer, 153, 186
    in sick infants, 110
Shouting, in temper tantrums, 125
Sick infants
    abnormal cry, 100, 108, 148
    acoustic cry analysis, 108–109, 110, 112–113
    cry types, 109–110, 112–113
    duration of crying, 108
    infant–caregiver interaction, 111–114
    jitter, 110
    pain cry, 116, 146
    parents, 113, 116, 117, 118
    pitch of cry, 100, 108, 113–114
    shimmer, 110
Sign
    crying as, 2, 211–213
    definition, 2
Signals
    confusing, from disabled children, 115–116
    crying as, 2, 3–4, 211–213
    definition, 2
    discrete, 8–9, 13

graded, *see* Graded signals
  pain, in infants, 31–32
Simple cry, *185*, 193
Sino-atrial (S-A) node, 14, 15
Sleep
  in chimpanzee infants, *164*, 165
  disturbances, excessive crying with, 100
  in infants with colic, 43, 44, 85, 86
Smiles, in chimpanzees, 158, *159*, 173
Social factors
  in excessive crying, 100
  expression of pain, 34
Soothing
  by chimpanzee mothers, observations, 163–167
  resistance, in infants with colic, 55–56, 69
Sound spectrography, 3–4, 141–142
  cry types, 9, 10
  history, 139–141
  in neonatal disease, 146–149
  neonatal outcome studies, 149–152
  in sick/disabled infants, 108–109
Soundless crying, 109, *110*
Source–filter theory, 143
Stamping, in temper tantrums, 125, 126
Startle cry, 12, 13
Stimuli, eliciting, 152
  in acoustic analyses, 138
  in colic studies, 56, 57
  in cry type discrimination studies, 9, 11, 12–13
  in neonatal disease, 147
Stress
  parental, 113
  responses, developmental changes, 51–52, 54
Subglottal air pressure, control of, 196, 197
Subjective analyses, cry types, 30–31, 36
Subjective–experiential system, *45*, 47
Sucrose taste responses, 32
  in colic studies, 58–59, *60*, 61
Sudden infant death syndrome (SIDS), 137, 148
Supine position, 199, 200
Supraglottal muscles, 143
Survival value, crying, 23–25
Swallowing, fetal, 189
Sweating, 122, 127
Sympathetic nervous system
  in cry production, 145, 149
  response to pain, 32
  in temper tantrums, 122, 130–131
Symptom
  crying as, 2, 3, 211–213
  definition, 2
Synchrony of arousal hypothesis, 20

T
Tears, *see* Lacrimation
Teeth, 198

Temper tantrums, 4–5, 121–134, 213
  cross-sectional survey, 123
  future research needs, 133–134
  model, 125–126
  narrative data/analysis, 123–125
  operational definition, 123
  visible autonomic activity, 121–122, 127–131
    acute *vs* chronic factors, 127–128
    post-tantrum mood and, 131
    sympathetic and parasympathetic tone, 130–131
    tantrum characteristics and, 127
    temporal locus, 129–130
Temperament
  difficult, *see* Difficult temperament
  infants with colic, 42–44, 81, 85, 86
  in nonhuman primates, 162
  responsivity concept, 45–46
  temper tantrums and, 134
Temporal analysis
  cry bouts, 17, 152
  cry types, 29–30
  pain cries, 25–27
  temper tantrums, 125, 129–130
Threshold, cry, in neonatal disease, 147
Throwing, in temper tantrums, 125, 126
Time × amplitude plot, 138–139
Toddler Temperament Scale, 43–44, 81
Toddlers
  expressions of pain, 35
  temper tantrums, *see* Temper tantrums
Tongue movements, 189, 198–199
Topical anesthesia, 26, 32
"Toxic" infant, 103–104
Toy removal, 56, 57, 133
Tracheostomy, 109, *110*
Training
  in identifying cry types, 30–31
  in sound spectrogram analysis, 142
Transient responsivity hypothesis, 42, 48–61, 213
  evidence for, 53–59, 61
  strong and weak versions, 51–53
  see also Reactivity; Regulation of responses; Responsivity
Trauma, causing excessive crying, 100, 101
Trisomy 21, *see* Down syndrome

U
Uncoordinated crying, *185*
Urinalysis/urine culture, 102
Urinary tract infections, 76, 102

V
Vagal tone
  age-related changes, 52
  in colic studies, 57
  emotional regulation, 14, 130, 144–146

in pain, 32
in stressful conditions, 14–15
Vagus nerve, 14, 144, 195
dorsal motor nucleus, 130, 145
Variables, continuous *vs* discontinuous, 214–215
Velum, 198, 200
Vocal intonation, vagal control, 14, 130, 145
Vocal tract
abnormalities, 116, 153
development, 195–199
models of cry production, 143–146
Vocalizations, in nonhuman primates, 13–14, 157–158, 159–161
Vomiting, 76, 77

W
Wessel's crying, 72
Wessel's plus crying, 69–70, 73
Wessel's "rule of threes", 3, 69–71
limitations, 69, 70–71
modified, 69
Wheezing, 101–102
Whimper face, in chimpanzee infants, 159, *160*
Whining, in tantrums, 125
Williams syndrome, 115
Wolff, P.H., 3–4, 184

X
X-rays, skeletal, 103